Practical Signal and Image Processing in Clinical Cardiology

Jeffrey J. Goldberger • Jason Ng (Eds.)

Practical Signal and Image Processing in Clinical Cardiology

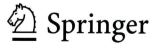

Jeffrey J. Goldberger
Jason Ng
Northwestern University
Feinberg School of Medicine
Division of Cardiology
251 East Huron
Feinberg Pavilion
Suite 8-503
60611 Chicago Illinois
USA

ISBN: 978-1-84882-514-7   e-ISBN: 978-1-84882-515-4

DOI: 10.1007/978-1-84882-515-4

Springer Dordrecht Heidelberg London New York

British Library Cataloguing in Publication Data
A catalogue record for this book is available from the British Library

Library of Congress Control Number: 2010929047

© Springer-Verlag London Limited 2010
Apart from any fair dealing for the purposes of research or private study, or criticism or review, as permitted under the Copyright, Designs and Patents Act 1988, this publication may only be reproduced, stored or transmitted, in any form or by any means, with the prior permission in writing of the publishers, or in the case of reprographic reproduction in accordance with the terms of licences issued by the Copyright Licensing Agency. Enquiries concerning reproduction outside those terms should be sent to the publishers.

The use of registered names, trademarks, etc. in this publication does not imply, even in the absence of a specific statement, that such names are exempt from the relevant laws and regulations and therefore free for general use.

Product liability: The publisher can give no guarantee for information about drug dosage and application thereof contained in this book. In every individual case the respective user must check its accuracy by consulting other pharmaceutical literature.

Cover design: eStudioCalamar, Figueres/Berlin

Printed on acid-free paper

Springer is part of Springer Science+Business Media (www.springer.com)

Foreword

Wikipedia states that "Signal processing is an area of electrical engineering, systems engineering and applied mathematics that deals with operations on or analysis of signals, in either discrete or continuous time to perform useful operations on those signals." How boring is that? But then, it goes on to say, "Signals of interest can include sound, images, time-varying measurement values and sensor data, for example, biological data such as electrocardiograms, control system signals, telecommunication transmission signals such as radio signals, and many others." Now that is getting interesting because if you stop to think about it, we live in an era surrounded by signals. In fact, we are assailed by them. These ubiquitous devices are attached to the jacket you tried on in the department store or the book you read while drinking the espresso to ensure that you don't leave without paying for each; they are in the windshield of the taxi as it automatically registers the bridge toll; they are a part of the identification system used to track your FedEx package and in the handheld credit card payment device to pay for the rental car. We are bombarded with signals from iPhones and BlackBerrys, from automobile dashboards warning that the trunk is open or the tires need air, from the GPS to make a left turn, and from the kitchen oven that the roast is cooked. The signals are processed, as the editors state in their preface, "for the purposes of recording, analysis, transmission, and storage." This is true whether you are an astronaut in a space ship or a physician evaluating a patient in the CCU or device clinic. So, all of a sudden signals take on a much more personal importance.

Imagine medicine without signals. Impossible! That hit home recently when I had an MRI after I tripped down a short flight of stairs, landing on my hip. In the magnetic tunnel with the whirring and growling rolling over me like undulating storm clouds, I reflected on the incredible advances of signal processing that would show I just had a bruised hip.

So, now we have a book to explain it all to us, thanks to Drs. Ng and Goldberger. In the first half, they provide an overview of general signal processing concepts and then turn to additional experts in the second half to tell us about the clinical application of these signals for cardiac electrical activity, hemodynamics, heart sounds, and imaging.

While reading this book will not make you a biomedical engineer, it will provide you with an insight into which signals to believe and which to ignore. A medical maxim is that the only thing worse than no data is wrong data. This book will help you make that distinction.

Douglas P. Zipes, MD
Distinguished Professor
Indiana University School of Medicine
Krannert Institute of Cardiology, suite E315
1800 North Capitol Avenue
Indianapolis, IN 46202, USA

Preface

Signal processing is the means and methodology of handling, manipulating, and converting signals for the purposes of recording, analysis, transmission, and storage. Signals, particularly in the context of the biomedical field, are recorded for the presentation and often the quantification of some physical phenomena for the purposes of directly or indirectly obtaining information about the phenomena. There may not be a medical specialty that relies on the acquisition, recording, and displaying of signals more than cardiology. We have come a long way from the days when stethoscopes and blood pressure cuffs were the only diagnostic equipment available to assess the cardiovascular system of a patient. Imagine modern cardiology without electrocardiograms, continuous blood pressure monitoring, intracardiac electrograms, echocardiograms, and MRIs. In fact, these technologies have become so ubiquitous that interpretation of these signals is often performed with little understanding of how these signals are obtained and processed.

Why then would the understanding of signal and image processing be important for a clinician, nurse, or technician in cardiology? Electrocardiograms, for example, can be practically performed with a touch of a button providing a near instantaneous report. Why does it matter how the machine was able to come to the conclusion that the patient had a heart rate of 65 beats/min or a QT interval of 445 ms? The effects of signal processing can appear mysterious and it is tempting to consider that this aspect is best left for engineers and researchers who have technical and mathematical backgrounds. One reason why a better understanding of signal processing would be beneficial is that these technologies used in cardiology all have their own strengths and limitations. For example, a surface electrocardiogram signal may look "noisy" because of motion artifact or poor electrode contact. Changing filter settings can make a signal look much cleaner. These settings, however, may also result in distortion or loss of important information from the signal of interest. Understanding of filters and the frequency content of signals may help determining the proper balance between acceptable noise and the acceptable amount of distortion of the waveform. This is only one example of the importance of understanding the process of obtaining the signal or image, as judging signal quality is often more important than how "clean" a signal or image looks.

More advanced signal processing is also essential in cardiovascular imaging and a variety of advanced electrocardiographic techniques, such as heart rate variability, signal-averaged ECGs, and T-wave alternans. The role of processing is to enhance, embellish, or uncover the signal of interest among a variety of other signals, both physiologic and non-physiologic. By definition, the more a signal is processed, the more deviation there will be from the raw signal. The interpreter must therefore be able to assess whether this deviation is desirable or undesirable. Understanding the signal processing used in these methods will allow the interpreter to understand the issues that are created with signal processing.

The aim of this book is to provide those in the cardiology field an opportunity to learn the basics of signal and image processing without requiring extensive technical or mathematical background. We feel that the saying "a picture is worth a thousand words" is particularly applicable for the purposes of this book. Therefore most of the concepts will be conveyed through illustrative examples. Although this book is geared towards the clinical cardiologist, a beginner in the biomedical engineering field may also find the review of concepts useful before requiring a more in-depth signal processing text. Signal processing is an extremely interesting and thought-provoking subject.

The first half of the book is an overview of general signal processing concepts. In Chap. 1, the architecture of a digital physiologic recording system will be described. The reader will understand the commonality in how all the main cardiology diagnostic systems are put together. In Chap. 2, the fundamentals of analog and digital signals, the reasons why we use them, and the advantages and disadvantages of both will be discussed. In Chap. 3, we will go through what it means to analyze signals in the time domain and frequency domain. In Chap. 4, we will discuss filters, why they are so important to recording systems, and the interpretation of signals. Chapters 5 and 6 discuss ways to detect events such as the heart beat and how the rate of events can be estimated. Chapter 7 then describes the technique of signal averaging, a common method used to improve signal quality. The topic of Chap. 8 is compression, which describes the methods by which digital data can be reduced in size to facilitate storage and transmission. And finally, Chap. 9 shows how the previously described concepts and techniques can be applied to two-dimensional images.

The second half of the book is devoted to discussions on how signal and image processing is used in the specific modalities of cardiac instrumentation. The modalities which utilize one-dimensional signals include the electrocardiogram, invasive and noninvasive blood pressure measurement, pulse oximetry, intracardiac electrograms, and stethoscope. The two (or three)-dimensional modalities include coronary angiograms, ultrasound, magnetic resonance imaging, nuclear imaging, and computed tomography.

We hope that this text will not only enhance the reader's knowledge for clinical and research purposes, but also provide an enjoyable reading experience.

Chicago, IL, USA				Jason Ng and Jeffrey J. Goldberger

Acknowledgments

The editors would like to acknowledge the following individuals who offered their assistance and support for this book: Grant Weston and Cate Rogers at Springer Publishing for their guidance through this whole process, the Cardiology division and section of Cardiac Electrophysiology at Northwestern, Valaree Walker Williams for her administrative support, Vinay Sehgal for his review, the Goldberger family including, Sharon, Adina, Sara, Michale, Akiva, and Mom and Dad and the Ng family, including Pei-hsun, Mary Esther, Mom, Dad, and Justin, for their wonderful support and patience during this project, and to the many colleagues and friends who provided their encouragement for both of us.

Chicago, IL, USA   Jason Ng and Jeffrey J. Goldberger

Contents

Part I Fundamental Signal and Image Processing Concepts 1

1 Architecture of the Basic Physiologic Recorder 3
Jason Ng and Jeffrey J. Goldberger

2 Analog and Digital Signals 9
Jason Ng and Jeffrey J. Goldberger

3 Signals in the Frequency Domain 17
Jason Ng and Jeffrey J. Goldberger

4 Filters 27
Jason Ng and Jeffrey J. Goldberger

5 Techniques for Event and Feature Detection 43
Jason Ng and Jeffrey J. Goldberger

6 Alternative Techniques for Rate Estimation 57
Jason Ng and Jeffrey J. Goldberger

7 Signal Averaging for Noise Reduction 69
Jason Ng and Jeffrey J. Goldberger

8 Data Compression 79
Jason Ng and Jeffrey J. Goldberger

9 Image Processing 89
Jason Ng and Jeffrey J. Goldberger

Part II Cardiology Applications 111

10 Electrocardiography 113
James E. Rosenthal

11 Intravascular and Intracardiac Pressure Measurement 133
Clifford R. Greyson

12	Blood Pressure and Pulse Oximetry 145
	Grace M.N. Mirsky and Alan V. Sahakian
13	Coronary Angiography 157
	Shiuh-Yung James Chen and John D. Carroll
14	Echocardiography 187
	John Edward Abellera Blair and Vera H. Rigolin
15	Nuclear Cardiology: SPECT and PET 219
	Nils P. Johnson, Scott M. Leonard and K. Lance Gould
16	Magnetic Resonance Imaging 251
	Daniel C. Lee and Timothy J. Carroll
17	Computed Tomography 275
	John Joseph Sheehan, Jennifer Ilene Berliner, Karin Dill, and James Christian Carr
18	ECG Telemetry and Long Term Electrocardiography 303
	Eugene Greenstein and James E. Rosenthal
19	Intracardiac Electrograms 319
	Alexandru B. Chicos and Alan H. Kadish
20	Advanced Signal Processing Applications of the ECG: T-Wave Alternans, Heart Rate Variability, and the Signal Averaged ECG 347
	Ashwani P. Sastry and Sanjiv M. Narayan
21	Digital Stethoscopes 379
	Indranil Sen-Gupta and Jason Ng

Index 391

Contributors

Jennifer I. Berliner
Department of Medicine,
Division of Cardiology,
University of Pittsburgh Medical Center,
Pittsburgh, PA, USA

John E.A. Blair
Department of Medicine,
Division of Cardiology,
Wilford Hall Medical Center;
Lackland, AFB, TX and
Uniformed Services University of
the Health Sciences, Bethesda, MD

James C. Carr
Department of Cardiovascular Imaging,
Feinberg School of Medicine,
Northwestern University,
Chicago, IL, USA

John D. Carroll
Department of Medicine,
Anschutz Medical Campus,
University of Colorado Denver,
Aurora, CO, USA

Timothy J. Carroll
Departments of Biomedical Engineering
and Radiology, Northwestern University,
Chicago, IL, USA

Shiuh-Yung James Chen
Department of Medicine,
Anschutz Medical Campus,
University of Colorado Denver,
Aurora, CO, USA

Alexandru B. Chicos
Department of Medicine,
Division of Cardiology,
Feinberg School of Medicine,
Northwestern University,
Chicago, IL, USA

Karin Dill
Department of Cardiovascular Imaging,
Feinberg School of Medicine,
Northwestern University,
Chicago, IL, USA

Jeffrey J. Goldberger
Northwestern University,
Feinberg School of Medicine,
Division of Cardiology,
Department of Medicine,
Chicago, IL, USA

K. Lance Gould
Department of Medicine,
Division of Cardiology, Weatherhead P.E.T.
Center For Preventing and Reversing
Atherosclerosis, University of Texas
Medical School and Memorial Hermann
Hospital, Houston, TX, USA

Eugene Greenstein
Division of Cardiology,
Feinberg School of Medicine,
Northwestern University,
Chicago, IL, USA

Clifford R. Greyson
Denver Department of Veterans
Affairs Medical Center,
University of Colorado at Denver,
Denver, CO 80220, USA

Nils P. Johnson
Department of Medicine,
Division of Cardiology,
Feinberg School of Medicine,
Northwestern University,
Chicago, IL, USA

Alan H. Kadish
Division of Cardiology,
Feinberg School of Medicine,
Northwestern University
Chicago, IL, USA

Daniel C. Lee
Division of Cardiology,
Feinberg School of Medicine,
Northwestern University,
Chicago, IL, USA

Scott M. Leonard
Manager Nuclear Cardiology Labs (FLSA),
Myocardial Imaging Research Laboratory,
Feinberg School of Medicine,
Northwestern University,
Chicago, IL, USA

Sanjiv M. Narayan
Division of Cardiology,
University of California San Diego and
VA Medical Center, La Jolla,
CA, USA

Jason Ng
Northwestern University,
Feinberg School of Medicine,
Division of Cardiology,
Department of Medicine,
Chicago, IL, USA

Grace M.N. Mirsky
McCormick School of Engineering,
Northwestern University, Evanston,
IL, USA

Vera H. Rigolin
Department of Medicine,
Division of Cardiology,
Feinberg School of Medicine,
Northwestern University,
Chicago, IL, USA

James E. Rosenthal
Department of Medicine,
Division of Cardiology,
Feinberg School of Medicine,
Northwestern University,
Chicago, IL, USA

Alan V. Sahakian
Department of Electrical Engineering and
Computer Science, Department of
Biomedical Engineering, McCormick
School of Engineering, Northwestern
University,
Evanston, IL, USA

Ashwani P. Sastry
Division of Cardiology,
Duke University Medical Center,
Durham, NC

Indranil Sen-Gupta
Division of Neurology,
Feinberg School of Medicine,
Northwestern University,
Chicago, IL, USA

John J. Sheehan
Department of Cardiovascular Imaging,
Feinberg School of Medicine,
Northwestern University,
Chicago, IL, USA

Part I

Fundamental Signal and Image Processing Concepts

Architecture of the Basic Physiologic Recorder

1

Jason Ng and Jeffrey J. Goldberger

1.1 Chapter Objectives

Signals are acquired from medical instrumentation of many different types. They can be as small as a digital thermometer or as big as a magnetic resonance scanner. In spite of the differences in size, cost, and the type of data these devices obtain, most biomedical devices that acquire physiologic data have the same basic structure. The structure of what we will call the basic digital physiologic recording system will be described in this section with the details of each of the processes in the following sections. A block diagram of the basic digital physiologic recording system is shown in Fig. 1.1.

By the end of the chapter, the reader should know and understand the functions of these general components found in most medical instrumentation used to acquire physiologic signals.

1.2 Transducers

The first element shown in the block diagram is the transducer. The transducer is an element that converts some physical measurement to a voltage and electrical current that can be processed and recorded by an electronic device. Table 1.1 provides some examples of physiologic recording systems, the type of transducers that are used, and the physical measurement that is converted to an electrical signal.

The physiologic recording systems can have from one to thousands of transducers in a single system. An important element in how transducers obtain signals is the reference. A reference is either a known value or a recording where a specific value, such as zero,

---

J. Ng (✉)
Department of Medicine, Division of Cardiology, Feinberg School of Medicine,
Northwestern University, Chicago, IL, USA
e-mail: jsnng@northwestern.edu

J.J. Goldberger and J. Ng (eds.),
Practical Signal and Image Processing in Clinical Cardiology,
DOI: 10.1007/978-1-84882-515-4_1, © Springer-Verlag London Limited 2010

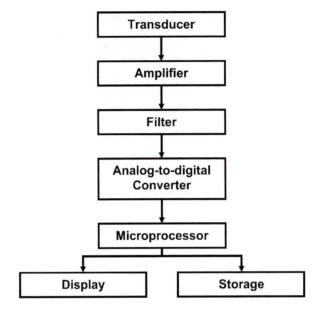

Fig. 1.1 Block diagram of basic digital physiologic recording system

Table 1.1 Examples of physiologic recording systems and the corresponding transducer and physiologic measurement

Physiologic recording system	Transducer	Measurement
ECG	Electrode	Voltage
Continuous blood pressure recorder	Piezoelectric pressure transducer	Pressure
Digital thermometer	Thermocouple	Temperature
CT	Photodiode	X-ray
Pulse oximeter	Photodiode	Light from light-emitting diode
MRI	Radiofrequency antennas	Radiofrequency electromagnetic waves
Echocardiogram	Piezoelectric transducer	Ultrasound

is assumed. The difference between the signal obtained by the transducer and the reference is the signal of interest. For modalities that measure potential or voltage, such as the ECG, recording from an electrode requires a reference potential from another electrode. Configuration of the recording electrode with the reference electrode can be close together or far apart depending on whether local or global measurements are desired. For modalities such as continuous blood pressure monitors or thermometers, the reference is determined by the same transducer that is used for recording. For blood pressure monitors, calibration is performed by recording atmospheric pressure prior to recording the arterial pressure for each use of the monitor. For digital thermometers, the calibration is usually performed where the device is made by applying the transducer to known temperatures (e.g., ice water or boiling water). The reference is then programmed into the device. Because temperature is an absolute measurement, no further calibration is needed. For imaging modalities, such as X-ray or CT, an array of detectors are used. Two levels of references are required. First, each detector element in the array must be identically calibrated, meaning the same level of X-ray exposure must produce the same output for each detector element. This calibration would be typically performed in the factory. Second, during the acquisition of the image, the output of the detectors by themselves does not provide very meaningful information when analyzed individually. However, when each detector output is referenced with that of every other detector, an image is formed that will allow differentiation of tissue.

1.3
Amplifiers

The electric signals produced with the transducer are typically very small continuous waveforms. These continuous signals are known as analog signals. Modern biomedical instrumentation converts analog signals to a discrete or digital form, so that signal processing and storage can be performed by microprocessors and digital memory. Because the small amplitude of the signals from the transducer may make it difficult to convert the analog signal into a digital signal without error or distortion, often the next step after the transducer is amplification to increase the amplitude of the signal closer to the range that is better handled by the analog-to-digital conversion circuitry. This amplification is usually performed by a group of transistors and resistors. Sometimes the device has variable resistors or switches that allow the user to manually adjust the amplification. At other times, however, the circuit can sense the amplitude of the signal and adaptively adjust the amplification. This is known as automatic gain control.

1.4
Filters

The analog-to-digital converter not only has a desired amplitude range, but also a desired frequency range that is dependent on the sampling rate of the converter. As a result, filtering is usually performed after amplification and before conversion to reject the frequencies that are too fast for the analog-to-digital converter to sample. This "low pass" filter is often called an "antialiasing" filter and will be discussed in further detail in the subsequent sections. A second type of filter that is sometimes used is a "high pass" filter, which rejects low frequencies. Rejecting low frequencies is done to prevent baseline wander by keeping the baseline signal near zero, thus also keeping the signal within range of the converter. For applications where the baseline value contains information in itself (temperature readings for example), a high pass filter is not used. High pass and low pass filters in this third stage of the digital physiologic recording system are implemented by a network of transistors, resistors, and capacitors.

1.5
Analog-to-Digital Convertors

The transducers, amplifier, and filters comprise the analog portion of the system. In this portion, the signal processing is performed through electronic components such as transistors, resistors, and capacitors usually without the aid of a microprocessor. The fourth stage of the system is the analog-to-digital converter. In this stage, the signal, whose information is contained in the voltage amplitudes and patterns, is converted into binary numbers at discrete instances of time.

1.6
Microprocessor

Once converted, the digital signal is now in a format which a microprocessor can understand. With the data in the system's memory, additional signal processing can be performed to additionally filter, detect features, or perform measurements. These operations are performed through "software" rather than "hardware" components. Performing operations through "software" means that instructions are provided to the microprocessor to read, write, add, and multiply the binary numbers. It is at this level where the majority of the digital signal processing operations that are covered in this book are performed. The microprocessor also controls how the data are displayed and stored.

Summary of Key Terms

- Physiologic recording system – Device that acquires physiologic measurements for the purposes of display, analysis, and storage.
- Transducer – A material or device that converts a physiologic parameter into another type of signal (typically voltage) that will allow signal processing by electronic circuits.
- Reference – A signal of known value or assumed value. The difference between the recording output and the reference is the signal of interest.
- Calibration – The procedure of mapping the output of a recording transducer to known values of the phenomena to be recorded.
- Antialiasing filter – A circuit that rejects high frequency components so that a signal may be digitized without distortion.
- Analog-to-digital converter – A circuit that takes samples from a continuous waveform and quantizes the values.
- Microprocessor – A digital device made up of transistors that are capable of performing mathematical operations (e.g., addition and multiplication) and reading, moving, and storing digital data.

Reference

1. Webster JG, ed. *Medical Instrumentation: Application and Design.* New York: Wiley; 1998.

Analog and Digital Signals

2

Jason Ng and Jeffrey J. Goldberger

2.1
Chapter Objectives

"Digital" has been the buzz word for the last couple of decades. The latest and greatest electronic devices have been marketed as digital and cardiology equipment has been no exception. "Analog" has the connotation of being old and outdated, while "digital" has been associated with new and advanced. What do these terms actually mean and is one really better than the other? By the end of the chapter, the reader should know what analog and digital signals are, their respective characteristics, and the advantages and disadvantages of both signal types. The reader will also understand the fundamentals of sampling, including the trade-offs of high sampling rates and high amplitude resolution, and the distortion that is possible with low sampling rates and low amplitude resolution.

2.2
Analog Signals

To say a signal is analog simply means that the signal is continuous in time and amplitude. Take, for example, your standard mercury glass thermometer. This device is analog because the temperature reading is updated constantly and changes at any time interval. A new value of temperature can be obtained whether you look at the thermometer 1 s later, half a second later, or a millionth of a second later, assuming temperature can change that fast. The readings from the thermometer are also continuous in amplitude. This means that assuming your eyes are sensitive enough to read the mercury level, readings of 37, 37.4, or 37.440183432°C are possible. In actuality, most cardiac signals of interest are analog by nature. For example, voltages recorded on the body surface and cardiac motion are continuous functions in time and amplitude.

J. Ng (✉)
Department of Medicine, Division of Cardiology, Feinberg School of Medicine,
Northwestern University, Chicago, IL, USA
e-mail: jsnng@northwestern.edu

J.J. Goldberger and J. Ng (eds.),
Practical Signal and Image Processing in Clinical Cardiology,
DOI: 10.1007/978-1-84882-515-4_2, © Springer-Verlag London Limited 2010

If the description of analog instrumentation and signals stopped here, it would seem like this would be the ideal method to record signals. Why then have analog tape players and VCRs been replaced by digital CD players and DVD players, if tape players can reproduce continuous time and amplitude signals with near infinite resolution? The reason is that analog recording and signals suffer one major drawback – their susceptibility to noise and distortion. Consider an audio tape with your favorite classical music performance that you bought in the 1980s. Chances are that the audio quality has degraded since the tape was purchased. Also consider the situation where a duplicate of the tape was made. The copy of the tape would not have the same quality as the original. If a duplicate of the duplicate of the duplicate was made, the imperfections of the duplication process would add up. In an analog system, noise cannot be easily removed once it has entered the system.

2.3
Digital Signals

Digital systems attempt to overcome the analog system's susceptibility to noise by sacrificing the infinite time and amplitude resolution to obtain perfect reproduction of the signal, no matter how long it has been stored or how many times it has been duplicated. That is why your audio CD purchased in the 1990s (assuming it is not too scratched up) will sound the same as when you first purchased it. The advantages can also be readily seen in the cardiology field. For example, making photocopies of an ECG tracing will result in loss of quality. However, printing a new copy from the saved digital file will give you a perfect reproduction every time. The discrete time and discrete amplitude nature of the digital signal provide a buffer to noise that may enter the system through transmission or otherwise. Digital signals are usually stored and transmitted in the form of ones and zeros. If a digital receiver knows that only zeros or ones are being transmitted and when approximately to expect them, there is a certain acceptable level of noise that the receiver can handle. Consider the example in the Fig. 2.1. The top plot shows a digital series of eight ones and zeros. This series could represent some analog value. The transmission or reproduction of the digital series results in noise being added to the series, such that the values now vary around one and zero as shown in the middle plot. If a digital receiver of the transmitted series uses the 0.5 level as the detection threshold, any value above 0.5 would be considered a one and any value below 0.5 would be considered a zero. With this criterion, all the ones and zeros would be detected correctly (bottom plot), despite the presence of noise. Thus the received digital signal provides a more accurate representation of the true signal of interest than would be if the analog signal itself was transmitted through the noisy channel.

Beyond the advantages of noise robustness during reproduction and transmission, digital signals have many other advantages. These include the ability to use computer algorithms to filter the signal, data compression to save storage space, and signal processing to extract information that may not be possible through manual human analysis. Thus there can be a large benefit in converting many of the signals that are used in cardiology to digital form.

Fig. 2.1 Illustration of a digital signal transmitted through a noisy channel. The top panel shows a plot of the eight binary digits (amplitude values 0 or 1). The middle panel shows the same eight digits after transmission through a noisy channel causing deviation from 0 and 1. The 0.5 level represents the threshold, above or below which a 0 or 1 is decided by the digital receiver. The bottom panel shows the results of the decisions, which are equivalent to the original digital signal. Transmitting a digitized signal through a noisy channel usually results in a more accurate representation of the true signal than transmitting the original analog signal

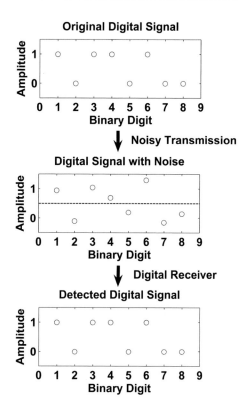

2.4 Analog-to-Digital Conversion

2.4.1 Sampling

The process of converting an analog signal to a digital signal has two parts: sampling and quantization. The sampling process converts a continuous time signal to a discrete time signal with a defined time resolution. The time resolution is determined by what is known as the sampling rate, usually expressing in Hertz (Hz) or samples per second. Thus if the sampling rate is 1,000 Hz, or 1,000 times/s, this means that the signal is being sampled every 1 ms. The sampling rate needed for a faithful reproduction of the signal depends on the sharpness of the fluctuations of the signal being sampled. An illustration of a sine wave with the frequency of 8 Hz or 8 cycles/s that is sampled 100 times a second (100 Hz) is shown in the top example of Fig. 2.2. As shown in the second panel, the 100 Hz sampling takes points from the sine wave every 10 ms. Connecting the points as shown in the third panel produces a good reproduction of the original sine wave.

The middle example of Fig. 2.2 shows the same sine wave with 25 Hz sampling. With 25 Hz sampling, the reconstructed signal is clearly not as good as when the sine wave was sampled at 100 Hz. However, the oscillations at 8 cycles/s can still be recognized. Decreasing

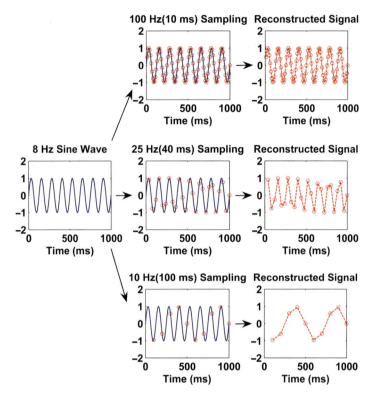

Fig. 2.2 Plots showing a sine wave with a frequency of 8 Hz sampled at rates of 100, 25, and 10 Hz. The reconstructed signal with 10 Hz sampling shows aliasing, the distortion resulting from undersampling

the sampling rate even further can result in a completely distorted reconstruction of the signal. The bottom example of Fig. 2.2 shows the sine wave sampled at 10 Hz. The reconstructed signal in this case resembles a 2-Hz sine wave, rather than an 8-Hz sine wave.

Distortion to the point where the original sine wave is unrecognizable because of undersampling is known as aliasing. Stated differently, if the signal is changing at a frequency that is faster than the sampling rate, important information about the signal will be lost. Consider the three signals in Fig. 2.3 – all three have the same sampled signal, but the original signals are not identical. This is because the signal contains high frequency components that are not detected by the relatively low sampling rate. To prevent aliasing, the Nyquist sampling rule states that the sampling rate must be at least twice the frequency of the sine wave. For our example of an 8-Hz sine wave, a sampling rate of at least 16 Hz is needed to prevent aliasing. Nonsinusoidal signals must be sampled at least 2 times the highest frequency component of the signal to avoid aliasing. Higher sampling rates are preferable in terms of the fidelity of the sampling. However, higher sampling rates come at the cost of additional size of the data. Thus, storage space is a consideration while determining an appropriate sampling rate.

Fig. 2.3 Illustration of aliasing due to undersampling. A sine wave, square wave, and an alternating positive and negative pulse function produce the identical triangle wave when sampled at the same rate. Sampling occurs at 20 Hz and is indicated by the open *red circles*

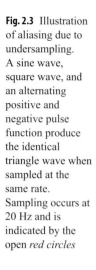
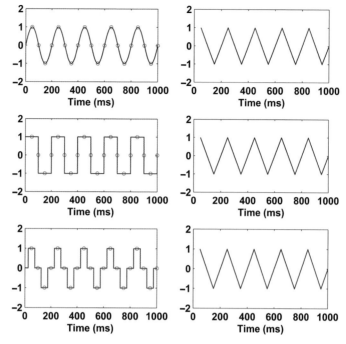

2.4.2 Quantization

The second aspect of analog-to-digital conversion is quantization. Quantization converts continuous amplitude signals to a signal with a finite number of possible amplitude values. Quantizing with a high amplitude resolution will allow representation of the original signal with the least amount of error. However, higher resolution also comes with the trade-off of requiring more storage space. Quantization occurs with a fixed range of voltage. Therefore, proper amplification is important to get the best resolution possible. Figure 2.4 shows a sine wave that is sampled by a nine-level quantizer with a sample rate of 100 Hz and an amplitude resolution of 0.25 units or one eighth of the peak-to-peak amplitude of the signal. The amplitude of the sine wave in this example is perfectly fit over the quantization range. Reconstruction of the sine wave after quantization shows a decent approximation of the original sine wave.

Quantization can be poor if the amplification of the signal is less than ideal. In Fig. 2.5, the same nine levels are used to quantize a signal with a peak-to-peak amplitude of 0.5 units. The amplitude resolution of 0.25 is now only half of the peak-to-peak amplitude.

The poor relative amplitude resolution in this example results in a reconstructed signal that resembles more like a trapezoidal wave than a sine wave since only three of the nine levels are being utilized.

Figure 2.6 shows an example of a sine wave that is amplified beyond the range of the quantizer (peak-to-peak amplitude of two). In this situation, the signal is clipped at −1 and 1.

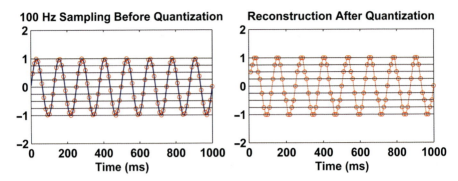

Fig. 2.4 Eight Hertz sine wave with 100 Hz sampling and nine-level quantization. The quantization levels are equally distributed over the amplitude range of the sine wave resulting in a good reproduction of the original signal. Note that the quantized signal takes on only the nine values indicated by the horizontal lines while the original signal spans over a range of values at the times sampled (indicated by the open *red circles*)

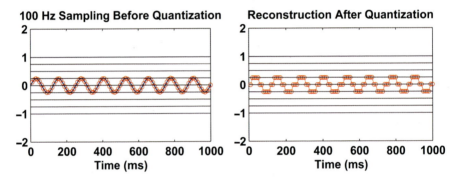

Fig. 2.5 Example of the sine wave that is underquantized leading to poor reproduction of the signal

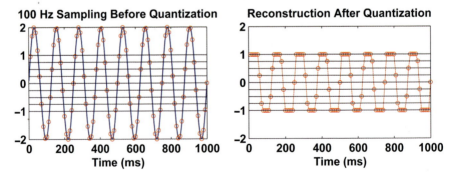

Fig. 2.6 Example of sine wave whose amplitude is beyond the range of the quantization. The result is a signal that is clipped at the upper and lower parts of the signal (also known as saturation)

This distortion is also known as "saturation" or "clipping." Thus even though the relative amplitude resolution of the quantization is high, the clipping of the signal cannot be undone.

2.4.3 Summary

In summary, the sampling rate and amplitude resolution of the sampling process are important qualities for digital signals to be a good representation of an analog signal. High sampling rates and amplitude resolution require more hardware complexity and storage space to store the signals. However, low sampling rates and amplitude resolution can result in distorted signals with loss of information. Proper amplification of the signal is also required to optimize the quantization process.

Summary of Key Terms

- Analog signal – Continuous time and continuous amplitude signal.
- Digital signal – Signal characterized by discrete time points and discrete amplitude values having a defined sampling rate and amplitude resolution.
- Sampling – The process of obtaining data points from an analog signal at defined intervals. The frequency of the sampling is known as the sampling rate.
- Quantization – The process of assigning sampled data points to discrete amplitude values of a defined resolution.
- Undersampling – Sampling at too slow of a rate which results in loss of information.
- Nyquist sampling rate – The rate of twice the highest frequency of a signal that is the minimum rate required to sample without loss of information.
- Aliasing – The distortion that occurs when a signal is undersampled (i.e., the Nyquist sampling criterion is not met).
- Saturation – The distortion of a signal that occurs when the amplitude of the signal is beyond the limits of the highest or lowest quantization amplitude. This is also known as clipping.

References

1. Oppenhein AV, Schafer RW. *Discrete-Time Signal Processing*. Englewood Cliffs, NJ: Prentice Hall; 1989.
2. Ziemer RE, Tranter WH, Fannin DR. *Signals and Systems: Continuous and Discrete*. New York, NY: Macmillan; 1993.

Signals in the Frequency Domain

3

Jason Ng and Jeffrey J. Goldberger

3.1 Chapter Objectives

Interpreting signals in the time domain is intuitively grasped by most people as time plots are commonly encountered in everyday life. Time domain plots represent the variable of interest in the y-axis and time in the x-axis. Stock charts show the up and down trends of your investment's value over time. Your electric company bill will show your power usage month-to-month over the course of the year. Signals in cardiology are also most commonly displayed in the time domain. ECG and blood pressure monitors, for example, continuously plot voltages or pressure vs. time.

Frequency domain plots, on the other hand, plot the variable of interest vs. frequency. The frequency domain is less commonly encountered in everyday life than the time domain, but is very important in the field of signal processing. Concepts such as filtering, sampling, and periodicity detection require at least a basic understanding of the frequency domain.

3.2 What is the Frequency Domain?

Audio and music are perhaps the applications where most people have experienced working in the frequency domain. A single tone or note (e.g., from a piano or guitar) corresponds primarily to a sine wave of a single frequency. The loudness of the tone would be reflected in the amplitude of the sound waves. When multiple notes are combined to yield a musical piece, the sine waves of different frequencies are summed together making it difficult to separate the different sine waves in the time domain. In the frequency domain, however, the different frequency components can be easily separated out.

J. Ng (✉)
Department of Medicine, Division of Cardiology, Feinberg School of Medicine, Northwestern University, Chicago, IL, USA
e-mail: jsnng@northwestern.edu

J.J. Goldberger and J. Ng (eds.),
Practical Signal and Image Processing in Clinical Cardiology,
DOI: 10.1007/978-1-84882-515-4_3, © Springer-Verlag London Limited 2010

Figure 3.1 shows the sine waves with frequencies corresponding to the musical notes "middle C," "E," and "G." When displayed individually, the frequencies are apparent both in the time domain and the frequency domain. In the time domain, the frequencies can be measured as the number of periods in a second or as 1/(duration of one period). In the frequency domain, the power spectrum plots the power (square of the amplitude of the sine wave) at each frequency. Thus, the frequency of a simple sine wave is simply the frequency where the peak in the power spectrum occurs. When "middle C," "E," and "G" are simultaneously played to form the "C chord," the different frequencies cannot be easily identified in the time domain, as the summation of the three sine wave combine to a more complex pattern. However, in the frequency domain, three distinct peaks for each frequency can be clearly identified.

Figure 3.2 shows an example of a Windows Media Player playing a more complicated piece of audio with the time domain signal (amplitude vs. time) on the left panel and the corresponding frequency domain bar plot on the right. The frequency spectrum simply displays the strength (loudness) of each pitch or frequency that is a component of the complete audio signal. For audio, the frequency domain display is useful when trying to adjust the balance between the low-frequency sounds (bass) and the high-frequency sounds (treble).

What do the frequency plots actually represent? Mathematically, it has been shown that any signal (such as our common examples of time domain signals) can be completely decomposed into a sum of sine waves of different frequencies. This mathematical operation is known as the Fourier transform named after French mathematician Jean Baptiste Joseph Fourier who pioneered this work in the early 1800s. The formula for the Fourier transform is:

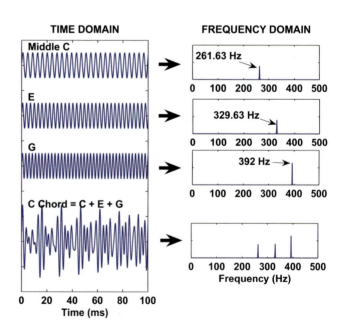

Fig. 3.1 Time domain and frequency domain representations of middle C, E, G and the C chord

3 Signals in the Frequency Domain

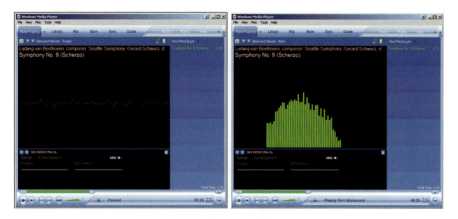

Fig. 3.2 Time and frequency domain plots of an audio signal displayed using Windows Media Player

$$X(f) = \int_{-\infty}^{\infty} x(t) e^{-i2\pi ft}\, dt,$$

where $X(f)$ is the frequency domain function and $x(t)$ is the time domain function.

In Fig. 3.2, each bar of the frequency domain plot would represent the amplitude of the sine wave for a particular frequency. In this example, the sine waves with the highest amplitude tend to occur in the middle of the band, while the sine waves with the lowest amplitude have the highest frequencies.

3.3
Uses of Frequency Domain Plots

Frequency domain analysis can provide a visual and quantitative sense of both a signal's morphology and periodicity. Let us take the example of the frequency domain analysis of atmospheric temperature readings. Figure 3.3 shows the time domain and frequency domain plots of daily temperatures in Chicago and Seattle in the years 2004–2006. Chicago is famous for its large variations in temperature, both on a seasonal and day-to-day scale. Seattle, on the other hand, is known for its moderate and steady temperatures due to its location on the Pacific coast. From the visual inspection of the time domain plots this appears to be true. Frequency domain analysis can be used to quantify these assumptions. The frequency domain plots in Fig. 3.3 are divided into two bands for each city: low frequency (0–0.1 cycles/day) and high frequency (0.2–0.5 cycles/day). Typically, frequency is measured in Hertz, which is equivalent to cycles per second. For daily temperature, it makes more sense to measure frequency in cycles/day. The y-axis of these plots depicts power with units of $(°F)^2$. The power at each frequency is simply the square of half the amplitude term associated with the sine wave of that frequency. Thus, these plots are known as power spectra. The area of the power spectrum, known as the total power of the

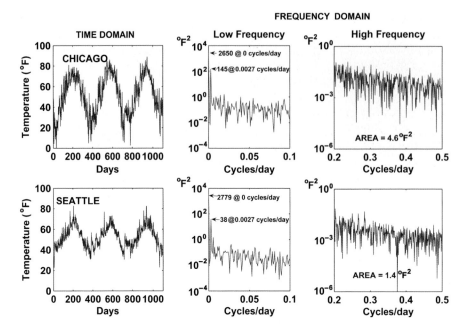

Fig. 3.3 Comparison of time and frequency domain plots of daily temperatures of Chicago and Seattle. Seattle shows higher power at 0 frequency, which is due to a higher mean temperature in Seattle vs. Chicago. Chicago shows higher power at 0.0027 cycles/day (or 1/356 days), which suggests larger seasonal changes in temperature. Chicago also shows more power at high frequencies, suggesting more day-to-day variability in temperature vs. Seattle

signal, is mathematically equal to the variance of the time domain signal (the variance is the square of the standard deviation).

The low-frequency power spectra contain a couple of features that highlight the differences in temperature between the two cities. The first is the large peak at the 0 cycles/day frequency. The zero frequency value of the power spectrum is equivalent to the square of the mean value of the entire signal. Chicago has a zero frequency power of 2,650 ($°F$)^2 which translates to a mean temperature of 51.5°F. Seattle has a zero frequency power of 2,779 ($°F$)^2 and therefore a mean temperature of 52.7°F.

The second largest peak occurs at 0.0027 cycles/day for both the cities. Another way of expressing this frequency is 1 cycle per 365.3 days or roughly 1 cycle/year. Thus, the power at this frequency reflects the seasonal variation of temperature. Except for the mean, the value at any particular frequency on the power spectrum is equivalent to the square of half the amplitude of the sine wave of that frequency. The Chicago value at 0.0027 cycles/day is 145 ($°F$)^2 vs. 38 ($°F$)^2 for Seattle. This translates to sine wave amplitudes of 24°F (48°F peak-to-peak) and 12°F (24°F peak-to-peak) for Chicago and Seattle, respectively. Thus, we have shown quantitatively that Chicago has larger seasonal variations in temperature than Seattle.

If we wanted to test the hypothesis that Chicago has greater short-term variations than Seattle without considering seasonal changes, we could compare the higher frequency components from one city to another. The frequency band that we would analyze would depend on what we considered to be "short-term." Seasonal fluctuations were shown to have a frequency of approximately 1 cycle/year. A reasonable band may be frequencies with cycle lengths of less than 5 days which is equivalent to frequencies greater than 0.2 cycles/day. Therefore, if the area in the band above 0.2 cycles/day is greater in Chicago than in Seattle, it would suggest that Chicago has greater short-term fluctuations in temperature than Seattle. The power spectra for the 0.2–0.5 cycles/day band are also shown in Fig. 3.3. The area under the defined high-frequency band is 4.6 ($°F$)^2 in Chicago and 1.4 ($°F$)^2 in Seattle. We have now quantitatively determined through frequency domain analysis that although Seattle had a higher average temperature, Chicago had higher seasonal and short-term fluctuations in temperature during this 3 year period.

For another example of the application of frequency domain analysis, let us assume that we do not know how many days there are in a year and want to obtain an estimate based on temperature data alone. One time domain approach might be to detect the day of highest temperature for each of the estimated summer seasons. This approach may give a reasonable estimate, but short-term fluctuations may make estimation in this way inaccurate. For Chicago, the number of days between the highest temperature day of the first year and that of the second year was 411. There were 373 days between the highest temperature day of the second year and that of the third year. Taking the average periods over many years will likely improve this estimate. The estimation can also be performed with the frequency domain. The seasonal changes in temperature have the strongest yearly trends. Therefore, there should be a prominent peak in the frequency corresponding to 1 cycle/year. This frequency can be determined from the frequency domain and used to estimate the number of days in a year. As we have shown previously, the largest peak aside from the zero frequency peak is at the frequency 0.0027 cycles/day or 1 cycle per 365.3 days, which provides an excellent estimate for the number of days in a year.

3.4
Transforming a Time Domain Signal to the Frequency Domain

Although we have now demonstrated the utility of frequency domain analysis, it may still be difficult to conceptualize how any signal can be decomposed into a sum of sine waves of different frequencies. This is understandable as most signals look nothing like sine waves. This concept might be best illustrated by summing the different sine waves one-by-one until the signal of interest is reconstructed. In Fig. 3.4, we will take this approach to reconstruct a single square wave. In the left panel of the figure are the individual sine waves that are being summed. The middle panel shows the cumulative sum. Thus, the first graph shows the first sine wave. The second graph shows the sum of the first and second sine wave. The third graph shows the sum of the first three sine waves, and so on. The last graph represents the sum of the many sine waves of different frequencies that finally reproduces the square wave. The right panel demonstrates the amplitudes and frequencies of the sine waves included in the cumulative sum in the corresponding middle panel. This is the frequency spectrum or frequency domain representation of the cumulative sum signal in the middle panel. As we can see in the figure, each sine wave that gets added makes the

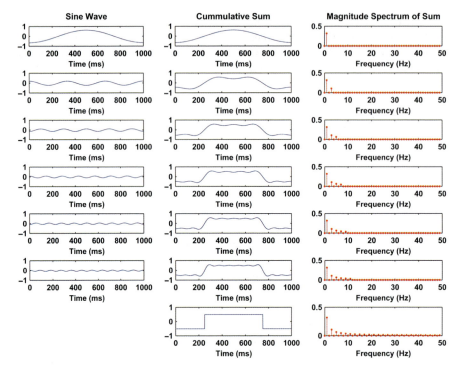

Fig. 3.4 Illustration of how sine waves of different frequencies can be summed together to form a square wave

sum more and more like a square wave. With all frequencies present, the edges of the square wave are sharp and the ripples of the incomplete sums are now eliminated. This process can be performed starting with the square wave to determine which sine waves (both frequency and amplitude) are required to constitute the square wave. Similar decomposition can be applied to a signal of any morphology.

3.5
Frequency Domain of Digital Signals

For the examples above, frequency domain plots were constructed from digital (discrete time) data. Where analog signals would be transformed to the frequency domain using the Fourier Transform, digital signals would be transformed with discrete Fourier Transform algorithms. The Fast Fourier Transform (FFT) is a commonly used discrete Fourier Transform algorithm. The result of the discrete Fourier Transform is the frequency response corresponding to sinusoids at discrete frequencies. The range of frequencies of these sinusoids will be from 0 Hz to half the time domain sampling rate. The FFT cannot detect frequencies above half the sampling rate as this exceeds the Nyquist limit discussed in Chap. 2.

The frequency resolution of the resulting transformed signal is the sampling rate divided by the number of samples in the time domain. A signal that is 10 s in duration with a sampling rate of 1,000 Hz will have 10,000 samples. Applying the FFT to this signal will result in a frequency domain signal that ranges from 0 to 500 Hz and a frequency resolution of 1,000/10,000 = 0.1 Hz.

The choice of the time domain signal length is an important consideration for frequency domain analysis, because it affects both the frequency resolution and the time resolution of the analysis. The top panel in the example shown in Fig. 3.5 displays a time domain signal which consists of the five different sine waves appended one after another. The sine wave segments are each 1 s in length and have frequencies of 4.2, 5.6, 6.3, 7.8, and 8.5 Hz. The sampling rate is 100 samples/s. The next five panels show the power spectra of each of the five 1-s segments. Because the segments have lengths of 100 samples with a sampling rate of 100 Hz, the frequency resolution from the FFT is 1 Hz (the sampling rate divided by the number of samples). The frequencies with the highest power, also known as the dominant frequency, were found to be 4.0, 6.0, 6.0, 8.0, and 8.0 Hz for the five 1-s segments. These estimates of the actual frequencies of the sine waves have some error because of the 1 Hz sampling resolution of the FFT.

The last panel of the figure shows the power spectrum of the entire 5-s window. The frequencies of the five highest peaks in the spectrum were 4.2, 5.4, 6.0, 7.6, and 8.2 Hz. Although these estimated frequencies were closer to the actual frequencies compared to the estimates using the shorter windows, there is no way to know when the different frequencies occurred within those 5 s or whether they occurred sequentially or simultaneously. This is what is meant by loss of time resolution.

If higher frequency resolution is required in situations where short time segments are necessary, frequency resolution can be increased using an additional step known as zero-padding prior to applying the FFT. Zero-padding essentially increases the length of the segment by appending zero values to the segment to obtain the desired frequency resolution without adding additional power to the signal. For example, if we take a 1-s window of the signal in Fig. 3.5 and append 9 s worth of zero values, the frequency resolution will improve from 1 to 0.1 Hz. Recalculating the FFTs for the five segments with 9 s of zero padding will result in dominant frequencies of 4.2, 5.6, 6.3, 7.8, and 8.5 Hz, the actual frequencies of the sine waves in those segments. A question one may have about this approach is that how are we able to gain information from the signal by just appending zeros. The answer to this, which is also a caveat to this approach, is that actually no information is gained, but is rather interpolated. So, while zero padding was found useful in this example when single sine waves were analyzed, in more complex signals that may have multiple closely spaced frequencies, zero padding will not overcome the initial lack of frequency resolution to exhibit multiple peaks corresponding to the different frequencies.

Another issue to consider when performing frequency analysis of short segments, particularly if zero-padding is applied is the discontinuity that occurs at the beginning and the end of the segment. Take for example the first segment of the signal in Fig. 3.6, in which the 4.2 Hz sine wave ends at a value close to one at 1,000 ms. If zeroes are appended to this segment, this signal would now have a steep drop from one to zero. Sine waves of other frequencies beside 4.2 Hz would be required to describe this abrupt change. For this example, the dominant frequency of 4.2 Hz still accurately reflects the frequency of the sine

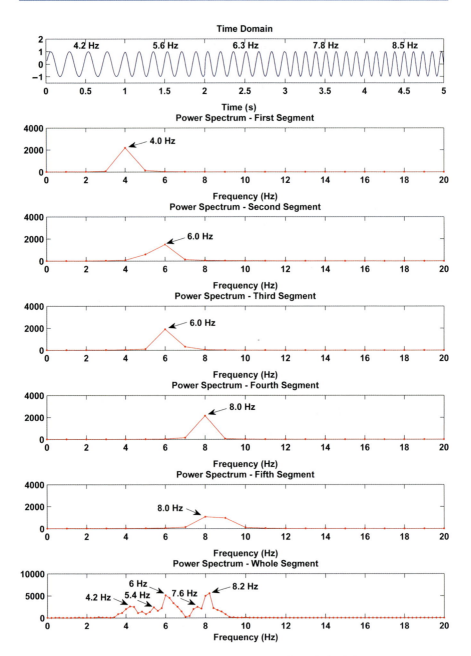

Fig. 3.5 A frequency-varying sine wave with frequency domain analysis of short segments and the whole segment

wave despite the discontinuity. However, if this signal had other noise present, the estimation of the frequency may be more difficult if the one-to-zero abrupt jump is present.

Windowing is a common processing step that is applied to short time segments prior to applying the FFT. The purpose of windowing is to lessen the effect of the edge discontinuities by gradually attenuating the edges. This gradual attenuation is accomplished by multiplying a rounded waveform to the signal as illustrated in Fig. 3.6. Hanning and Hamming windows are two commonly used windows. As shown in Fig. 3.6, the power spectrum of a sine wave multiplied with the rectangular window, a window with no attenuation, shows ripples adjacent to the main peaks while the power spectrum of the sine wave multiplied with a Hanning window has a power spectrum with a single peak without ripples.

Because windows that attenuate the edges of the segment by design place greater weight on the middle portion of the segment, this can distort the frequency spectrum, particularly for signals where frequencies are constantly changing. Thus, it is important when using windowed segments that the middle portion of the segment is representative of the entire segment (i.e., has stable periodicity).

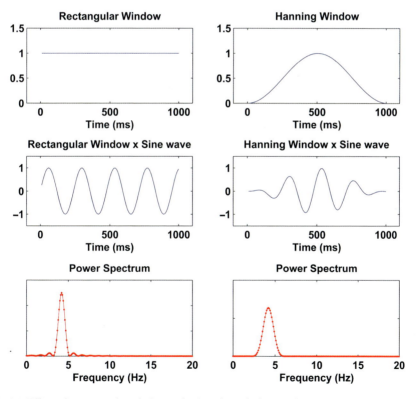

Fig. 3.6 Effect of a rectangular window and a Hanning window on the power spectrum of a sine wave. The rectangular window captures a segment of a sine wave without attenuation of the edges of the segment. In contrast, the Hanning window captures a segment of the sine wave with attenuation of the edges of the segment

3.6 Summary

In summary, frequency domain analysis can provide valuable information that may be difficult to obtain with time domain analysis. The choice of segment length is important in frequency domain analysis as there are tradeoffs between time and frequency resolution. Thus, it is important to have a general idea of the dynamic properties of the signal on which the analysis is performed.

> **Summary of Key Terms**
>
> - Time domain – A representation of a signal with time in the x-axis and amplitude in the y-axis.
> - Frequency domain – A representation of a signal with frequency in the x-axis and amplitude in the y-axis. Each point on the plot corresponds to the frequency, amplitude, and phase of the sine waves that make up the signal.
> - Fourier transform – A mathematical operation used to transform a time domain signal to the frequency domain and vice versa.
> - Fast Fourier Transform (FFT) – An algorithm used to convert a discrete time domain signal to a discrete frequency domain signal.
> - Zero padding – A technique used to increase the frequency resolution of the result obtained by the FFT by increasing the length of the time domain signal.
> - Windowing – A technique that emphasizes the center of the signal and attenuates the beginning and end of a signal to eliminate the effect of the edge discontinuity on the frequency domain.

References

1. Harris FJ. On the use of windows for harmonic analysis with the discrete Fourier transform. *Proc IEEE*. 1978;66(1):51–83.
2. Ng J, Goldberger JJ. Understanding and interpreting dominant frequency analysis of AF electrograms. *J Cardiovasc Electrophysiol*. 2007;18:680–685.
3. Oppenhein AV, Schafer RW. *Discrete-Time Signal Processing*. Englewood Cliffs, NJ: Prentice Hall; 1989.
4. Ziemer RE, Tranter WH, Fannin DR. *Signals and Systems: Continuous and Discrete*. New York, NY: Macmillan; 1993.

Filters

4

Jason Ng and Jeffrey J. Goldberger

4.1
Chapter Objectives

A transfer function is a mathematical description of how an input signal is changed into an output signal. Transfer functions can be expressed in either the time or frequency domain. Filtering is perhaps the most common type of transfer function and possibly the most common type of signal processing operation. The aim of filtering is to reject (attenuate) unwanted parts of the recorded signal and enhance (amplify) the part of the signal that contains the information of interest. The mathematical description of these changes in the signal is the transfer function of the effects of the filter. Filtering can be performed on both analog and digital signals and can be operated in both the time and frequency domains. In this chapter we will discuss how filtering is performed for the purposes of improving signal-to-noise ratio, prevention of aliasing when sampling, and reconstruction of digital signals into analog form.

4.2
Noise

Any discussion of filtering to improve signal-to-noise ratio should first begin with an understanding of what is noise. The noise is any unwanted signal that interferes with the detection and analysis of the signal of interest. Noise can have various characteristics and comes from physiologic or nonphysiologic sources. Some common sources of noise in the context of cardiovascular instrumentation include 50/60 Hz power line interference, myopotentials, motion, poor electrode contact, and ambient electromagnetic radiation.

J. Ng (✉)
Department of Medicine, Division of Cardiology, Feinberg School of Medicine, Northwestern University, Chicago, IL, USA
e-mail: jsnng@northwestern.edu

J.J. Goldberger and J. Ng (eds.),
Practical Signal and Image Processing in Clinical Cardiology,
DOI: 10.1007/978-1-84882-515-4_4, © Springer-Verlag London Limited 2010

4.3 Filtering to Improve Signal-to-Noise Ratio

Filtering can be an effective tool to increase the ratio of signal power to noise power. The more that is known about the characteristics of the signal and noise, the more effective the filters can be. We will illustrate this point using a very common source of electrical noise – 60 Hz power line interference. The illustration in Fig. 4.1 shows a square wave with cycle length of 100 ms, a pulse width of 30 ms, and sampling rate of 1,000 samples per second or 1 kHz. In the frequency domain, this signal has peaks in the power spectrum every multiple of 10 Hz from 0 to 500 Hz. Adding a 60-Hz sine wave results in distortion of the square wave in the time domain and a significantly larger 60-Hz peak in the frequency domain.

Reducing or eliminating the effect of the 60-Hz sine wave on the square wave can be approached in a few ways. Ideally, one would like to be able to subtract the sine wave from the original signal. Unfortunately, in real world applications and especially in the biomedical field, the characteristics of the signal and noise can be estimated but not precisely determined. In the current illustration, for example, both the signal and noise have power at the 60-Hz frequency. If we do not precisely know the cycle length, pulse width, and amplitude of the signal, we cannot know how much of the 60-Hz power is from the signal and how much of the noise to subtract. A more practical approach would be to attenuate a band of frequencies that includes 60-Hz and assume that distortion due to the attenuation of the frequency band of the original signal would be minimal.

The two most common types of filters are low-pass filters and high-pass filters. Low-pass filters attenuate frequencies above a defined cut-off point, while high-pass filters attenuate frequencies below a defined cut-off point. If we use a high-pass filter to attenuate the 60 Hz noise, a filter with a cut-off of 70 Hz (attenuate frequencies below 70 Hz and allow frequencies above 70 Hz) may be a reasonable choice. From the standpoint of the percentage of the frequency band that is modified, the high-pass filter only affects approximately 70 Hz (14%) of the 500-Hz band, which includes the 60 Hz that we are trying to eliminate. Therefore, this approach may seem reasonable. Figure 4.2 shows the results of filtering the signal with a high-pass filter with a 70-Hz cut-off.

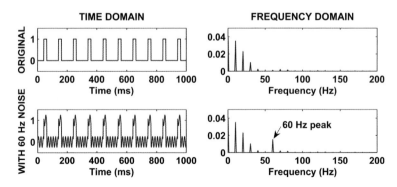

Fig. 4.1 Illustration of time and frequency domain representations of a repeated pulse wave with and without 60 Hz interference. In the frequency domain, the 60 Hz interference adds a peak at 60 Hz

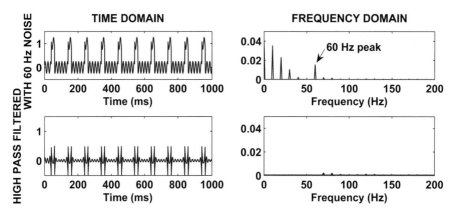

Fig. 4.2 Time and frequency domain plots of a pulse wave with 60-Hz interference before and after high-pass filtering with a cut-off of 70 Hz. The high-pass filter significantly attenuates the 60-Hz noise. Because the pulse wave is comprised of large low-frequency components, the high-pass filter also results in significant distortion of the pulse wave

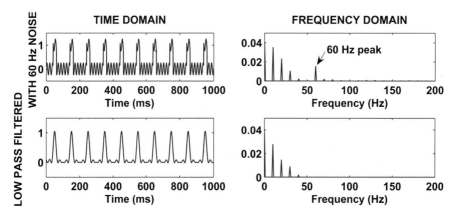

Fig. 4.3 Time and frequency domain plots of a pulse wave with 60-Hz interference before and after low-pass filtering with a cut-off of 50 Hz. Like the high-pass filter, the low-pass filter is effective in attenuating the 60-Hz noise. Although the pulse wave is more rounded than the original pulse wave, there is much less distortion compared to the high-pass filtered signal

Although the high-pass filter attenuated the 60-Hz noise, as is evident in both the time and frequency domains, the square wave has become unrecognizable with the filter leaving only a couple of deflections that occur at times corresponding to the sharp rise and fall of the square wave. The signal is significantly distorted despite attenuation of only 14% of the band, because the first 70 Hz contained 99% of the power in the original signal before noise was added. Thus, a high-pass filter to combat the 60-Hz noise was not a good choice as there was too much "collateral damage" to the original signal. A low-pass filter that attenuates frequencies above 50 Hz may, therefore, be a better choice than the high-pass filter. Figure 4.3 shows the results of low-pass filtering.

Following low-pass filtering with a 50-Hz cut-off frequency, the added 60-Hz sine wave is almost completely eliminated, while the square wave, although more rounded, retains more of its original shape. Again, the amount of power that was sacrificed from the original signal with the low-pass filter was much less than what was sacrificed with the high-pass filter. However, if we could narrow the attenuation to the band around the 60 Hz frequency, we could expect even less distortion. This can be accomplished with what is known as a notch filter. A notch filter does what its name suggests – it rejects a small frequency band but allows all other frequencies to pass.

Figure 4.4 shows the results of notch filtering. Although there is still some distortion, the notch filtered waveform maintains much more of the original shape compared to the high-pass or low-pass filters.

Another common type of noise is wandering of the baseline of the signal. Baseline wander typically occurs in electrode recordings with unstable contact (e.g., ECG). This type of noise generally has low-frequency characteristics. Thus, high-pass filters are often effective in minimizing baseline wander. Figure 4.5 below shows the square wave example with a parabolic function added to it to simulate baseline wander. The increase in low-frequency power due to the baseline wander can be noticed in the power spectrum.

Applying the high-pass filter almost eliminated the baseline wander, although some distortion of the signal occurs. One outcome of the filtering that should be noticed is that the baseline of the signal, although stable, is no longer at zero as it was for the original signal. The high-pass filter rejects the 0-Hz frequency component that defines the offset of the signal. No power at 0-Hz frequency corresponds to a mean of zero in the time domain. Thus for signals where the offset contains information (e.g., continuous blood pressure waveforms), high-pass filters cannot be used. Filtering out the zero frequency removes the mean value of the signal. High-pass filters are ideal for signals where timing and relative amplitudes are the important characteristics (e.g., ECG).

Unfortunately, not all types of noise have such a defined frequency band where the choice of filter could be so easily made. For example, ambient electromagnetic noise is often

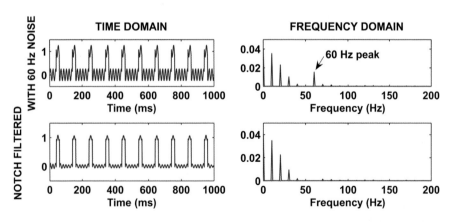

Fig. 4.4 Time and frequency domain plots of a pulse wave with 60 Hz interference before and after 60 Hz notch filtering. Notch filtering attenuated the 60 Hz noise, but distorted the pulse wave less than either the high-pass or low-pass filters

4 Filters

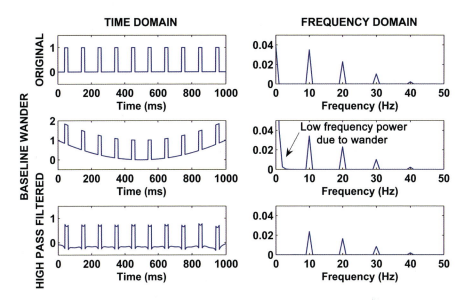

Fig. 4.5 Illustration of the effect of baseline wander and high-pass filtering on time and frequency domain plots

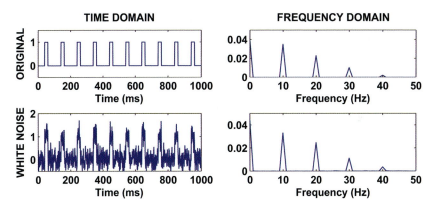

Fig. 4.6 Effect of white noise on time and frequency domain plots of a pulse wave signal

modeled as a random signal with power distributed equally over all frequencies. Noise with uniform power over all frequencies is known as white noise. Figure 4.6 shows the same square wave signal with added Gaussian white noise. Gaussian white noise is commonly used for white noise simulations and simply means that each value of the noise is randomly generated with a Gaussian (also known as normal) distribution. In Fig. 4.6 the white noise has a Gaussian distribution with a mean value of 0 and standard deviation of 0.25.

The addition of the white noise is apparent in the time domain. However, the effect of noise is barely noticeable in the frequency domain. A low-pass filter would probably be the best choice to improve the signal-to-noise ratio, since most of the power of the signal is in

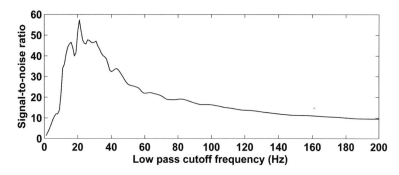

Fig. 4.7 A plot of signal-to-noise ratio vs. low-pass filter cut-off frequency for a pulse wave signal with added white noise. The optimal low-pass filter had a cut-off around 20 Hz

the lower frequencies. However, the choice of cut-off frequency that would maximize signal-to-noise ratio is not obvious. Figure 4.7 plots signal-to-noise ratio against the low-pass cut-off frequency.

As the low-pass cut-off frequency decreases from 200 Hz, the signal-to-noise ratio initially increases as expected. At around 20 Hz, the signal-to-noise ratio peaks and begins to fluctuate. Below 15 Hz, the signal-to-noise ratio decreases dramatically. Figure 4.8 demonstrates the effect of different low-pass cut-off values on the signal. A cut-off of 200 Hz already shows improvement over the signal shown in Fig. 4.7. Noise is further reduced when the cut-off is reduced to 100 Hz and even more when the cut-off is 40 and 20 Hz. It is important to realize that even though signal-to-noise ratio is optimized, the original signal can be distorted. The rounding of the square wave can be seen in Fig. 4.8. Thus the need for improved signal-to-noise ratio must be balanced with the amount of information that can be sacrificed to achieve the signal-to-noise ratio. The optimum low-pass filter has a cut-off frequency of 20 Hz. Below this frequency, the relative attenuation of the signal is greater due to the high-frequency content of the signal in the low-frequency range. Above 20 Hz, the filter allows proportionally more noise to pass through the filter leading to a reduction in the signal-to-noise ratio.

4.4 Filtering to Prevent Aliasing

In addition to improving signal-to-noise ratio, filtering is an important step in the analog-to-digital conversion process. As was discussed in the chapter about analog and digital signals, aliasing is the result of undersampling that occurs when the sampling rate is less than twice the highest frequency component of a signal. We showed in that chapter how a reconstruction of an 8-Hz sine wave after sampling with a 10-Hz rate results in a signal that looks nothing like the original 8-Hz sine wave. Distortion can also occur with signals that are not sinusoidal, but have power at frequencies above twice the sampling rate.

Figure 4.9 shows an example of square waves with 5 ms pulse widths and variable cycle lengths. When the square wave signal is sampled with a 100-Hz rate or every 10 ms,

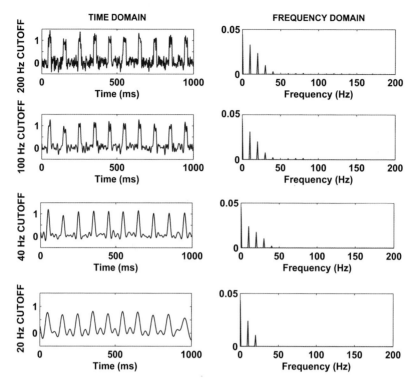

Fig. 4.8 Time and frequency domain plots of the pulse wave signal with added white noise after low-pass filtering with cut-off frequencies of 200, 100, 40, and 20 Hz. The optimal signal-to-noise ratio was obtained with the 20 Hz low-pass filter

only five of the ten square pulses were captured. The third panel shows the original signal after 50-Hz low-pass filtering. When this signal is sampled at 100 Hz (bottom panel), each impulse is identified. Even though all the filtered impulses were captured, the reconstructed signal does not look exactly like the signal that was sampled. Because of sampling and quantization, the signal will look like a sequence of step functions when outputted by a digital-to-analog converter. As you can imagine, the sharp changes of the step function would have high-frequency components that did not occur in the filtered signal. However, the same 50-Hz low-pass filter that was used for antialiasing can be applied on the reconstructed signal to obtain a signal that closely approximates the original.

4.5
Analog Filters

How are filters implemented? Filtering can be performed both on analog and digital signals. Analog filtering is typically performed using electronic components such as resistors, capacitors, and amplifiers. The orientation, size, and number of these components can be

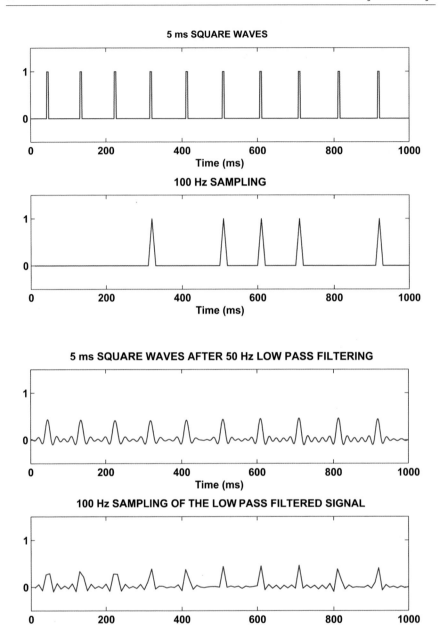

Fig. 4.9 Illustration of the need for low-pass filtering prior to sampling to prevent aliasing

designed to achieve a particular frequency domain response of the filter. Without going into detail into the physics and the electrical engineering of these components, we can briefly discuss how these components can be used to form a low-pass filter. A capacitor is a device that holds charge. A special property of capacitors that makes them useful components in filters is that it takes some time to charge. The amount of time it takes to charge depends on the size of the capacitor and the amount of current available to charge it. Thus if a signal is passed through the capacitor, the amount of charge that is stored in the capacitor cannot keep up with the signal if the signal changes very fast. The result is that high frequencies will be attenuated. A resistor is a component that limits the amount of current that will pass through it for a given voltage. Making a signal go through a resistor before the capacitor will decrease the current flow to the capacitor, allowing it more time to charge. Therefore, increasing both resistance and capacitance when the two components are configured this way will lower the cut-off frequency of the low-pass filter. Filters designed this way often are attenuated over all frequencies and require amplification to boost the signal back to its original level.

4.6
Digital Filters

Unlike analog filters, digital filters do not directly use electronic components such as resistors and capacitors, but rather use instructions that are performed by a computer processor. Digital filters can be used to perform a number of different operations such as moving averages, differentiation, integration, as well as frequency domain manipulation. Digital filters are often defined as a set of coefficients that are multiplied for each sample of the digital signal and then summed. A moving average filter will replace the value at each time point by the average of a fixed number of surrounding points. Thus a three-point moving average will multiply the preceding data point, the index data point, and the following data point by 1/3 and sum the result. Similarly, a five-point moving average would have coefficients of (1/5 1/5 1/5 1/5 1/5). Figure 4.10 is an illustration of the calculations involved in the use of the three-point moving average filter. Each set of three values displayed in the columns represents the preceding value ($N-1$), the index value (N), and the following value ($N+1$). At the bottom is the average of the three values. The bottom panel is a plot of the signal after the application of the three-point moving average filter. Note how the signal has been smoothed.

Changing the filter coefficients to (-1, 1) would cause the filter to act as a differentiator as it would subtract from each sample the value of the previous sample (example shown in Fig. 4.11). In each column are the values of the index point (N) and the previous point ($N-1$). This filter is implemented by multiplying the $N-1$ point value by -1 and adding it to the N point value. The sum is shown in the bottom row. The bottom graph demonstrates the result of this differentiator filter. Note that when the signal is increasing in value, the differentiator takes on positive values, and when the signal is decreasing, it takes on negative values.

Beyond just averaging and differentiation, one of the most useful aspects of digital filters is the ability to select coefficients to filter with specific frequency domain characteristics.

Low-pass, high-pass, band-pass, and notch filters with different cut-off frequencies are possible. The number of coefficients determines how good an approximation of the desired frequency response the digital filter will be. Figure 4.12 shows how different combinations of 11 coefficients can produce different filter frequency responses. Low-pass, high-pass, and band-pass filters are illustrated.

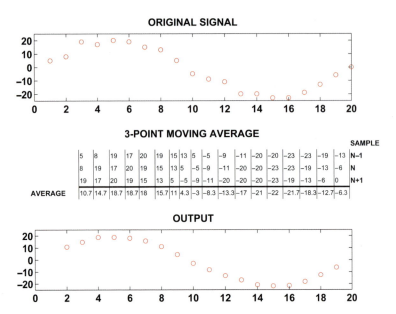

Fig. 4.10 Example of a three-point moving average digital filter

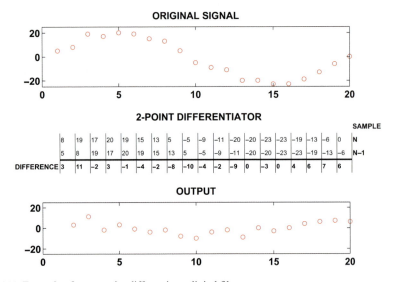

Fig. 4.11 Example of a two-point differentiator digital filter

These filters that multiply the sample values by the indicated coefficients and use the sum in the filtered signal are known as linear filters as they use linear operations. Sometimes it is advantageous to use nonlinear filters. One example of a nonlinear filter is the median filter. The median filter works similarly to the moving average filter except that the average of the moving window is replaced by the median. Median filtering is particularly effective in

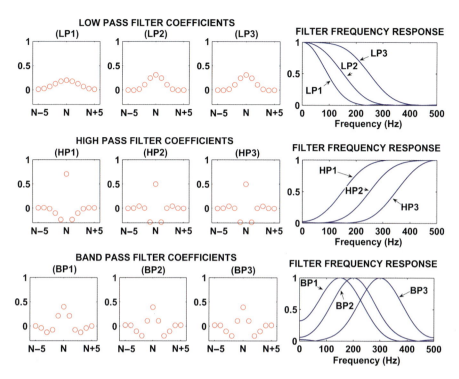

Fig. 4.12 Example of low-pass, high-pass, and band-pass digital filters. The filter frequency response defines the attenuation level over the whole frequency range. Thus the low-pass filter allows frequencies below a certain frequency to pass through unattenuated, followed by a range of frequencies in which there is progressive attenuation (values between 0 and 1), and then complete attenuation. The cut-off frequency increases from LP1 to LP2 to LP3. The high-pass filters operate similarly, but attenuate low frequencies and allow the higher frequencies to pass through. Finally, the band-pass filter attenuates both low and high frequencies and allows the frequencies within the specified ranges to pass through

signals with stray impulses as artifacts as shown in Fig. 4.13. While moving averages may attenuate these impulses, median filters can seemingly eliminate them. The trade-off is that information contained in the more subtle changes of the signal may be lost due to the non-linear distortion. Figure 4.14 shows an illustration of the median filtering operation. Using a five-point median filter, the filtered signal consists of the median value of the index point (N), the two preceding points ($N-1$, $N-2$), and the two following points ($N+1$, $N+2$). Below each point in the top panel, these five points are listed and the median value is shown at the bottom. The bottom graph is the median-filtered signal. Note the high-frequency fluctuations in the signal have been eliminated. If these are not desirable, then the filtering is effective. However, if these high-frequency oscillations carry significant information, the filtering is not appropriate as it causes a loss of information.

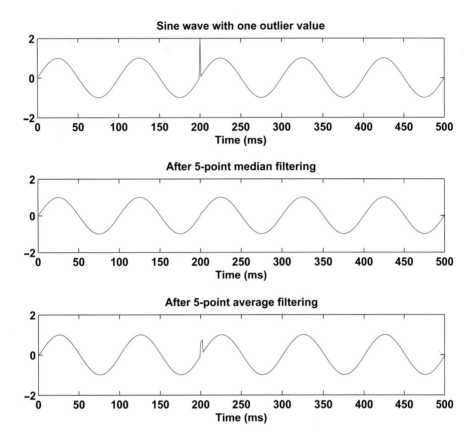

Fig. 4.13 Example of median and average filtering applied to a sinusoid with a single outlier value. The outlier is almost completely eliminated by median filtering. With average filtering, the outlier is significantly attenuated but a significant remnant exists

4.7
Phase Distortion

In this chapter we have seen how filtering frequencies important to the signal can cause distortion to the waveform. In addition to the attenuation of power at specific frequencies, filters can also modify the phase characteristics of a signal. This modification of phase can also be a source of distortion of a signal after filtering. In Chap. 3, we demonstrated that a waveform can be decomposed into a series of sinusoids with different amplitudes, frequencies, and phases. In Fig. 4.15, a square wave is approximated by summing five sinusoids.

4 Filters

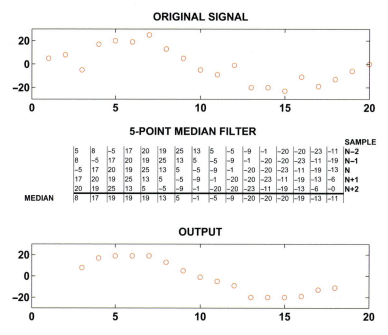

Fig. 4.14 Example of a five-point median digital filter

After phase shifting the second and fourth sinusoids by 180°, the summation no longer resembles a square wave, even though the magnitude spectra for both waveforms are identical. Therefore, an important characteristic for either an analog or digital filter to have is a linear phase response, at least for the frequencies of interest. A linear phase response simply means that all frequency components must be delayed the same amount of time after going through the filter. If any of the frequency components are delayed more than the others, distortion similar to what we saw in Fig. 4.15 can occur.

4.8
Summary

In summary, filters are basic signal processing techniques that can be used in many ways. When using filters, it is important that the characteristics of the desired signal, the noise, and the filters themselves are known to be sure that important information from the signal is not lost or distorted.

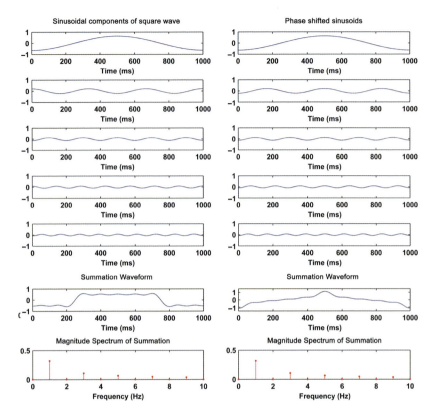

Fig. 4.15 Sinusoidal components to an approximate square wave before and after phase distortion. In the distorted waveform, the second and fourth sinusoidal components are phase shifted 180°

Summary of Key Terms

- Filters – Signal processing for the purpose of enhancing certain characteristics (usually frequency bands) of a signal and rejecting other parts.
- Noise – An unwanted addition to a signal of interest.
- Signal-to-noise ratio – The ratio of the desired signal power to the noise power.
- Low-pass filter – A filter that rejects high-frequency components of a signal above a defined cut-off frequency.
- High-pass filter – A filter that rejects low-frequency components of a signal below a defined cut-off frequency.
- Band-pass filter – A filter that rejects frequencies outside a defined frequency band.
- Notch filter – A filter that rejects a narrowly defined frequency band.
- Antialiasing filter – A low-pass filter with a cut-off at or below one half of the sampling rate of the analog-to-digital converter used to prevent distortion due to undersampling.
- Analog filter – A filter typically designed with electronic components such as resistors, capacitors, and amplifiers that operate on an analog signal.
- Digital filter – A mathematical operation typically performed by a microprocessor that performs filtering on digital signals.

References

1. Oppenhein AV, Schafer RW. *Discrete-Time Signal Processing*. Englewood Cliffs, NJ: Prentice Hall; 1989.
2. Ziemer RE, Tranter WH, Fannin DR. *Signals and Systems: Continuous and Discrete.* +New York, NY: Macmillan; 1993.

Techniques for Event and Feature Detection

5

Jason Ng and Jeffrey J. Goldberger

5.1
Chapter Objectives

Event and feature detection are important aspects of signal processing in cardiology. Knowledge of the rate and rhythm of the heart are critical aspects of patient monitoring. Even within a single beat, the different phases of the cardiac cycle provide important information of the physiology. Although this information could be gleaned manually from the electrocardiogram, continuous blood pressure, or respiratory signals, having automatic calculations of the rates, rhythms, and amplitudes of these different signals nearly instantaneously saves precious time that could be used to save a patient's life. These real-time measurements are often also linked to visual or audio alarms that alert hospital staff when something is going wrong. Cardiac gating for image acquisition requires accurate identification of electrocardiographic features. Automatic event and feature detection is also useful in off-line analysis and in automated analysis for cardiac imaging (i.e., determining the heart's boundaries). This chapter will discuss common signal processing techniques that are used for event and feature detection.

5.2
Purpose and Challenges of Event and Feature Detection

The typical electrocardiographic signal has a systolic and diastolic phase. The major event of interest that is to be detected is contained in the systolic phase. The diastolic phase is also important as it provides the baseline signal to which the systolic signal can be referenced. The challenge of event detection is to avoid missing events (undersensing) while not falsely calling something an event that is not (oversensing). Because of the importance

J. Ng (✉)
Department of Medicine, Division of Cardiology, Feinberg School of Medicine, Northwestern University, Chicago, IL, USA
e-mail: jsnng@northwestern.edu

in accurate determination of rate and rhythm of heart beats, the criteria for event detection often also include being able to detect a precise point on the waveform to minimize error in calculation of intervals.

5.3
Event Detection by Amplitude

We will begin the illustration of event detection with a repeated waveform shown in Fig. 5.1. The waveform is a rounded bell-shaped curved with an amplitude of one and a width of 200 ms. The signal that we will analyze repeats this waveform once every second for 5 s. The baseline of this signal is at zero.

Detection of the waveforms in this signal is quite simple when done visually. Measuring intervals is also straightforward as we can position calipers from one peak to the next. Whether the waveforms are being detected in real time or off-line will determine what methods we can use. For either of the two situations, we will need to assume that we know a couple of things about the waveform. One is the amplitude of the waveform. The amplitude is necessary for defining a threshold level to distinguish the waveform from the baseline. The second necessary parameter is the width of the waveform. The width will determine the window in which we would not anticipate another waveform to occur.

In real-time monitoring, data are processed as they are acquired. Figure 5.2 shows the threshold level to detect a waveform set at 0.5 or 50% of the maximum amplitude. Starting from time zero, the signal begins at baseline or amplitude of 0. The threshold is first crossed at 149 ms from the beginning of the signal. The first waveform is now detected.

Because we know that the waveform is 200 ms in duration, we will employ a 200-ms blanking period beginning at the threshold crossing. This means that all amplitudes in this window will be ignored even though they may be above the threshold. The next time the amplitude crosses the threshold is at time 1.149 s.

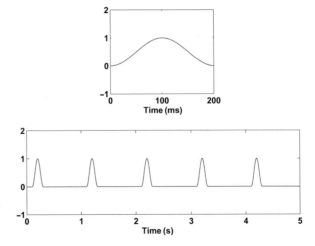

Fig. 5.1 A rounded waveforms with amplitude of one and duration of 200 ms (*top*) that is repeated once per second for 5 s (*bottom*)

5 Techniques for Event and Feature Detection

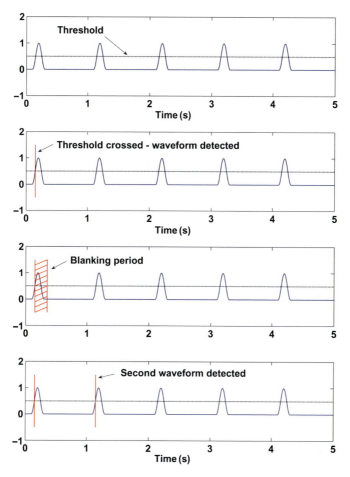

Fig. 5.2 Example of an event detection algorithm using an amplitude threshold of 0.5. The *top row* shows the signal with the threshold at 0.5. The second row shows where the signal first crosses the threshold line. The third row illustrates a 200-ms blanking period during which no other events are to be detected. The last row shows next time point where the waveform crosses the amplitude threshold

Let us consider a second scenario. Instead of being constant, the amplitude of the waveform varies a little bit as seen in Fig. 5.3. The width of the waveform is kept constant at 200 ms. Although each waveform is properly detected, we note that the point at which each waveform crosses the threshold is different for each waveform depending on its amplitude. For the first to fifth waveform, the times between the onset of the waveform and the threshold crossing point are 49, 61, 44, 81, and 41 ms – a range of 40 ms. The uncertainty or imprecision in detecting the onset of the waveform (or some other common point) is often called "jitter." If precise timing of these signals is important, this method for event detection may be inadequate. One way to overcome jitter is to find a landmark or landmarks from which all the waveforms can be aligned. These common reference points are called "fiducial points."

Fig. 5.3 Example of event detection for an amplitude-varying waveform using an amplitude threshold of 0.5. Using the threshold level of 0.5, each waveform is detected. However, the point on the waveform where the signal crosses the threshold is different for each of the five events

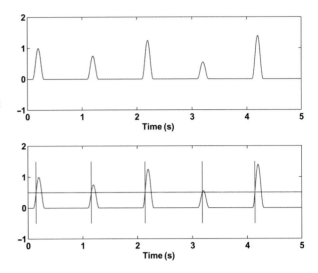

Ideally, the onset of the signal would be chosen as the fiducial point. For this example, the onset would be the first nonzero point. However, this would not be practical in real-world situations as the baseline would not be noise-free as it is in this simulation. The peak amplitude above the threshold value is a better choice as a fiducial point than the threshold point or the waveform onset as it is consistently located in the same point in the waveform despite variation in amplitude and can be easily identified. A possible algorithm to detect the peak would be to first detect when the amplitude crosses the threshold and then choose the maximum amplitude point for the next 200 ms.

5.4
Event Detection by Slope

Addition of noise in the signal may alter the maximum amplitude point. However, as long as the signal-to-noise ratio is relatively high, the detected maximum should not deviate too much from the actual maximum in this single-peaked waveform. This is not to say that the peak amplitude is always the best fiducial point to use. Consider the next example shown in Fig. 5.4. The signal used in this example is similar to the previous example except that the waveform in Fig. 5.4 has a double peak. The amplitude at both peaks is one and the duration of the waveform is 300 ms. The two peaks are 105 ms apart. Therefore, introduction of any noise can make either the first or the second peak the largest amplitude peak. Jitter of 105 ms would be unacceptable in most cardiology standards.

The double-peaked waveform does have other characteristics that can be more reliably detected. One is the steep upslope and the second is the steep downslope. Examine the derivative or the instantaneous slope of the signal in Fig. 5.5. Notice that the steepest part of the upslope corresponds to the maximum positive peak in the instantaneous slope plot. This peak can be detected using a similar algorithm to that used to find the peak amplitude.

5 Techniques for Event and Feature Detection

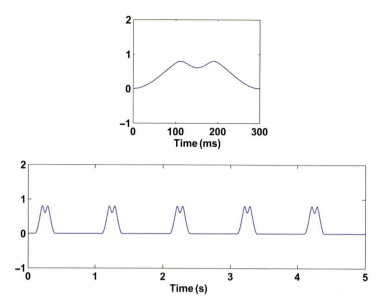

Fig. 5.4 Waveform with a double-peaked morphology

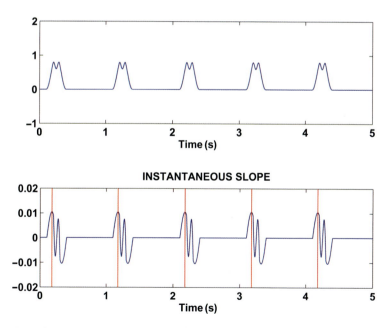

Fig. 5.5 Event detection of the double-peaked waveform using a maximum slope criterion

As with amplitude, variations in the amplitude scaling will not change the time of the point of steepest upward slope and thus is a robust feature that can be used as a fiducial point without the potential jitter of the maximum amplitude.

The differential signals have advantages over the raw amplitude signal in other scenarios as well. In cardiology and other applications, the polarity of the waveforms cannot be guaranteed, meaning that positive, negative, and biphasic waveforms are possible. Thus, setting an amplitude threshold to detect events may cause waveforms to be missed. However, these signals typically have steep slopes either at the onset, offset, or during the transition between polarities for biphasic waveforms. Figure 5.6 shows examples of a negative and biphasic waveform and their corresponding instantaneous slope plots. The maximum positive slopes in both cases are easily detected.

A second scenario is when baseline wander is present in the signal. Baseline wander can be a serious obstacle to event detection if amplitude thresholds are used as criteria. Undersensing can occur if the baseline drops below the normal level and oversensing can occur if the baseline rises above the normal value. Figure 5.7 provides an illustration of the addition of a 0.5-Hz sine wave to the signal with biphasic waveforms. Although the baseline wander drastically altered the amplitude values of the signals, the instantaneous slopes were only mildly affected – not enough to prevent the maximal slope points from being detected.

5.5
Event Detection by Template Matching

Despite the advantages of using maximum slope as detection criteria, using only a single point of any kind as the fiducial point will make accurate identification of the timing of the waveform susceptible to high-frequency noise. The amount of noise typically correlates with the amount of jitter in the fiducial point detection that can be expected. Consider the biphasic waveform in Fig. 5.8 before and after the addition of noise.

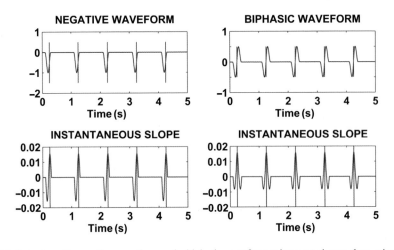

Fig. 5.6 Detection of a negative waveform and a biphasic waveform using a maximum slope criterion

Fig. 5.7 Detection of biphasic waveforms in the presence of baseline wander using maximum amplitude and slope criteria. The top panel shows the detection of peak amplitudes of the waveforms (marked by the red lines). The middle panel shows how some of the waveforms could be missed by peak amplitude detection if baseline wander is present. The third panel shows the detection of the peak instantaneous slopes of the signal with baseline wander

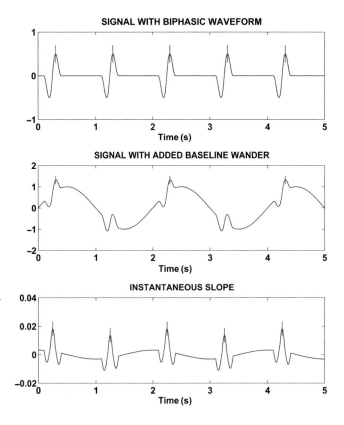

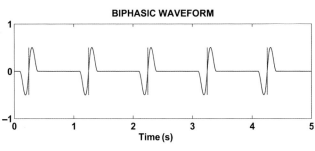

Fig. 5.8 Detection of biphasic waveforms in the presence of white noise using a maximum slope criterion. Jitter in the detection points of each waveform can be seen

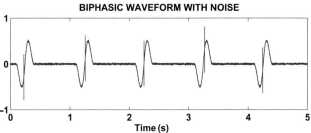

In the top panel, using the maximum slope criteria, the waveforms are detected at 0.2, 1.2, 2.2, 3.2, and 4.2 s. In contrast, in the bottom panel where a small amount of noise is evident, the waveforms are detected at 0.18, 1.22, 2.15, 3.17, and 4.25 s. This small amount of noise has created a maximum of 50 ms error in the correct timing of the signal. It may be difficult to conceptualize why the addition of so little noise can throw off the detection of the true maximum slope point. Visually for us the point appears to be easily determined if we were to select the point manually. The reason for this is that we look for this point in the context of the entire waveform. Our brain processes the signal and recognizes the downward and upward pattern of each biphasic waveform, even allowing us to visually filter the noise.

The signal processing technique that probably best approximates how the brain recognizes signal patterns is template matching. Template matching works very similarly to our digital filtering examples from chapter 4. Instead of designing the filter to have coefficients that when multiplied with the signal results in averaging or a desired frequency operation, the waveform amplitude values themselves are used as the filter coefficients. In other words, a template waveform is selected and all other waveforms are compared to this template. This is done by positioning the template at various locations in the signal and using this as the "filter." The aligned values of the template and the waveform are multiplied and then summed. The template is then moved forward over the signal and the process is repeated. For this reason, these templates are also called matched filters. The result from applying the matched filter to the signal produces an output where the highest values generally occur at the time when the template is best aligned with the waveform in the original signal. Figure 5.9 traces the matched filter output as the template is moved from the beginning of the signal to the end. For the first two positions of the template, the output is zero as the template is multiplied by the zero values of the signal. In the third position, there is overlap between the negative part of the signal and the positive portion of the template; multiplying the values and summing them provides a negative value that is shown in the

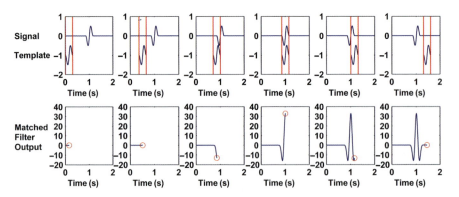

Fig. 5.9 Detection of a waveform using template matching (also known as matched filtering or cross-correlation). The maximum matched filter output occurs when the waveform and the template are perfectly aligned

5 Techniques for Event and Feature Detection

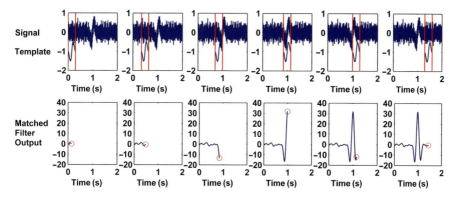

Fig. 5.10 Template matching to detect a waveform within a noisy signal. Despite the noise, a clear maximum can be seen when the waveform and the template are perfectly aligned

matched filter output. In the fourth position, the template and the signal are aligned perfectly. Thus, the output is equal to the sum of the squares of the template values and is mathematically the highest output possible with this combination of template and signal. The output becomes negative again when the template and signal lose alignment in the fifth position and back to zero in the sixth position.

The highest amplitude of the matched filter output can be used to locate the waveform to a high degree of precision. The method to locate the matched filter output peak can be the amplitude peak detector discussed earlier, with a defined threshold and blanking period.

Figure 5.10 demonstrates the application of the matched filter to the signal with a significant amount of noise added. The matched filter output remains very similar to that of the noiseless signal. The time of the maximum output corresponds to the same maximum point of the noiseless example.

Although template matching has definite advantages to amplitude and slope detection algorithms, it also has some limitations. First, a good quality template is required. For signals with relatively low levels of noise any representative waveform from the signal would work. For signals with more noise such as the example in Fig. 5.10, a template can be obtained through signal averaging – a concept to be discussed later in this book. However, such algorithms are possible for off-line analysis but not so for real-time detection. A second limitation is that the method is dependent on consistency of the waveform morphologies. Any aberration of the signal may cause missed detections.

5.6 Waveform Onset and Offset Detection

In addition to detecting events, an important part of analyzing signals in cardiology is the ability to measure durations of waveforms. Measuring durations requires the detection of onset and offset of waveforms. We define the onset and offset as the beginning and end of the waveform where the signal reaches the baseline. Although this detection would not be complicated for signals with abrupt changes in amplitudes at the onset and offset (e.g., a square wave), signals in cardiology often have rounded waveforms that make determination of these points more challenging. We will examine some commonly used algorithms for onset and offset detection.

5.7
Offset Estimation by Amplitude

Perhaps the simplest algorithm is the use of amplitude thresholds. Detecting the offset of a waveform with an amplitude threshold first requires the detection of the peak amplitude and knowledge of the baseline amplitude. Attempting to detect the offset using the time the waveform reaches the baseline is problematic, as the actual time to reach baseline can be highly variable depending on the noise level. Thus, using a percentage of the amplitude above the baseline as a surrogate to the true offset sacrifices accuracy for precision if the threshold is above the noise level. The offset will always be underestimated with this method. Higher noise levels would require higher thresholds. In fact, some algorithms use a factor above the noise level to define the offset. Amplitude thresholds are a reasonable approach to detecting offsets as long as the signal is monophasic with a known polarity. To increase robustness, the offset can be estimated as the first point that falls below the threshold for a defined amount of time. That would prevent estimation that is too early if the waveform fluctuates near the threshold line before decreasing. The example in Fig. 5.11 demonstrates detection using a 90% amplitude threshold.

5.8
Offset Estimation by Tangent Line Projection

A second method addresses the underestimation of the offset by the amplitude threshold. This method takes the point of the maximum descending slope, draws a tangent line at this point, and projects the line to the baseline. The point where the projected tangent line

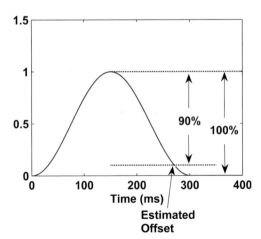

Fig. 5.11 Detection of a waveform offset using a 90% maximum amplitude threshold. Using this criterion, the offset is detected at 270 ms while the true offset is at 300 ms.

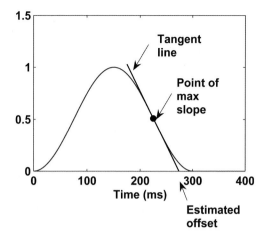

Fig. 5.12 Estimation of waveform offset using the projection of the tangent line at the point of negative descending slope to the baseline. Using this criterion, the offset is detected at 275 ms

intersects with the baseline is the estimated offset. The assumption of this technique is that the maximum slope point is above the noise level and that the descending amplitude is mostly linear. If these properties are met, then the estimated offset will be close to the true offset. In the case where the slope of the waveform gently tapers to zero, the tangent will still underestimate the offset, but often is still a better approximation than the amplitude threshold. In addition to maximum slope, projections using linear regression have also been used. An example of the tangent method to detect the waveform offset is shown in Fig. 5.12.

5.9
Offset Estimation by Slope

Limitations of the previous two methods are the need to have a monophasic waveform and a known polarity. A third method that attempts to overcome these limitations is the use of slope thresholds. In this method, the instantaneous slope is evaluated (using the differential filter) and the absolute value is taken (so that the polarity of the signal becomes irrelevant). An amplitude threshold is then applied; a percentage of the maximum absolute slope is used as the cutoff point to estimate the offset. As with using amplitude thresholds, the algorithm is made more reliable by requiring that the absolute slope fall below the threshold for a given amount of time. Figure 5.13 demonstrates this technique for a positive, negative, and biphasic waveform using a 90% threshold slope to detect the offset.

5.10
Offset Estimation by Cumulative Area

The final method of determining offset that will be discussed is the computing of area under the waveform by integration. The rationale for this approach is that the offset will be located at the time where the contribution of the signal beyond the offset to the total area

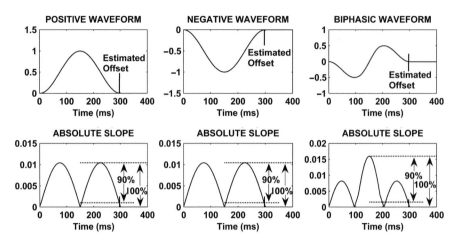

Fig. 5.13 Illustration of offset detection of a positive, negative, and biphasic waveform using a 90% slope threshold criterion. Using this criterion, the offsets are detected at 296, 296, and 295 ms, respectively

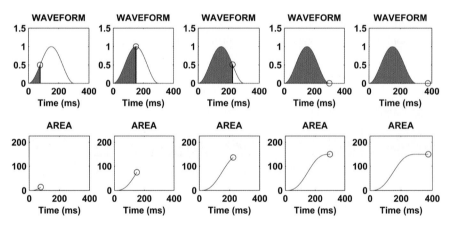

Fig. 5.14 Plot of waveform area vs. time for a positive waveform (also known as integration)

is negligible. Figure 5.14 demonstrates the progression of the cumulative area at different points of the waveform. The cumulative area increases monotonically until it reaches the offset at 300 ms. Afterward the area is constant at 150. The offset is again typically chosen to be a percentage of the maximum area.

The point chosen as the offset again depends on the defined threshold level for the area. As before, this technique will also underestimate the time offset. The advantage of this method is that it can be used for waveforms of different polarities and morphologies as long as the baseline is at zero (see Fig. 5.15). The area method is also generally most robust against noise compared to the other methods discussed.

5 Techniques for Event and Feature Detection

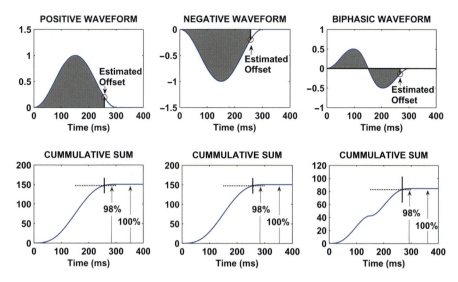

Fig. 5.15 Using absolute area calculation to detect waveform offset for a positive, negative, and biphasic waveform. Using this criterion, the offsets are detected at 257, 257, and 267 ms, respectively

5.11 Summary

Event and feature detection algorithms are an important, yet challenging, part of signal processing in cardiology. As computer hardware and software become more sophisticated, we may see new ways to improve on the algorithms for sensitivity, specificity, precision, and accuracy.

Summary of Key Terms

- Fiducial point – A time corresponding to a feature of a waveform that can be used as a common reference point for repeated signals.
- Jitter – The imprecision in timing in the detection of a waveform.
- Template matching – Event detection using a template of the waveform to be detected. Also known as matched filtering.

References

1. Pan J, Tompkins WJ. A real-time QRS detection algorithm. *IEEE Trans Biomed Eng.* 1985; 32(3):230-236.
2. Spach MS, Barr RC, Serwer GS, Kootscy JM, Johnson EA. Extracellular potentials related to intracellular action potentials in the dog Purkinje system. *Circ Res.* 1972;30:505–519.
3. McLaughlin NB, Campbell RW, Murray A. Comparison of automatic QT measurement techniques in the normal 12 lead electrocardiogram. *Br Heart J.* 1995;74(1):84–89.
4. Xue Q, Reddy S. Algorithms for computerized QT analysis. *J Electrocardiol.* 1998;30 suppl:181–186.

Alternative Techniques for Rate Estimation

6

Jason Ng and Jeffrey J. Goldberger

6.1
Chapter Objectives

Chapter 5 discussed different algorithms that might be used to detect cardiology related waveforms. The sequence of time intervals between the detected waveforms can be used to calculate the rate of the cardiac cycle. Cardiac rates are typically expressed as the number of beats per minute or as an average cycle length – the time interval between consecutive beats. These are reciprocally related:

Rate (in beats/min) = 60 divided by average cycle length (in seconds)

The accuracy of determining rate depends on the ability to detect the waveforms accurately. However, this process may be complicated by various factors. Changing amplitude, polarity, and morphology of the waveforms can complicate automated detection as demonstrated in the chapter 5. Artifacts, noise, and baseline wander are sources of interference for detection. Sometimes waveforms blend into each other so that no identifiable onset or offset exists. In these cases, a proper baseline cannot be defined as a reference for the detection algorithm. In this chapter, we will discuss alternative techniques to estimate rates without detection of the individual waveforms.

6.2
Autocorrelation

We will start with an example signal where rate estimation would be difficult with waveform detection. Figure 6.1 shows a 4 Hz sine wave with the amplitude modulated at 1 Hz. This signal has no definable baseline and the changing amplitude will confound most waveform detection algorithms. Yet, the 4 cycles per second rate or cycle length of 250 ms is apparent.

J. Ng (✉)
Department of Medicine, Division of Cardiology, Feinberg School of Medicine,
Northwestern University, Chicago, IL, USA
e-mail: jsnng@northwestern.edu

J.J. Goldberger and J. Ng (eds.),
Practical Signal and Image Processing in Clinical Cardiology,
DOI: 10.1007/978-1-84882-515-4_6, © Springer-Verlag London Limited 2010

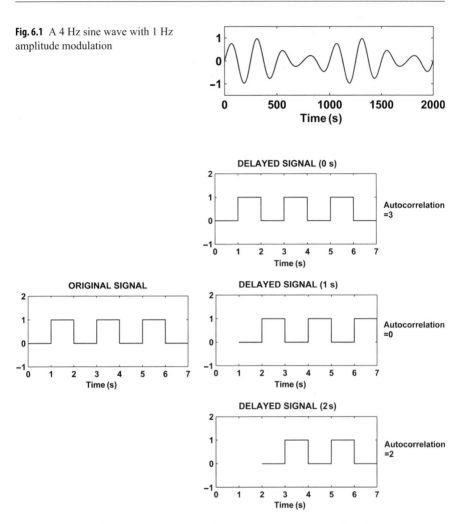

Fig. 6.1 A 4 Hz sine wave with 1 Hz amplitude modulation

Fig. 6.2 Example of autocorrelation of a simple square wave delayed at 0, 1, and 2 s

The first method we will introduce is called autocorrelation. Autocorrelation is a time domain method to estimate cycle length that is similar to the template matching method discussed in chapter 5. Instead of aligning a template with different parts of the signal, in autocorrelation a copy of the signal is aligned with itself with different delays. Consider the simple square wave shown in Fig. 6.2. The value is 0 from 0–1, 2–3, and 4–5 s. The value is 1 from 1–2, 3–4, 5–6 s. When this signal is multiplied by itself with a time delay of 0, the autocorrelation value is 3. When the signal is multiplied by itself with a time delay of 1 s, the autocorrelation value is 0 because when the original signal has a value of 0, the delayed signal has a value of 1 and when the original signal has a value of 0, the delayed signal has a value of 0; thus the product is always 0. When the delay is 2 s the square waves overlap again and the value of the autocorrelation is 2. For each delay, the product of the two signals is summed. The nonzero delay that results in the next largest peak in the output is chosen as the estimate of the cycle length. The autocorrelation method applied to the more complex signal in Fig. 6.1 is illustrated in Fig. 6.3.

The autocorrelation starts out at its maximal value (the sum of square of all the points) when the delay is zero and the two signals are perfectly aligned. As the "test signal" is delayed, the autocorrelation declines in value. With a delay of 125 ms the peaks of the first signal line up with the troughs of the second signal and vice versa resulting in a negative autocorrelation value. At 250 ms the peaks are aligned with peaks and the troughs are aligned with troughs. At 375 ms the two signals are out of phase again. The complete autocorrelation is shown in Fig. 6.4. The second peak occurs at 250 ms corresponding to the 4 Hz sine wave (4 cycles/s = 1 cycle/250 ms).

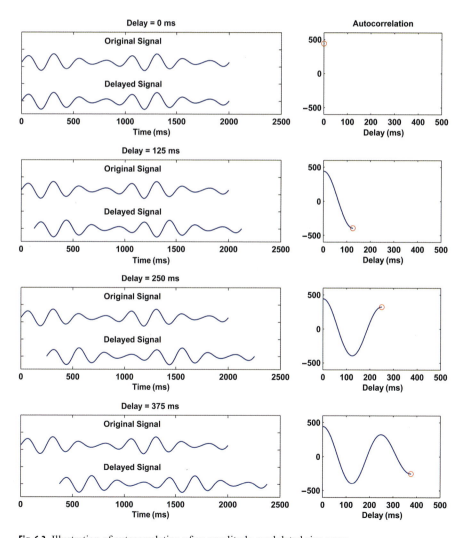

Fig. 6.3 Illustration of autocorrelation of an amplitude-modulated sine wave

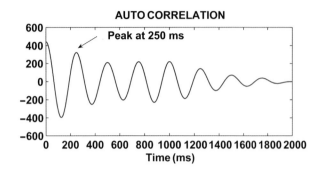

Fig. 6.4 The complete autocorrelation for the example in Fig. 6.3. The second peak occurs at 250 ms corresponding to the 4 Hz sine wave

6.3
Frequency Domain Estimation of Rate

A second common technique for rate estimation is through frequency domain analysis of the signals. As discussed in chapter 5, the premise of frequency domain analysis is that a signal can be decomposed to a set of sine waves, which when summed together will constitute the original signal. If a strong periodic element exists in the signal, in most cases there will be one sine wave component that will have an amplitude that is greater than that of the other sine waves that comprise the signal. The frequency of this sine wave is commonly referred to as the "dominant frequency." Like autocorrelation, dominant frequency analysis is used in situations where event detection is difficult because of amplitude variability, complex morphology, and noise.

Using the same example that was used for autocorrelation, the power spectrum of the 4 Hz sine wave with amplitude modulation was computed and is shown in Fig. 6.5. The peak of the power spectrum is located at 4 Hz as expected.

In the remainder of this chapter, we will examine some factors that may make event detection difficult and how they would affect rate estimation with autocorrelation and frequency domain analysis.

6.4
Noise

Noise was shown in chapter 5 to be a significant confounder in event detection, as a potential source of jitter, undersensing, and oversensing. In the setting of noise, template matching was shown in chapter 5 to be more robust than event detection techniques that attempt to detect a specific point. Autocorrelation similarly has advantages with noisy signals compared to computing intervals between waveforms. Because autocorrelation attempts to locate the strongest periodic element within a signal, it will be largely unaffected by white noise that has no dominant periodic elements. Autocorrelation of the amplitude modulated 4 Hz sine wave with added noise is shown in the middle row of Fig. 6.6. The estimated cycle length of the signal was found to be 231 ms, a 19 ms difference from the actual cycle length.

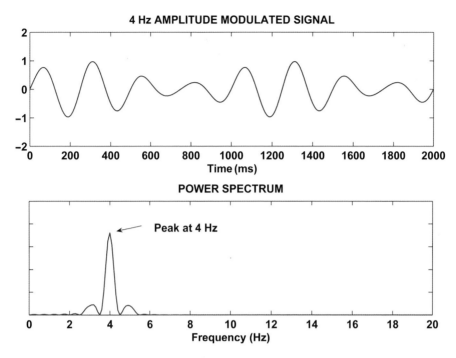

Fig. 6.5 Time and frequency domain plots of the 4 Hz amplitude-modulated sine wave. The peak of the power spectrum at 4 Hz corresponds to the frequency of the sine wave

Frequency domain analysis also has advantages over event detection in the presence of noise. The assumption is that the periodic element due to the repeated waveform will be much greater than any single frequency component due to noise. The bottom row of Fig. 6.6 shows that the power spectrum was largely unaffected by the noise, although the amplitude of the noise was roughly that of the signal. The dominant frequency of 4 Hz could be easily detected. Comparing this power spectrum to Fig. 6.5 without noise, the explanation for this seemingly difficult observation becomes apparent. The spectrum in Fig. 6.5 has no power at all above 6 Hz. The spectrum in Fig. 6.6 shows low levels of power up to 20 Hz. In addition, the side lobes off the peak frequency are clearly larger. Thus, although the noise has a high amplitude in the time domain relative to the signal, in the frequency domain this "amplitude" is distributed among many frequencies while the signal of interest remains concentrated at 4 Hz.

6.5 Frequency Variability

The previous examples demonstrate the effectiveness of autocorrelation and frequency analysis in situations where noise and amplitude variability are present. However, in these examples the signal had stable periodicity of 4 Hz. In other words, the intervals between

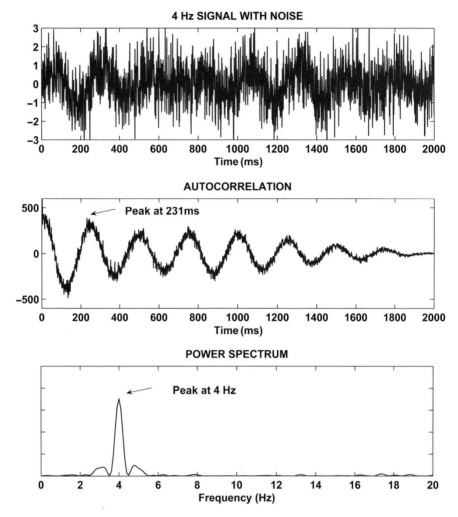

Fig. 6.6 Autocorrelation and power spectrum of the 4 Hz amplitude-modulated sine wave with noise. The noise changed the autocorrelation peak from 250 to 231 ms while the peak of the power spectrum was unchanged at 4 Hz

successive peaks were constant at 250 ms. The next example, shown in the first column of Fig. 6.7, tests autocorrelation and frequency domain analysis on a signal with variable intervals between waveforms. The cycle lengths were randomly generated with a mean and standard deviation of 222±32 ms. The estimated cycle length by autocorrelation is 222 ms. The dominant frequency of this signal is 4.6 Hz, which is equivalent to a cycle length of 217 ms.

The average rate of a signal with varying cycle length is calculated by an arithmetic average. If the order of the intervals were shuffled, the average rate would not change.

6 Alternative Techniques for Rate Estimation

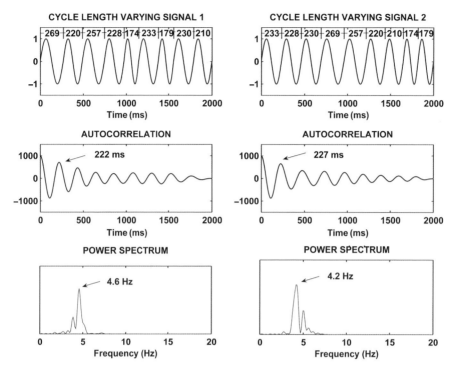

Fig. 6.7 Two sinusoidal-like signals and their corresponding autocorrelation plot and power spectrum. Each signal has the same set of cycle lengths but arranged in different orders, which results in differing autocorrelation and dominant frequency peaks

However, the autocorrelation and dominant frequency analysis are dependent upon the order or sequence of the intervals being evaluated. The effect of the order of the intervals can be assessed by shuffling the waveforms so that the same cycle lengths are present but in different orders. Consider the example in the second column of Fig. 6.7, which has the same set of cycle lengths as in the first column of Fig. 6.7. Thus, the mean and standard deviation remains 222 ± 32 ms. The estimated cycle lengths by autocorrelation and dominant frequency were 227 and 238 ms, respectively. Random shuffling of waveforms 100 times produced signals whose estimated cycle lengths from autocorrelation ranged from 225 to 240 ms with mean and standard deviation of 231 ± 3 ms. The narrow range of 15 ms was bounded by the range of intervals. The dominant frequencies ranged from 3.8 to 4.7 Hz (213–263 ms) with mean and standard deviations of 4.4 ± 0.2 Hz. The range of 50 ms was much larger than that of autocorrelation and exceeded the range of intervals. However, both methods had mean rates/cycle lengths that closely approximated the mean intervals. Therefore, in cases where the signal has variation in frequency, averaging the autocorrelation or dominant frequency results is recommended.

6.6 Phase Change

The reason that shuffling the intervals of the waveforms affects dominant frequency in particular is due in part to the importance of the relative timing (also known as "phase") of the waveforms with each other. It should be remembered that the dominant frequency analysis identifies the sine wave that best approximates the entire signal. Thus, changes in phase may make the prediction of the dominant frequency difficult. The example in Fig. 6.8 illustrates this point. The signal is a 4 Hz sine wave. At 1 s, the signal is inverted creating an

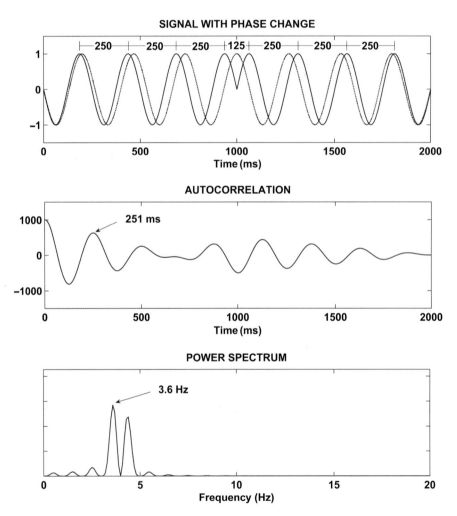

Fig. 6.8 A 4 Hz sine wave with a phase change at the half way point of the signal. The phase change did not significantly change the autocorrelation peak but changed the power spectrum peak from 4 to 3.6 Hz

interval that is 125 ms, half of the 250 ms intervals of the rest of the signal. The dominant frequency of this signal is 3.6 Hz, which is slower than the expected rate of 4 Hz or greater based on the intervals. The dotted line in the first panel represents the 3.6 Hz sine wave superimposed on the signal.

Autocorrelation on the other hand still provides a good estimate of the cycle length with the largest peak at 251 ms. The reason, autocorrelation is less susceptible to phase shifts, is that the result of the shifting process is more dependent on each waveform's distance to its adjacent waveform. Except for the waveform at 1 s, the intervals between waveforms were constant.

6.7
Waveform Morphology

The waveforms used in the examples thus far were all sinusoid-like waveforms. Sinusoidal waveforms are optimal especially for frequency domain analysis since this technique aims to deconstruct signals into sinusoidal components. Sinusoidal waveforms also are beneficial for autocorrelation as both the peaks and troughs of the signals provide references for alignment. The next portion of this chapter will look at some nonsinusoidal waveforms and how autocorrelation and dominant frequency analysis perform in this situation.

The first waveform we will examine is a narrow positive deflection (duration of 50 ms). This morphology produces obvious changes in both the autocorrelation and the power spectrum as seen in Fig. 6.9. In the autocorrelation, the discrete peaks are seen at multiples of 250 ms. The second largest peak after the zero delay peak is at 250 ms, the estimated cycle length. The frequency domain shows similar characteristics with peaks at multiples of 4 Hz. The dominant (nonzero) frequency is 4 Hz, the frequency of the signal. Because of the peaks at multiples of the fundamental value that occur in both methods, there are factors that may cause underestimation of rate with autocorrelation and overestimation of rate with dominant frequency analysis. Amplitude modulation is one factor that can cause a multiple to be chosen in the autocorrelation plot. Figure 6.10 shows how the 500 ms peak in the autocorrelation plot is chosen as the estimated cycle length in the amplitude-modulated 4 Hz signal. The dominant frequency remains accurately reflected at 4 Hz. Performing additional simulations showed that autocorrelation is sensitive to alterations of estimated cycle length with amplitude modulation while dominant frequency analysis is not.

Figure 6.10 also shows the effect of white noise on the signal with narrow waveforms. The estimated cycle length by autocorrelation is unaffected by the noise, however the dominant frequency is 8 Hz, double the expected 4 Hz rate. Additional simulations with this noise level showed that multiples or "harmonics" of the rate can be chosen as the dominant frequency. However with autocorrelation, the estimated cycle lengths were consistently around 250 ms.

Sharp biphasic waveforms are also commonly seen in cardiology. A biphasic morphology also presents its own challenges for the techniques described in this chapter. Figure 6.11 shows an example of a signal with a biphasic waveform again with a rate of 4 Hz. Autocorrelation of the signal produces a result with a peak every 250 ms. The peak

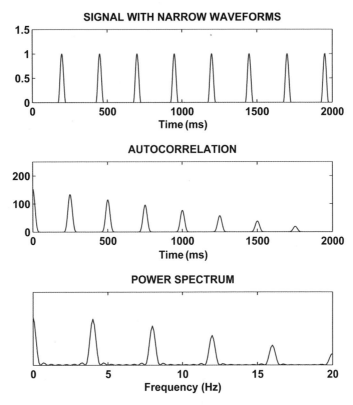

Fig. 6.9 Autocorrelation and power spectrum of a periodic signal with narrow waveforms. The autocorrelation also has narrow peaks while the power spectrum has peaks at harmonics of the frequency of the signal

autocorrelation is at the expected 250 ms. The frequency domain of the biphasic waveform is significantly different than that of the positive waveforms. The dominant frequency is at 16 Hz rather than the expected 4 Hz.

The biphasic morphology has such an effect on the frequency domain because it makes fitting a single sine wave with a frequency corresponding to the rate of the signal difficult. The rate of a signal with biphasic waveforms can be estimated with dominant frequency analysis by performing rectification, which is taking the absolute value of the signal. Rectification transforms the biphasic waveform to a double-peaked positive waveform. This allows a sine wave with a frequency corresponding to the rate of the signal to better approximate the signal. Thus, the dominant frequency of the rectified signal, as shown in Fig. 6.11, is at the expected 4 Hz. The results of autocorrelation and dominant frequency analysis on a rectified biphasic signal are similar to those for positive narrow waveforms.

6 Alternative Techniques for Rate Estimation

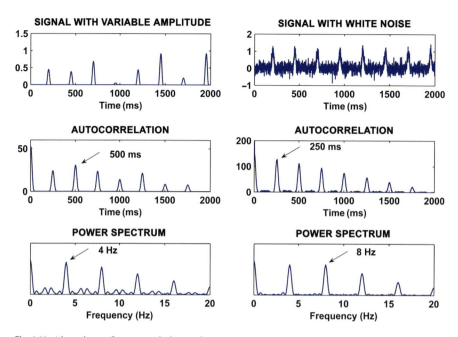

Fig. 6.10 Alterations of autocorrelation and power spectrum peaks of a signal with narrow waveforms when amplitude variation or white noise is introduced

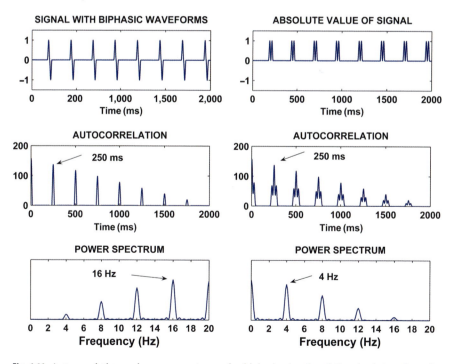

Fig. 6.11 Autocorrelation and power spectrum of a biphasic signal and the absolute value of a biphasic signal

6.8 Summary

Autocorrelation and dominant frequency both offer advantages over event detection in estimating the frequency of events. This is particularly true for signals with large variation of amplitude where a fixed threshold detection algorithm would likely miss events or for signals with a high degree of noise. Autocorrelation tends to have advantages over dominant frequency analysis for noisy signals, signals with different morphologies, and signals with variable frequency of events and change of phase. Dominant frequency analysis has advantages for signals with large amplitude variation. Both methods are ideally performed using multiple repeated measurements to overcome the limitations described in this chapter.

Summary of Key Terms

- Autocorrelation – A time domain method to estimate a signal's cycle length by determining the nonzero delay required for a copy of the signal to have the best alignment with itself. The computation is similar to that used in template matching.
- Dominant frequency analysis – A frequency domain method of estimating rate of a signal. This method chooses the frequency of the maximum point in the power spectrum as the estimate of the frequency of the signal.

References

1. Welch PD. The use of fast fourier transform for the estimation of power spectra: a method based on time averaging over short, modified periodograms. *IEEE Trans Audio Electroacoustics*. 1967;AU-15:70–73.
2. Oppenhein AV, Schafer RW. *Discrete-Time Signal Processing*. Englewood Cliffs, NJ: Prentice Hall; 1989.
3. Ng J, Kadish AH, Goldberger JJ. Effect of electrogram characteristics on the relationship of dominant frequency to atrial activation rate in atrial fibrillation. *Heart Rhythm*. 2006; 3:1295–1305.
4. Schwartz M, Shaw L. *Signal Processing: Discrete Spectral Analysis, Detection, and Estimation*. New York: McGraw-Hill, Inc; 1975.

Signal Averaging for Noise Reduction

7

Jason Ng and Jeffrey J. Goldberger

7.1
Chapter Objectives

In stable conditions, signals in cardiology contain a great deal of redundancy. If everything is working right, one beat should be very similar to the beats that occur around the same time. This redundancy can be used for the purposes of improving the accuracy of estimated values in the presence of noise. In this chapter, we will explore how this redundancy is used to improve signal-to-noise ratio in the signal processing technique of signal averaging.

7.2
Dart Board Example

A dart board can be used as our first illustration of how signal averaging works. The dart thrower aims for the center of the dart board. However, his hand is shaky and cannot hit exactly where he wants to throw. Figure 7.1a shows the results of the dart thrower's ten attempts to hit the bull's-eye. Some attempts are closer than others with some more left of the target, some more right, some above, and some below.

Consider the challenge of guessing where the bull's-eye is located with the dart board not visible and knowing only the locations of the darts (see Fig. 7.1b). Each dart can in itself be considered an estimation of the bull's-eye location. The distances of the darts from the center ranged from 2.4 to 20 cm. The average distance from the center was 7.3 cm. This means that even though our best estimate would have an error of only 2.4 cm, the average error would be 7.3 cm. Without knowing where the true center is, there is no way to know which single dart would provide the best estimate. However, we can take advantage of the fact that we have ten attempts, the assumption that the direction of error is completely random, and that the error is not biased in any direction. If we take the

J. Ng (✉)
Feinberg School of Medicine, Northwestern University, Chicago, IL, USA
e-mail: jsnng@northwestern.edu

J.J. Goldberger and J. Ng (eds.),
Practical Signal and Image Processing in Clinical Cardiology,
DOI: 10.1007/978-1-84882-515-4_7, © Springer-Verlag London Limited 2010

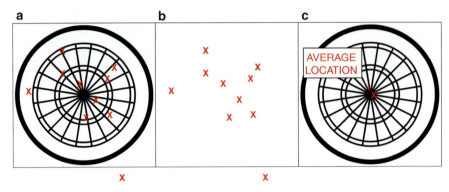

Fig. 7.1 Illustration of signal averaging using a dart board. Using the average location of the darts, the location of the bull's-eye can be predicted

average location of the ten darts, as shown in Fig. 7.1c, we obtain an estimate that is only 0.2 cm from the true center.

How good of an estimate of the location of the bull's-eye can we expect from taking the average location of the dart? The answer depends on two factors. The first factor is the amount of variation expected from the person throwing darts. The second factor is the number of darts thrown. If the amount of variation is small then only a few number of darts need to be thrown to get a good estimate. Conversely, a larger variation would require more darts to be thrown to be confident about the estimate.

Using the dart-board analogy for signal averaging, the signal of interest is the bull's-eye. Any deviation of that signal due to noise is analogous to the imprecision of the dart thrower. If there is repetition of the signal, it would be analogous to having multiple throws. Assuming that the noise is random, without bias, and completely uncorrelated with the signal itself, then taking averages of the signals will theoretically bring us closer to the true signal, thus improving the signal-to-noise ratio.

7.3
Signal Averaging

Figure 7.2 shows an example of a repeated signal before and after the addition of noise. The high level of noise that was added to the signal makes it difficult to ascertain the actual morphology of the signal. The first step of signal averaging is to choose a window, which defines the beginning and end of each waveform. For this example, we will take the window starting from 100 ms before each waveform to 100 ms after the waveform. The markers delimiting the beginnings (B) and ends (E) of the window are shown in Fig. 7.3.

The next step is to align the ten waveforms such that the first point for each window corresponds to the first point of every other window. Figure 7.4 shows the ten waveform windows aligned and then overlaid. Averaging the ten waveforms at each sample point produces the signal-averaged waveform.

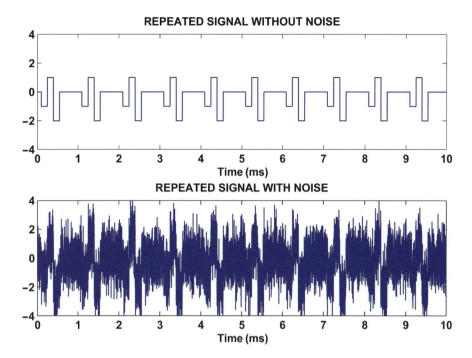

Fig. 7.2 A signal with repeated waveforms with and without white noise

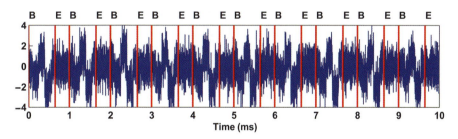

Fig. 7.3 Lines mark the beginning (B) and end (E) of each of the ten waveforms in the noisy signal

The signal-averaged result in Fig. 7.4 shows that the noise is significantly reduced, making the shape of the waveform much more apparent. However, the noise is not completely eliminated as ten redundant waveforms may not be enough to overcome the level of noise that was added to the system. Figure 7.5 shows the improvement in the signal quality that is possible by increasing the number of waveforms from 10 to 20 to 50 to 100. Increasing the number may improve the result even more but may not be practical in real-life situations, particularly in cardiology. However, signals with smaller noise levels may not require as many redundant waveforms to obtain the desired signal-to-noise ratio. The reduction in noise is inversely proportional to the square root of the number of waveforms. Thus, increasing the number of waveforms from 1 to 100 results in a tenfold reduction in

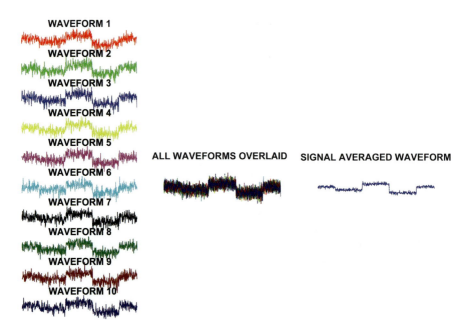

Fig. 7.4 The ten noisy waveforms displayed individually, overlaid, and then signal averaged

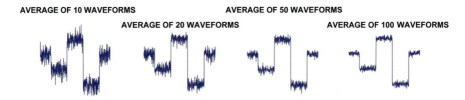

Fig. 7.5 Illustration showing the improvements to signal quality as the number of waveforms increase from 10 to 20 to 50 to 100

noise. To achieve a further tenfold reduction in noise, 10,000 waveforms would need to be averaged. It is therefore important to minimize the noise level in the original signal, as it may be impractical to expect to achieve 100-fold reductions in noise.

7.4 Limitations of Signal Averaging

Signal averaging is a powerful tool for the purposes of improving signal-to-noise ratio. Strict criteria, however, need to be met to prevent distortion of the signal of interest. First, there must be minimal intrinsic variability of the waveform. This means that without noise the signal must have a high degree of reproducibility. Consider the following example in Fig. 7.6. The signal in Fig. 7.2 was modified so that the waveform incrementally increased

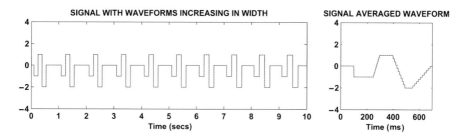

Fig. 7.6 The result of signal averaging for waveforms that are increasing in width. The signal-averaged waveform appears more trapezoidal rather than rectangular

in width from 450 ms for the first waveform to 585 for the tenth waveform. Performing signal averaging for this signal assuming all the waveforms are lined up at the first downward deflection produces the result shown in the right plot of Fig. 7.6. The morphology of this signal-averaged waveform is considerably distorted, showing a more trapezoidal shape than the original rectangular shape. This highlights the limitations of using this signal processing technique for dynamically changing waveforms.

A second important criterion for signal averaging is that the waveforms are lined up as perfectly as possible when the windows are determined. This criterion can be harder to fulfill than it sounds, particularly when noise is in the signal or if the waveform does not contain a clearly detectable feature that can be used as a reference or fiducial point. Figure 7.7 demonstrates the distortion misalignment can have on the signal-averaged result. In this example, the maximum misalignment is 40 ms.

A final criterion for signal averaging is that the noise cannot be synchronized with the signal. In other words, the timing of the noise must be completely independent from the timing of the waveform. Synchronization of the waveform and the noise will negate the ability of averaging to improve the signal-to-noise ratio. Consider the two examples shown in Fig. 7.8. The same waveform morphology is used; however, 60 Hz noise is added to the signal. On the left, the 60 Hz noise is dyssynchronous with the waveform. Averaging significantly decreased the effect of noise on the waveform. On the right, the 60 Hz noise is in synchrony with the waveform. Averaging in this case had no effect in reducing the amount of noise in the waveform.

Noise that contains large outlier values can have a profound effect on a signal. Although the absence of such outliers is not a requirement for signal averaging, it may take a large number of repeated waveforms to overcome the outlier values. We will examine an example shown in Fig. 7.9 in which a signal is almost completely free of noise. The only exceptions are ten large spikes that occur at different points of each of the waveforms. Signal averaging in this case reduces the amplitude of all the spikes but spread all ten over the signal-averaged waveform.

7.5
Median Waveforms

In Fig. 7.9, spurious spikes occur at various times throughout the signal. However, even though any one waveform may be distorted by this spike, the other nine waveforms contain the true value of the waveform at that particular time. It would be advantageous in cases like

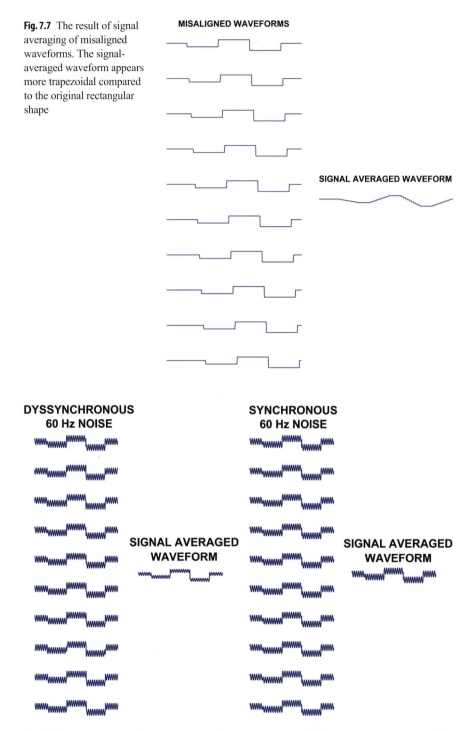

Fig. 7.7 The result of signal averaging of misaligned waveforms. The signal-averaged waveform appears more trapezoidal compared to the original rectangular shape

Fig. 7.8 Signal averaging of ten waveforms with dyssynchronous 60 Hz noise and synchronous 60 Hz noise. Signal averaging of the signal with dyssynchronous 60 Hz noise showed an attenuation of the 60 Hz noise while signal averaging of the signal with synchronous 60 Hz noise showed no attenuation

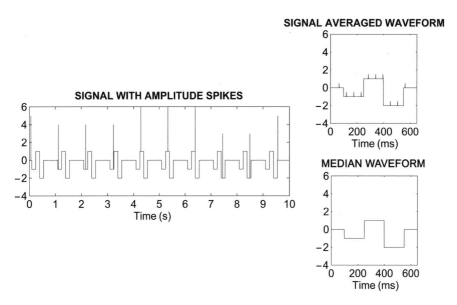

Fig. 7.9 Average and median waveform from a signal with added amplitude spikes. Although the amplitude spikes are attenuated in the signal-averaged waveform, residuals of the spike are scattered throughout the waveform. The spikes are completely eliminated in the median waveform

this to be able to take the correct value rather than incorporate the waveform that contains the outlier value. An alternative to averaging is using the median. The median is less susceptible to outliers, yet approximates the mean for most common types of random noise signals. For the example in Fig. 7.9, the time point with the first amplitude spike would have a value of 5 for the first waveform and 0 for the next nine waveforms. The median of ten values is the mean of the fifth and sixth largest values, which would be 0 in this example. The amplitude spikes, therefore, will be completely eliminated in the median waveform.

Median waveforms are also useful in noisy signals such as the example in Fig. 7.2. However, in situations where the signal contains occasional changes in morphology or occasional poor alignment of the waveforms, the median may have an advantage over the average. Examples comparing the median waveform to the average waveform in each of these cases are illustrated in Fig. 7.10. The median operation in general works best with high-frequency noise and has trouble with low-frequency noise such as baseline wander. A comparison between averaging and taking a median waveform in this situation is illustrated in Fig. 7.11.

The reasoning behind the difference in results for the signal with baseline wander is the nonlinearity of the median operation. In other words,

average (signal + noise) = average (signal) + average (noise)
however
median (signal + noise) ≠ median (signal) + median (noise)

Because the average of the noise is approximately zero, the average of the signal plus noise will approximately be the average of the signal. However, the median of the signal plus noise is not as predictable.

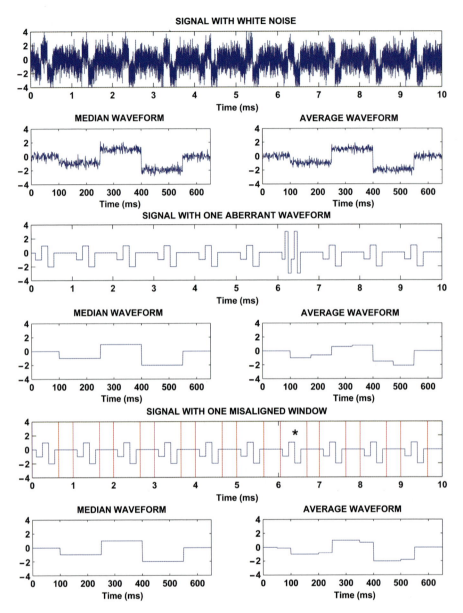

Fig. 7.10 Comparison between median waveforms and signal-averaged waveforms for three conditions: with white noise, with one aberrant waveform, and with one misaligned window

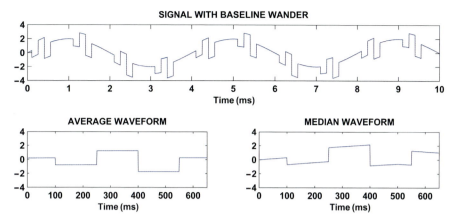

Fig. 7.11 Comparison between a signal-averaged waveform and a median waveform for a signal with baseline wander

7.6 Summary

For all the reasons discussed in this chapter, it is important that the characteristics of both the signal and noise be known when choosing between the mean and median operation for a noise reduction technique. Both can be effective tools in the right circumstances, but can also introduce unwanted distortion that can adversely affect measurements made to the signal.

Summary of Key Terms

- Signal averaging – A method of improving signal-to-noise ratio by lining up and calculating the mean waveform of multiple repeated waveforms.
- Fiducial point – A feature of a waveform that can be detected and used as a reference time point when analyzing multiple waveforms (e.g., for signal averaging).
- Median waveform – Similar to signal-averaged waveform except a median operation replaces the mean operation. Median waveforms have advantages over signal-averaged waveforms in signals with sporadic outliers.

References

1. Oppenhein AV, Schafer RW. *Discrete-Time Signal Processing*. Englewood Cliffs, NJ: Prentice Hall; 1989.
2. Simson MB. Use of signals in the terminal QRS complex to identify patients with ventricular tachycardia after myocardial infarction. *Circulation*. 1981;64:235.

Data Compression

8

Jason Ng and Jeffrey J. Goldberger

8.1
Chapter Objectives

Data compression is an important aspect of signal processing that affects almost all cardiology signal and image recording techniques. One of the big advantages of digital signal and image acquisition is that these files can be easily accessed from computer workstations. The need for large filing cabinets and physical archiving of the signals and images are lessened. Digital storage is relatively inexpensive and the prices are continuously dropping as technology for these devices improve. Despite this, digital storage space is still finite and efficient use of this space is required to handle the large amount of data that is constantly being generated. As discussed in the earlier chapters, choice of sample rates, amplitude resolutions, and spatial resolutions are important factors for the efficient use of digital storage space. This chapter will discuss how data compression can be used to store data in a more efficient manner.

8.2
General Concepts

Most data compression algorithms take advantage of an identified redundancy that is contained in the signal. Most algorithms fit into two categories: loss-less and lossy compression. In loss-less compression, data are transformed to a version that is smaller than the original, but contains all the information of the original data. With loss-less compression, the compressed data can be transformed back to the original form with no differences. With lossy compression, compressed data cannot be transformed back exactly to the original data. However, the differences between the compressed signal and the original

---

J. Ng (✉)
Department of Medicine, Division of Cardiology, Feinberg School of Medicine,
Northwestern University, Chicago, IL, USA
e-mail: jsnng@northwestern.edu

J.J. Goldberger and J. Ng (eds.),
Practical Signal and Image Processing in Clinical Cardiology,
DOI: 10.1007/978-1-84882-515-4_8, © Springer-Verlag London Limited 2010

may be small enough to not affect the ability to interpret the data. Thus, both types of algorithms are commonly used and the situation will determine which is most appropriate.

8.3
Downsampling

Downsampling is perhaps the most basic compression algorithm. Downsampling of a signal involves retaining a fraction of samples and discarding the rest. Although samples are being thrown away, downsampling can be both lossy or loss-less depending on the original sampling rate, the new sampling rate, and the frequency content of the signal. At first glance, it may not seem intuitive that downsampling can be a loss-less process. However, if we go back to the concepts of analog-to-digital conversion discussed earlier, the same conditions for loss-less analog-to-digital conversion are required for loss-less downsampling – the sampling rate must be twice the highest frequency component of the signal. However, when downsampling is used as a compression algorithm, it is typically a lossy process. Figure 8.1 shows an example of two signals that are downsampled: a lower frequency signal on the left and a higher frequency signal on the right. Despite downsampling of the lower frequency signal by a factor of 10 or 20 times, most of the shape information

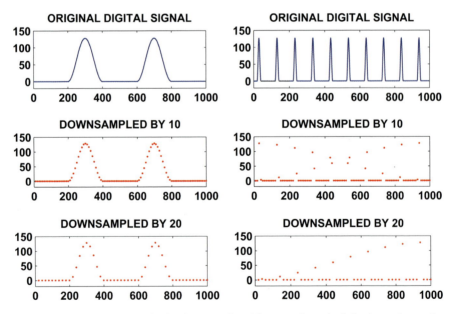

Fig. 8.1 Example of data reduction by downsampling. The example on the *left* column shows adequate approximation of the original digital signal after downsampling by factors of 10 and 20. The example on the *right* shows significant distortion of the original digital signal after downsampling by factors of 10 and 20

of the signal is retained. In contrast, downsampling the higher frequency signal by the same factors distorts the signals considerably.

8.4 Quantization

Quantization was also discussed earlier in this book for the conversion of analog signals to digital signals. The same process can be applied to a digital signal with given amplitude resolution to a new signal with a lower amplitude resolution to reduce the size of the data. Quantization to a lower amplitude resolution is almost always a lossy process. The reconstructed signal may look more "blocky" than the original. Figure 8.2 shows an example of a signal with amplitude resolution that is first reduced four times and then again for a total of 16 times the original amplitude resolution. In this example, a four-times reduction changes the signal slightly but the waveform still manages to retain most of its shape information. When the signal undergoes 16-times reduction, the signal no longer has smooth slopes but instead looks very "blocky."

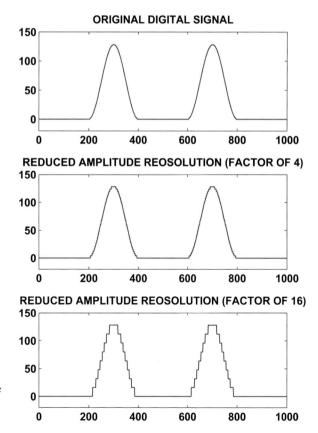

Fig. 8.2 Example of data reduction by reducing amplitude resolution. Decreasing the amplitude resolution by a factor of 4 and a factor of 16 makes the signal appear progressively more "blocky"

8.5 Variable Length Codes

One compression strategy takes advantage of the fact that some data values occur more frequently than others. By assigning the more frequent values with shorter codes and the more rare values with longer codes, the overall length of the coded signal can be shorter than if all the values were coded with the same length. To illustrate this point, we can consider coding the alphabet with the binary digits, where each letter in the alphabet is assigned a sequence of ones and zeros. At least five digits are required to encode all 26 letters with an equal length code. An example coding is shown below:

A: 00000	F: 00101	K: 01010	P: 01111	U: 10100	Z: 11001
B: 00001	G: 00110	L: 01011	Q: 10000	V: 10101	
C: 00010	H: 00111	M: 01100	R: 10001	W: 10110	
D: 00011	I: 01000	N: 01101	S: 10010	X: 10111	
E: 00100	J: 01001	O: 01110	T: 10011	Y: 11000	

To encode the Chinese proverb:

"The superior doctor prevents sickness; the mediocre doctor attends to impending sickness; the inferior doctor treats actual sickness," using the above code, 565 binary digits are required to represent the 113 letters in this text. The frequency of each letter is shown in Fig. 8.3.

Morse code is a well-known variable length code. Although the Morse code is typically expressed as a series of dots and dashes, we can replace the dots with zeros and the dashes with ones as shown below:

A: 01	F: 0010	K:101	P: 0110	U: 001	Z: 1100
B: 1000	G: 110	L: 0100	Q: 1101	V: 0001	
C: 1010	H: 0000	M:11	R: 010	W: 011	
D: 100	I: 00	N: 10	S: 000	X: 1001	
E: 0	J: 0111	O: 111	T: 1	Y: 1011	

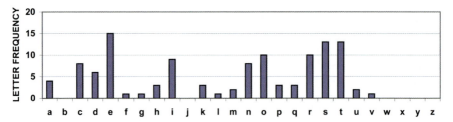

Fig. 8.3 Histogram of the frequency of the letters represented in the Chinese proverb – "the superior doctor prevents sickness; the mediocre doctor attends to impending sickness; the inferior doctor treats actual sickness"

8 Data Compression

Translating the Chinese proverb into Morse code resulted in 290 binary digits, roughly half of the fixed length code. Despite the obvious reduction of data, Morse code is not practical for digital data streams. The reason for this is that a code for one letter can be a portion of another letter. For example, a code of 0000 could either mean the letter H, two consecutive I's, or four consecutive E's. Morse code was able to be applied in telegraph because pauses could be used to separate letters. However, for a digital data stream this is not practical. The following is an alternative variable length code, called the Huffman code, which is derived using the specific letter frequency of the Chinese proverb. In the Huffman code, no individual code is the beginning of any other code.

A:11101	G:1110011	M:100101	S: 001	Y:1110010010
B:1110010011111	H:01111	N:1010	T: 000	Z:111001000
C:1111	I:1011	O:1000	U: 100100	
D:10011	J:11100100011110	P:01101	V: 1110000	
E:110	K:011110	Q:01100	W:111001001110	
F:11100101	L:1110001	R:010	X:11100100110	

The variable code length of this example ranges from 3 to 14 digits long. Overall, the resulting coded sequence of the proverb is 459 digits long, a reduction of roughly 12% from that of the fixed length code.

How does compression of encoded alphabet relate to the compression of signals? The letters of the phrase are analogous to the possible amplitude levels of a signal. A signal that spends most of the time at the baseline level with occasional deviations from the baseline is more able to be compressed using a variable length code than a signal with a more uniform distribution of amplitudes.

8.6
Differencing

Differencing is a loss-less compression technique that can be applied to signals with relatively small changes from sample-to-sample. Consider the following sequence of numbers:

33034	33025	33011	33001	32999	33008	33020	33028

The number of binary digits required to encode each number into binary form is determined by the smallest power of two that is greater than the largest number. The largest number 33034 is less than 2^{16} but greater than 2^{15}; therefore, the number of binary digits required is 16. The total number of binary digits is 128 (16 binary digits × 8 numbers) for the entire sequence. One thing that should be noticed about this sequence of numbers is that although the numbers are relatively large (and thus requiring 16 binary digits), the difference between the numbers are actually quite small in comparison. Taking the successive differences between the numbers, we get

−9	−14	−10	−2	9	12	8

The seven differences are indeed much smaller than the actual numbers. The number of binary digits required to encode the difference is five bits ($2^4 = 16$, times 2 for positive and negative numbers). Therefore, this sequence can be encoded beginning with the 16-digit binary number representing the first number and then the five digit binary numbers representing the difference for the next seven numbers. The total number of binary numbers for this sequence will be $16 + 5 \times 7 = 51$, a reduction of roughly 60%. Even if the difference is encoded as a more standard eight binary digits rather five binary digits, the reduction is still a significant 44%. Decompression of the signal would be accomplished by cumulatively summing the numbers.

The differencing method of compression is effective for signals that have relatively small sample-to-sample changes. However, signals with very fast fluctuations may require more binary digits to encode the difference than what is required for the original signal. Consider the following sequence as an example:

−100	100	−100	100	−100	100	−100	100

The successive differences would then be

200	−200	200	−200	200	−200	200

The original sequence requires eight binary digits per number (a total of 64 digits). Each of the differences, however, requires nine binary digits and thus the sequence would require 71 binary digits.

8.7
Template Subtraction

Signals in cardiology generally have a good deal of redundancy in the time domain because the cardiac cycle is a fairly reproducible process. This characteristic can be used to reduce the amount of data required to represent the signal. Template subtraction is a loss-less compression algorithm where the events/beats are detected and a template of the events/beat is created using signal averaging (see chapter 7). The template is subtracted from the original signal and the remainder, having a much smaller range than the original signal, can be encoded with a smaller number of binary digits. Figure 8.4 shows an example of a pulsed waveform with variable amplitude. A template was created by averaging the ten pulses and then the template was subtracted from the original pulses leaving a residual waveform.

8.8
Curve Fitting

Lossy compression may be acceptable if the amount of distortion in the compressed signal is approximately the level of noise. Curve fitting is a method of compression where the signal is approximated by a function such as a line or polynomial. This method is appropriate

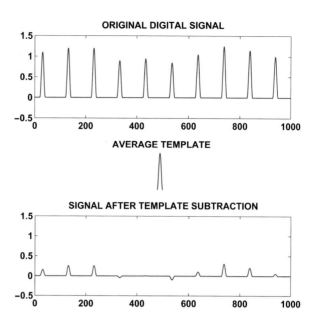

Fig. 8.4 Example of data reduction by means of average template subtraction

for waveforms that are not completely random but follow certain trends. For example, if a signal is comprised of long linear segments, each of the segments can be represented by the starting point of the segment, the slope of the segment, and the length of the segment. Storing these three numbers for each segment instead of the raw data can save a significant amount of space. Higher order approximations are also possible.

The amount of compression that this technique provides depends largely on the amount of error that is allowed in the approximation. If a high amount of error in the approximation is tolerated, then the approximated curves can fit longer segments of data. However, if little or no error is tolerated, then the amount of compression would probably be minimal or could even require more information than the original signal.

Figure 8.5 shows an example of a signal that is approximated by nine linear segments. The approximation was set so that any of the linear segments would not have an error greater than 0.05 at any single point.

8.9
Data Transformation

Some signals in the time domain may not benefit from the above methods but may benefit after transformation of the data. For example, a high-frequency sine wave would not benefit too much from variable length codes since the amplitudes are fairly evenly distributed over the amplitude range of the signal. Differencing would also not significantly help with reducing the data. Transforming the sine wave signal into the frequency domain would result in a spectrum with a peak at a single frequency. Thus, this signal could be completely

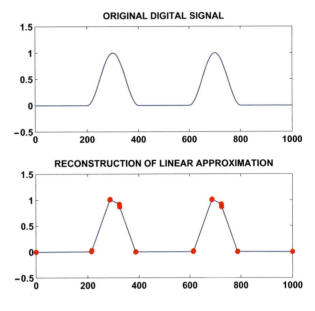

Fig. 8.5 Example of data reduction by linear approximation of segments of the signal

described by the amplitude and phase of the sine wave. Although signals rarely can be described with a single sinusoid, information from some signals can be well approximated using only a portion of the frequency band or reduced resolution of some of the frequencies. Data transformation can also be used in combination with the other compression methods discussed above.

8.10 Summary

The appropriateness of any of the compression algorithms mentioned above depends primarily on the characteristics of the data that is to be compressed and the amount of error that is tolerated. The proper balance between the amount of data reduction required and fidelity needed must be determined when choosing an algorithm.

Summary of Key Terms

- Compression – Signal processing for the purpose of reducing the size of data.
- Lossless compression – Type of compression where all original data can be reproduced from the compressed data.
- Lossy compression – Type of compression where an approximation of original data can be obtained from the compressed data.

- › Downsampling – A lossy compression technique where data are reduced by resampling a digital signal to a lower sampling rate.
- › Quantization – A lossy compression technique where data are reduced by resampling a digital signal to a lower amplitude resolution.
- › Variable length codes – A lossless compression technique where data values are encoded with binary numbers of different lengths. Shorter codes are reserved for more frequently occurring data values while longer codes are reserved for more infrequently occurring data values.
- › Differencing – A lossless compression technique where differences between successive data values are taken to reduce the range of the data values. Differencing is useful in situations where data values have gradual changes from sample to sample.
- › Template subtraction – A lossless compression technique where a template waveform is subtracted from the actual waveform to reduce the range of the data values. This technique is effective when repeated waveforms are present in the signal.
- › Curve fitting – A lossy compression technique where segments of the signal are approximated with a function, such as a line or a curve. The parameters for the functions are saved rather than the data values themselves. This technique is effective in situations where some error is acceptable.

References

1. Hamilton PS. Compression of the ambulatory ECG by average beat subtraction and residual differencing. *IEEE Trans Biomed Eng*. 1991;38(3):253–259.
2. Huffman DA. A method for construction of minimum-redundancy codes. *Proc IRE*. 1952; 40: 1098-1101.
3. Cox JR, Nolle FM, Fozzard HA, Oliver GC. AZTEC: a preprocessing program for real time ECG rhythm analysis. *IEEE Trans BME*. 1968;15:128–129.
4. Reddy BRS, Murthy ISN. ECG data compression using Fourier descriptor. *IEEE Trans Biomed Eng*. 1986;33:428–434.
5. Jalaleddine SMS. ECG data compression techniques–a unified approach. *IEEE Trans Biomed Eng*. 1990;37(4):329–343.

Image Processing

9

Jason Ng and Jeffrey J. Goldberger

9.1 Chapter Objectives

Multiple imaging modalities are used in cardiology for diagnostic purposes. Thus, familiarity and understanding of image processing is very important in the use and interpretation of the images produced by these modalities. The previous chapters examined signal processing concepts and techniques for time domain signals, which are considered one-dimensional signals where amplitude is plotted on the y-axis vs. time on the x-axis. In this chapter, we will explore images, which are two-dimensional signals where amplitude is plotted on the z-axis vs. space in the x- and y-axes. The amplitudes of a two-dimensional signal can be displayed in a three-dimensional plot, as seen in Fig. 9.1a. However, images are more commonly displayed as an intensity map where the colors of each point, known as a pixel, correspond to an amplitude value for that particular x and y value. Figure 9.1b shows the corresponding image of the three-dimension plot of Fig. 9.1a. The color of the image is scaled so that a z amplitude value of zero corresponds to black and one corresponds to white. The opposite of this scaling where black represents the highest amplitude values is also commonly seen. Different colors can also be used to represent different amplitude values.

Many of the signal processing concepts and techniques that were discussed for time-domain signals are also applicable in image processing. Images also have their own unique set of challenges. Although our focus in this chapter will be on two-dimensional images, three-dimensional (volume) images, time-varying two-dimensional images (movies), and time-varying three-dimensional images are commonly used clinically as imaging modalities are becoming more sophisticated.

J. Ng (✉)
Feinberg School of Medicine, Northwestern University, Chicago, IL, USA
e-mail: jsnng@northwestern.edu

J.J Goldberger and Jason Ng (eds.),
Practical Signal and Image Processing in Clinical Cardiology,
DOI: 10.1007/978-1-84882-515-4_9, © Springer-Verlag London Limited 2010

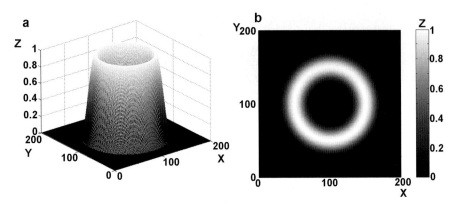

Fig. 9.1 A three-dimensional plot (**a**) displayed as a two-dimensional image (**b**)

9.2 Sampling

Many aspects of acquiring digital images are similar to acquiring time-domain signals. One of the key similarities is that both types of acquisition utilize analog-to-digital converters. The difference is that instead of taking multiple samples in time, images require multiple samples in space that are often taken simultaneously using multiple sensors and analog-to-digital converters. As adequate sampling rates are important in the time domain to prevent undersampling and aliasing, spatial resolution for images (analogous to the sampling period (1/sampling rate) of time-domain signals) is a major factor in the quality of images. Aliasing in images is characterized by jagged edges and missing details. Figure 9.2 illustrates aliasing using an image of circles with different sizes. This image is sampled with a resolution of 5 mm. Aliasing is evident in the reconstructed signal in a few different ways. First, the large circle when reconstructed has jagged edges that make it less circular. For the second and third largest circles, each circle was captured by sampling. However, the morphologies of each circle not only look less circular but are different from each other despite having identical shapes and sizes before sampling. Finally, for the smallest circles, only 6 of 16 were detected. The ones that were detected are represented by only a single 5 × 5 mm pixel.

In the time domain, aliasing can be prevented by sampling at a rate greater than twice the highest frequency component of the signal (Nyquist sampling criterion). Low-pass anti-aliasing filters applied to the signals before sampling will ensure that the Nyquist criterion will be met. These sampling rules also apply in image processing. Low-pass filtering before sampling, however, is not usually practical to implement in most imaging modalities. Alternatively, to reduce the aliasing effects, the average intensity around the area closest to the sampling pixel can be obtained and used as the intensity of the sample rather than a single point. Most detectors intrinsically perform averaging in this way. Figure 9.3 shows the reconstruction of the image with the average value of each grid. The tapering of the intensities allow for better approximation of the original shapes of the

9 Image Processing

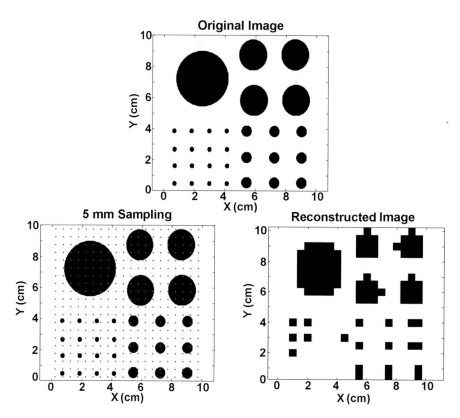

Fig. 9.2 Sampling and reconstruction of an image of different sized circles. The sampling was performed at points spaced 5 mm apart

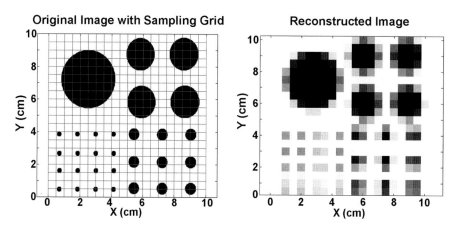

Fig. 9.3 Sampling and reconstruction of an image of different sized circles. The sampling was performed by taking the average value of each 5 × 5 mm grid

circles. Despite this method of approximation, the only way to really improve the quality of the obtained image is to improve the resolution of the sampling.

9.3
Quantization

As with the time domain, the quantization process is just as important as the sampling process for imaging. Poor amplitude resolution and suboptimal amplitude range can result in loss of important information from the image. The example in Fig. 9.4 illustrates the effects of poor amplitude resolution during quantization. There are a few things to notice from this example. One is that a few of the circles are lost in the background. Once information is lost like this in the quantization process, there is no signal processing that can be done to recover the information. The second thing to notice is that each circle of a common size originally had different shades of gray. After quantization, the circles that did not get lost to the background only have two shades for each size. Again, this loss of differentiation cannot be recovered.

9.4
Image Resizing

Images often need to be resized in order to fit on the computer screen or reduced in size to save storage space. Similar to interpolation in one-dimension, interpolation increases the image size by making reasonable "guesses" as to what values should occur between the known pixels. Figure 9.5 show an example grayscale image of a rock formation with image

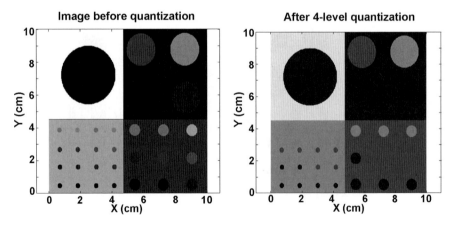

Fig 9.4 Effect of quantizing an image with poor amplitude resolution

9 Image Processing 93

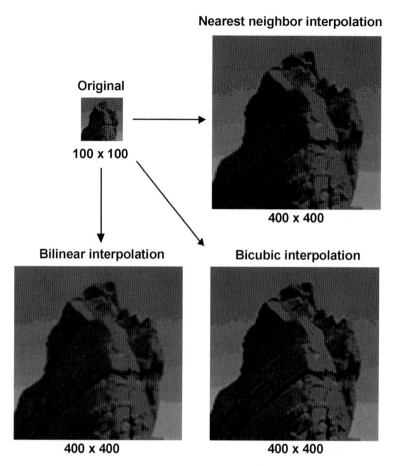

Fig. 9.5 Example of an 100 × 100 image that is resized to 400 × 400 using nearest neighbor interpolation, bilinear interpolation, and bicubic interpolation

dimensions of 100 by 100 pixels that is resized to 400 by 400 pixels with three different methods of interpolation.

The upper right image shows the original image resized with nearest neighbor interpolation. Nearest neighbor interpolation is the simplest to compute out of the three methods. Each interpolated point is simply replaced by the value of its nearest neighbor. For our example, this action results in the replacement of each of the original pixels with 4 × 4 pixels of the same value. Thus, the resized image has a "blocky" look to it. The lower left image of Fig. 9.5 is resized with bilinear interpolation. Bilinear interpolation replaces every point with a weighted sum of four points of the nearest 2 × 2 set of pixels of the original image. The weights used for the sum are determined by the distance from the location of the interpolated point to the location of the four points, where a closer distance corresponds to a larger weight. We notice in the example that the resized image is less blocky than the nearest neighbor interpolated image. Lastly, the lower right shows the image resized with bicubic interpolation. Bicubic interpolation works similarly to bilinear interpolation, except that bicubic interpolation replaces every point with a weighted sum of 16 points of the nearest 4×4 set of pixels of the original image. Although bicubic interpolation has much more computational requirements than nearest neighbor or bilinear interpolation, the result is often a sharper image than those of the other two methods. These interpolation techniques can also be used to shrink images.

It is important to note that although these resizing techniques can enhance viewing the images on the computer screen, no new information from the original image can be gained from resizing no matter how many times the image is magnified. For example, if we knew that there was a fly sitting on the rock formation, no amount of resizing with interpolation will allow us to see that fly since the fly was much smaller than the original resolution of the image. The typical digital camera often has optical and digital zoom as features. With optical zoom, additional detail from objects far away can actually be gained. However, digital zoom uses the resizing and interpolation techniques that allow the picture to be magnified in the desired area, but no additional detail is actually gained.

9.5
Contrast and Brightness

The ability to adjust brightness and contrast are important features for the viewing of images. Our eyes (and sometimes our display screens) have limited ability to distinguish shades of very similar colors. Thus, adjusting brightness and contrast can help us detect subtle differences in pixel intensity values. Adjusting brightness is comparable to amplifying the intensity values. Increasing the intensity values will make dark areas appear lighter on a black (zero intensity) background. Contrast is an image property that defines how easy it is to differentiate pixels of similar but different intensities. Adjusting contrast is accomplished by changing the width of the range of image pixel values that are mapped from dark to bright. Figure 9.6 demonstrates the usefulness of being able to adjust both contrast and brightness. Row A shows a 400×400 pixel image, which appears to be half black and half white. The histogram on the right of the image shows the number of pixels of the image that exists for each intensity value (from 0 to 255). The scale above the histogram shows how the gray scale is mapped to the intensity values, with black at 0, 50% gray at 127.5, and white at 255. A closer inspection of this histogram shows that all the pixels have intensity values near the upper and lower ends of the range. Furthermore at each end of the range, there is a distribution, albeit narrow, of pixel values. Yet, the image appears to be pure black and pure white, with no shades of gray to represent these narrow range of pixel values near 0 and near 255.

In the second row of Fig. 9.6 is the same image as the top row but with a change in the color mapping to focus on the upper end of the intensity values. Now, intensity values of 248 and below are mapped to black. Fifty percent is mapped to 251.5 and white remains at 255. The resulting image shows new detail (different colored circles and ovals) in what previously looked completely white. This new detail was made possible

9 Image Processing

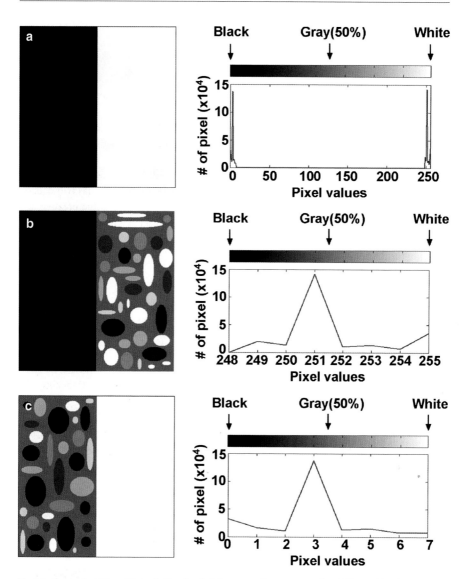

Fig. 9.6 Example of the effect of adjusting brightness and contrast on the ability to identify features that have similar color values

by increasing brightness (50% gray was shifted from 127.5 to 251.5) and by increasing contrast (grayscale range from black to white reduced from 256 to 8). The third row of Fig. 9.6 shows how additional detail can be obtained from the black side of the image. In this example, brightness is reduced and the contrast remains the same as the second example in Fig. 9.6.

9.6 Images in the Frequency Domain

Just like with one-dimensional signals, two-dimensional images can also be analyzed and manipulated in the frequency domain. Images in the frequency domain contain information of the sinusoidal components in both the horizontal and vertical directions which comprise the image. Figure 9.7 shows three examples of 2D frequency domain plots. The left image consists of vertical stripes which are constructed by mapping the amplitude values of a sine wave (shown on top left) to intensity values of the image. The intensity values are then replicated vertically. The resulting frequency domain plot has two dots on the left and right of the center of the plot at locations corresponding to the positive and negative frequency of the sine wave. The middle image consists of a pattern of horizontal lines which was similarly constructed using the sine wave in the top middle plot. The FFT

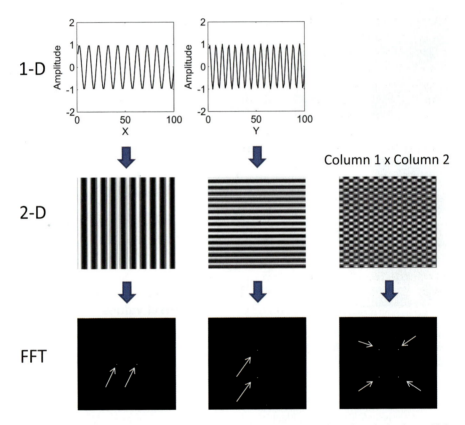

Fig. 9.7 Examples of 2D frequency domain plots. The left image consists of vertical stripes which results in a Fast Fourier Transform (FFT) with two dots on the left and right of the center of the plot. The middle image consists of a pattern of horizontal lines. The FFT of this image shows two dots above and below the center point. The right image was created by multiplying the left image with the middle image. The result is an image with a checkerboard pattern. The FFT of this image consists of four dots, symmetrically surrounding the center point

of this image shows two dots above and below the center point again corresponding to the positive and negative frequency of the sine wave. The right image was created by multiplying the left image with the middle image. The result is an image with a checkerboard pattern. The FFT of this image consists of four dots, symmetrically surrounding the center point, where the vertical distance of each dot from the center is the frequency of the vertical sine wave component and the horizontal distance of each dot is the frequency of the horizontal sine wave component.

To further illustrate how an image is reflected in the frequency domain, we can examine the image of the rock formation in Fig. 9.8 and its corresponding FFT. The symmetric FFT plot includes high intensity values at the center of the FFT plot which represent low frequency power, while points closer to the periphery represent higher frequencies. The rows labeled "Low pass 1" and "Low pass 2" demonstrate progressive smoothing as high frequency components are removed from the image. Low pass filtering images can be used to improve signal-to-noise ratio, but over-filtering can blur an image beyond recognition as seen in "Low pass 2" of Fig. 9.8. Similarly, Fig. 9.9 illustrates the effect of removing low frequency components from the image. High pass filtering has the effect of enhancing the boundaries of an object or any transitions between different intensity values. Thus, high pass filtering can be a useful step in edge detection, a concept further explored later in this chapter. Although boundaries are enhanced by high pass filtering an image, the color information of the object can be lost as seen in Fig. 9.9.

In Chapter 4, it was discussed how manipulation of the phase information in the frequency domain can significantly distort the morphology of a signal in the time domain. The same is true for images. Specifically, to restore a spatial domain image from the frequency domain, both the magnitude and phase spectra are needed. To illustrate the importance of the phase information, consider the images that result from phase distortion with the intact magnitude spectrum. The left panel of Fig. 9.10 shows the rock formation image after back transformation using both the magnitude and phase spectra (identical to the original image from which the magnitude and phase spectra were derived). The middle panel shows the back transformed image with the identical magnitude spectrum for the original image, but with phase distortion. Although, the magnitudes of the FFTs of both images are identical, yet the images in the spatial domain are completely different. Finally, the right panel shows the back transformed image with the identical phase spectrum for the original image, but with the magnitude spectrum uniformly set to one (i.e. the magnitude spectrum is ignored). Interestingly, this image using only the phase spectrum information has a greater likeness to the original image. This highlights the necessity to consider phase when performing filtering or other processing on an image.

9.7
Noise

Signal-to-noise ratio is as important a quality for images as it is for one-dimensional signals. Ambient noise in images is usually characterized by a grainy look. Low signal-to-noise ratio can make detection of small or faint elements or boundaries of elements in the image difficult. Fig. 9.11 shows a previous example before and after adding white noise. The noise for each pixel

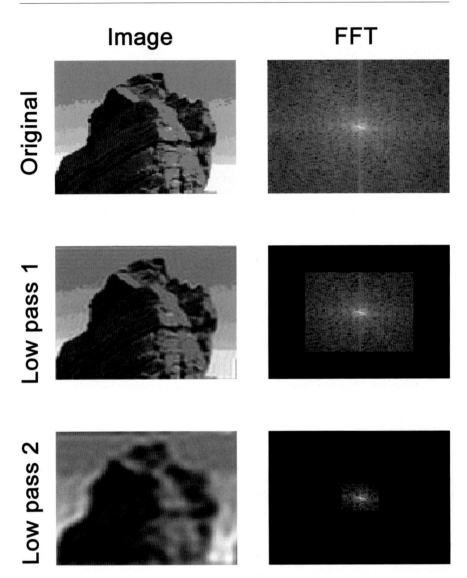

Fig. 9.8 Image and its corresponding FFT plot before and after removal of high frequency components. The top plot shows the original image of a rock formation and the complete FFT. The intensity values at the center of the FFT plot represent low frequency power, while points closer to the periphery represent higher frequencies. The rows labeled "Low pass 1" and "Low pass 2" demonstrate progressive smoothing/blurring as high frequency components are removed from the image

was independently generated with a Gaussian distribution. We can observe from this example that although the noise characteristics are uniform across the entire image, the effect of the noise is different for each circle. The largest circle has the greatest amount of contrast with its background. Therefore, the added noise does not interfere much with our ability to clearly identify the circle and its boundaries. For some of the other circles that have intensity values that are similar to that of the background, these circles are almost completely hidden by the noise.

9 Image Processing

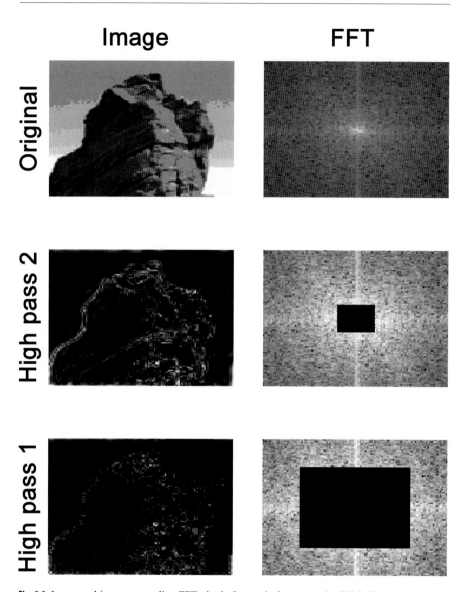

Fig. 9.9 Image and its corresponding FFT plot before and after removal of high frequency components. The top plot shows the original image of a rock formation and the complete FFT. The rows labeled "High pass 1" and "High pass 2" demonstrate enhancement of the object borders as the low frequency components are removed from the image. However, much of the color information is lost

Ambient noise that is picked up by the detectors used for imaging can be modeled by the Gaussian white noise shown in this example. Noise can have other characteristics as well. Another common source of noise is from dust particles that can come between the image source and the detector. This type of noise is characterized by spots of low or no intensity in the image. These white spots are shown in the example in Fig. 9.12, where 10% speckled noise was added to the image.

Original Phase Distortion Magnitude Distortion

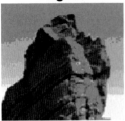 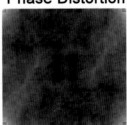 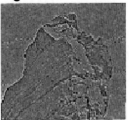

Fig. 9.10 The spatial domain images with either phase or magnitude distortion. The left image is the back-transformed image using both the magnitude and phase spectra which provides the original, starting image. In the middle panel, the original image magnitude spectrum is used, but the phase is distorted. The resultant image bears no resemblance to the original image. In the right panel, the original image phase spectrum is used, but the magnitude is distorted (all values set to 1). The resultant image bears some resemblance to the original image. This illustrates the importance of the phase spectrum when recreating (back-transforming) an image from the frequency domain

9.8 Filtering

Filtering is one common tool used to improve signal-to-noise ratio of images after acquisition. Digital filtering is performed in images in a similar fashion as it is performed in two-dimensions. The only difference is that the filtering coefficients are in the form of a two-dimensional matrix. For example, a 3 by 3 averaging filter and a 5 by 5 averaging filter would have the following coefficients:

$$\begin{vmatrix} \frac{1}{9} & \frac{1}{9} & \frac{1}{9} \\ \frac{1}{9} & \frac{1}{9} & \frac{1}{9} \\ \frac{1}{9} & \frac{1}{9} & \frac{1}{9} \end{vmatrix} \quad \begin{vmatrix} \frac{1}{25} & \frac{1}{25} & \frac{1}{25} & \frac{1}{25} & \frac{1}{25} \\ \frac{1}{25} & \frac{1}{25} & \frac{1}{25} & \frac{1}{25} & \frac{1}{25} \\ \frac{1}{25} & \frac{1}{25} & \frac{1}{25} & \frac{1}{25} & \frac{1}{25} \\ \frac{1}{25} & \frac{1}{25} & \frac{1}{25} & \frac{1}{25} & \frac{1}{25} \\ \frac{1}{25} & \frac{1}{25} & \frac{1}{25} & \frac{1}{25} & \frac{1}{25} \end{vmatrix}$$

The averaging filter essentially replaces each point with the average of itself and its neighbors. The filter does not need to be symmetric as in the above example. For images

9 Image Processing

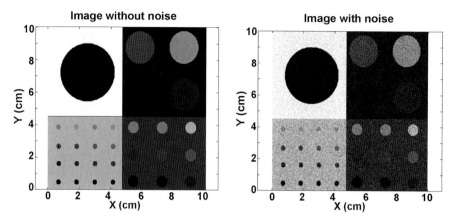

Fig. 9.11 Example of image with and without added white noise

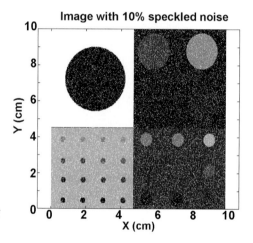

Fig. 9.12 Example of an image with 10% of pixels randomly replaced by white dots

with different spatial resolutions for the x and y directions a filter of unequal dimension may be preferred. The following example in Fig. 9.13 shows the effect of averaging filters of size 3 by 3, 9 by 9, and 15 by 15 on the noisy image of Fig. 9.11. The signal-to-noise ratio of the images increases with size of the averaging filter evidenced by increased smoothing of the image in the areas where there should be solid colors. Although increasing the filter size improves the signal-to-noise ratio, the sharpness of the original image is degraded. For the 15 by 15 filter, some of the smaller circles are blurred almost beyond recognition. Thus, for applications that require the accurate measurement of dimensions or size or require detection of fine details, the choice of filter must be carefully considered.

A median filter is also commonly used in imaging. Median filtering is used for situations where it is important to retain high contrast. For a 3 by 3 median filter, each pixel of the image is replaced by fifth largest (or fifth smallest) value in the 3 by 3 window. The

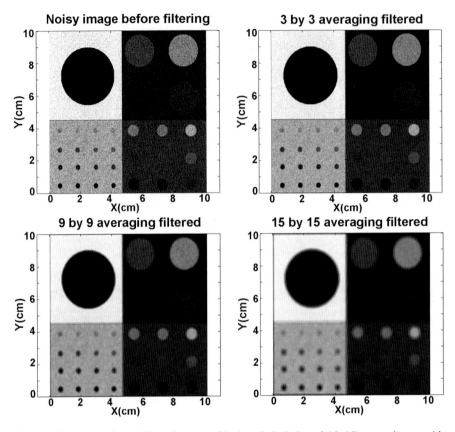

Fig. 9.13 Illustration of the effect of average filtering (3×3, 9×9, and 15×15) on an image with added white noise

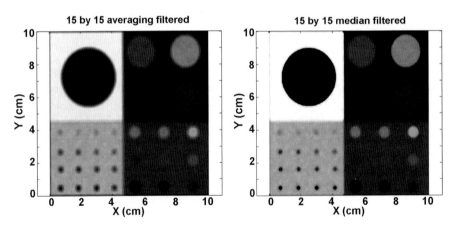

Fig. 9.14 Comparison between 15×15 average filtering and 15×15 median filtering on the image from Figure 9.4 with added white noise

9   Image Processing   103

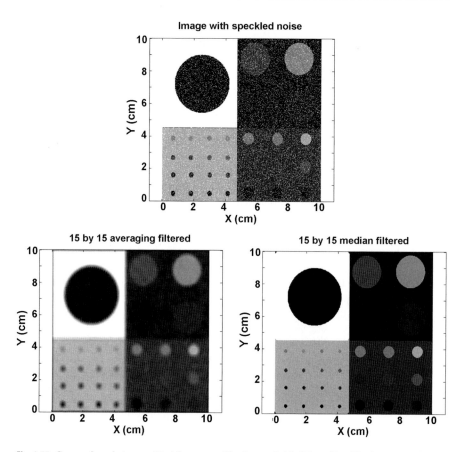

Fig. 9.15 Comparison between 15×15 average filtering and 15×15 median filtering on an image with added speckled noise

choice of the size of the median filter depends on the characteristics of the noise and the signal. The result of 15 by 15 averaging filtering on the image with white noise is compared with the result of 15 by 15 median filtering is shown in Fig. 9.14. Although both filters appear to reduce the amount of noise in the solid portions of the images, the most striking difference is the smaller amount of blurring at the edges of the circles. The amount of blurring is reduced the most for the circles with high contrast with the background. The circles with similar intensities with the background still show some blurring of the edges.

The maximal difference between the two types of filters can be seen in images with speckled noise. Figure 9.15 shows how the 15 by 15 averaging filter reduces the speckled noise but some grainy quality still remains. At the same time, the edges of all the circles are blurred. The 15 by 15 median filter, on the other hand, nearly eliminated all traces of the noise while leaving the edges without blurring. The only noticeable distortion by the median filter is the reduction of size of the smallest circles. This occurred because the diameters of the circles were less than 15 pixels long.

9.9 Signal Averaging

Signal averaging is another effective tool to improve signal-to-noise ratio. In the time domain, repeated waveforms are detected, aligned with each other, and averaged to produce a signal composite result so that the random occurrence of noise will cancel while the signal of interest repeats and remains intact with the averaging process. In some ways signal averaging for imaging is a simpler process. No detection or alignment of a specific element of the image is required if the source of the image and the detector are stable. The average of the entire image repeated multiple times is taken. Figure 9.16 shows the results of averaging ten images with noise.

The number of repeated images required depends on the level of noise and the desired signal-to-noise ratio. Signal averaging has the advantage over average filtering in that it improves signal-to-noise ratio without blurring the desired image. Signal averaging also has the advantage over median filtering where fine details do not get distorted or eliminated. However, the advantage over averaging and median filtering does have an important caveat. The object to be imaged has to be completely stable, which is often easier said than done in cardiology applications. Trying to perform signal averaging in situations where the object is moving is like taking a picture of a moving object with a slow shutter-speed

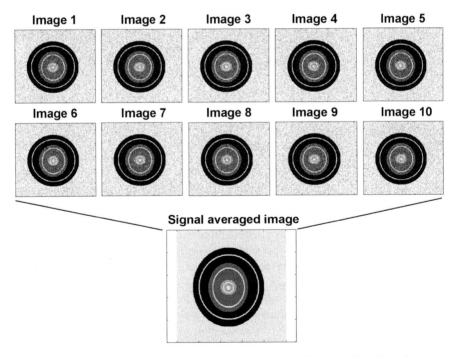

Fig. 9.16 Example of signal averaging of multiple perfectly aligned images with white noise

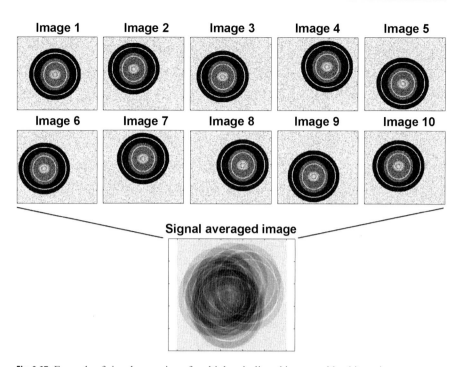

Fig. 9.17 Example of signal averaging of multiple misaligned images with white noise

camera. Figure 9.17 demonstrates signal averaging of an object that is moving within the acquisition window and the blurring that results.

9.10
Template Matching

Template matching in cardiology is a useful technique in imaging for the purposes of detecting the existence and locations of specific patterns within an image. In addition, it can be used to perform image stabilization (e.g., for cardiac motion) or to optimize signal averaging. The concept of template matching for images is similar to that for one-dimensional signals. A two-dimensional template is shifted though each x and y value of the image. For each position, the intensity values of each pixel of the template are multiplied with those of the image in the corresponding window and then summed. The maximum point of this matched filter output is the location where the alignment is the greatest.

The example shown in Fig. 9.18 demonstrates template matching of the letter "A." The template is aligned with the "A" in the image and moved from left to right in the x direction. The peak of the matched filter output is located at the position where the template and the "A" in the image are completely overlapped.

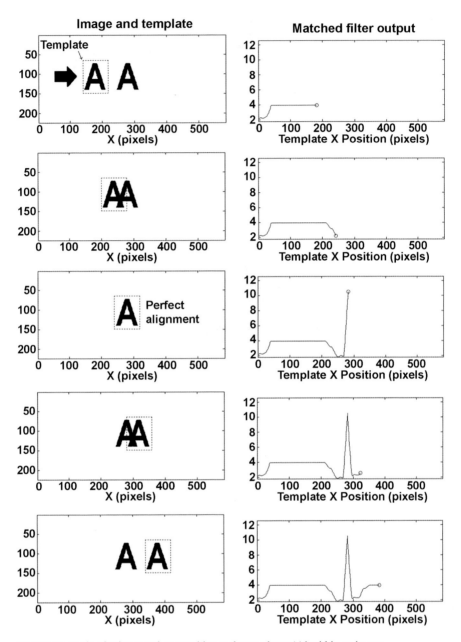

Fig. 9.18 Example of using template matching to detect a letter 'A' within an image

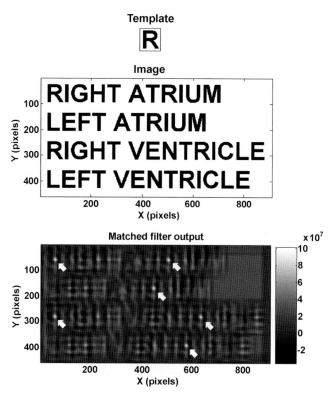

Fig. 9.19 Example of using template matching to detect multiple letter 'R's within an image with many other letters

A more interesting example is shown in Fig. 9.19, in which a template with the letter "R" is applied as a matched filter to an image with the names of the four chambers of the heart. An intensity map of the two-dimensional matched filter output is shown below the image. The brightest spots on the map show the locations of the highest matched filter output (indicated by arrows) and correctly identify the locations of the "R's."

9.11
Edge Detection

In most real-life situations, feature detection using template matching is not possible because there is no prior information of what the desired feature exactly looks like. There may be significant variability in shape and size of the feature that would prevent template matching to catch the feature. Edge detection is another image processing technique that can be used for feature detection. The simplest method of edge detection involves the use of gradients. Gradients are essentially slopes or the quantification of the rate of change in intensity values going from one pixel to another. Unlike the slope obtained by the derivative of a one-dimensional signal, a gradient has both a magnitude and a directional component. Using the magnitude of the gradient, edge detection works in similar fashion to the onset and offset detection using slope threshold criteria for one-dimensional signals as described in Chapter 5.

Figure 9.20 demonstrates edge detection using the same image shown in Fig. 9.1. The bottom left image is the gradient magnitude of the top image. The whiter parts of the gradient images correspond to the areas of the original image during the either transition from black to white or white to black. The darker parts of the gradient image correspond to area with little detectable change in intensity. The lower right image shows results of the edge detection using a gradient threshold of 0.06 to delimit an edge. Edge detection through this process is quite susceptible to noise and therefore the threshold must be carefully chosen. A threshold too low can lead to false detection of edges while a threshold too high will be prone to missed edges.

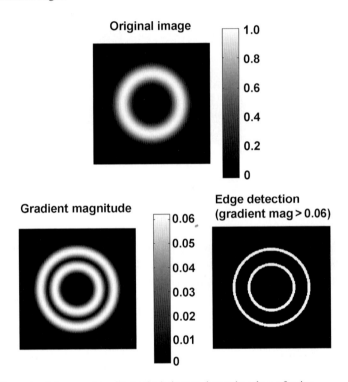

Fig. 9.20 Example of the use of gradient calculations to detect the edges of a ring

9.12
Color Images

Up to this point grayscale images have been used for all the illustrations in this chapter. Color images can provide additional information not possible in grayscale images. In addition, photographic images use color for realistic depiction of what we see visually. A practically ubiquitous way of representing different colors through electronic means is using the red–green–blue (RGB) color model. Televisions, computer monitors, digital cameras, and scanners all utilize the RGB color model. This model is capable of representing a majority of colors visible to the human eye by displaying a combination of different intensity levels of red, green, and blue. Whereas grayscale images provide three-dimensional data, RGB images can be considered four-dimensional data. Figure 9.21 shows how certain colors can be broken up into RGB components. The intensity components are scaled from 0 to 100%, where 100% represents pure red, green, or blue and 0% represents black.

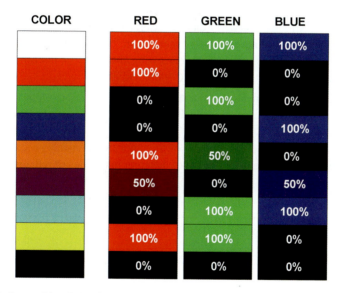

Fig. 9.21 Red-green-blue (RGB) breakdown of nine different colors

Summary of Key Terms

- Image – Two-dimensional representation of three-dimensional data with the third dimension expressed as intensity or color.
- Pixel – One sample point of a two-dimensional digital image.
- Sampling (spatial) – Acquisition of intensity or color information at equally (or non-equally) spaced pixels to achieve a given spatial resolution.
- Nearest neighbor interpolation – A method to resize an image by assigning interpolated pixels with the values of the nearest neighbor.
- Bilinear interpolation – A method to resize an image by assigning interpolated pixels with a weighted sum of the four closest points of the original image. The weights are determined by the distance to each of the four points.
- Bicubic interpolation – A method to resize an image that is similar to bilinear interpolation. Interpolated pixels are assigned with a weighted
- sum of the 16 closest points of the original image.
- Brightness – An image property that defines how visible pixels with low intensity values are against a dark background.
- Contrast – An image property that defines the ease in which objects within an image with similar intensity values can be visually differentiated. Increased contrast is achieved by narrowing the range of intensity values above and below that are considered white and black.
- Edge detection – An image processing operation that attempts to locate boundaries between objects, usually by detecting areas with large local gradients.
- RGB – A color model where most of the color in the visible spectrum can be reproduced from a combination of different intensities of red, green, and blue.

Reference

1. Kim JS. *Two-Dimensional Signal and Image Processing*. Englewood Cliffs, NJ: Prentice-Hall, Inc; 1990.

Part II

Cardiology Applications

Electrocardiography

10

James E. Rosenthal

10.1 Electrical Activity of the Heart: The Action Potential and Its Propagation

The electrocardiogram (ECG) records the electrical activity of the heart by means of electrodes attached to the surface of the skin. Electrical activity in the heart arises from the transmembrane movement of ions between the extracellular compartment and the intracellular space of myocardial cells. The intracellular compartment of resting cardiac cells is electrically negative when compared to the extracellular compartment, with a potential difference of about −90 mV when the cell is at rest. To maintain this potential difference, cells expend energy to "power" the so-called sodium–potassium ATPase pump, which maintains ionic concentration differences between the intracellular compartments such that Na^+ is more concentrated extracellularly and K^+ is more concentrated intracellularly. It also provides the thermodynamic energy for another exchange mechanism that maintains a higher concentration of Ca^{2+} in the extracellular compartment. Channels in the cell membrane that selectively conduct Na^+, K^+, or Ca^{2+} open and close in a systematic, cyclical manner. They are triggered to do so mainly by specific changes in voltage. When the K^+ channels open (as they do when the cell is at rest), K^+ diffuses down its concentration gradient from the intracellular compartment to the extracellular compartment. This carries positive charge out of the cell, leaving the inside (which contains nondiffusible, negatively charged protein moieties) relatively negative compared to the outside. Conversely, since Na^+ and Ca^{2+} are more concentrated outside the cell, they move into the cell when the Na^+ and Ca^{2+} channels open. This carries positive charge into the cell, making the intracellular compartment relatively more positive than the extracellular compartment. Since this process of channels opening and closing is sequential and systematic, it generates a repetitive sequence of voltage changes between the intracellular compartment and the extracellular compartment. The non-resting, relatively positive portion of this repetitive sequence is called that *action potential*. The transmembrane voltages created by the ionic currents can be measured using electrodes with microscopic tips that penetrate the cell membrane and measuring the potential difference between the

J.E. Rosenthal
Department of Medicine, Division of Cardiology, Feinberg School of Medicine,
Northwestern University, Chicago, IL, USA
e-mail: jer@northwestern.edu

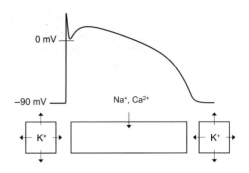

Fig. 10.1 A cardiac action potential. The duration is about 250 ms. The rectangles represent the cell. During diastole, membrane potential of about −90 mV is due to outward movement of potassium, which carries positive charges out of the cell. During systole, the more positive potential is due to inward movement of sodium and calcium carrying positive charges into the cell. The mechanism, as depicted, is highly simplified

intracellular compartment and a reference electrode in the extracellular compartment (Fig. 10.1). The action potential initiates the heartbeat and transports calcium into the heart, which triggers contraction. Propagation of the action potential from one cell to the next and, on a larger scale, from one part of the heart to the other, maintains a sequence of contraction that leads to efficient "milking" of blood from the heart to the aorta.

Automaticity, the property that allows the automatic, spontaneous, cyclical generation of an action potential, leads to the initiation of a heartbeat. Several portions of the heart are automatic and therefore can function as pacemakers. Normally, the predominant pacemaker is the sinus node, located in the right atrium. The rate at which impulses occur is largely dependent upon autonomic input to the sinus node and normally varies from 60 to 100 beats/min., but under conditions such as sleep and exercise can be well below 60 or above 100 beats/min. Other structures with pacemaker properties include the atria, atrioventricular node, and the specialized ventricular conduction system. As the distance from the sinus node of these potential pacemakers increases, the rate at which they "fire" progressively decreases. Thus, before they can reach their threshold for activation, they are depolarized by the wavefront emanating from faster pacemakers. However, when those faster pacemakers such as the sinus node fail, they can initiate an impulse and therefore function as a crucial back-up mechanism that prevents the heart from stopping if the dominant pacemaker fails.

For a normally activated sinus beat, the impulse propagates from the sinus node to the rest of the heart via low-resistance intercellular gap junctions. Propagation normally occurs from the sinus node to the right and left atria as well as to the atrioventricular node. The propagating wavefront is delayed in the atrioventricular (AV) node, typically by about 120–200 ms. This delay allows time for blood in the contracting atria to empty into the ventricles. Conduction then continues into a rapidly conducting specialized ventricular conducting system, which branches and forms electrical connections to the ventricular myocardium, resulting in the initiation of ventricular systole.

10.1.1
Recording of the Heart's Electrical Activity by Electrodes Located on the Surface of the Heart

Since the cardiac activation sequence described above results in sequential activation of cells as the impulse propagates down the conduction system and to myocardium, cells located more distally are still in the resting state, with a transmembrane voltage of about −90 mV, when more proximal cells are already activated and are at a voltage of about 10 mV. This creates potential differences between the resting and activated parts of the heart, resulting in extracellular current flow. Figure 10.2a shows a pair of recording electrodes located directly on the cardiac surface. The electrode on the left, labeled (−), is over a resting cell (intracellularly −) while the exploring electrode on the right, labeled (+), is over a cell that has just been activated (intracellularly +). The exploring electrode records a large potential difference and generates (by convention) a positive deflection. Figure 10.2b shows the same situation, but now the pair of electrodes measure the potential difference between two sites, one of which is activated a bit earlier (labeled endocardium) than the other (labeled epicardium). Note that the difference tracing between the two recordings generates a waveform, shown just above the two action potentials, that represents the ventricular portions (QRS complex, ST segment, and T-wave) of the ECG. Since the ECG is generated because of potential differences between action potentials that are registered at slightly different times, its shape is close to the first derivative of the action potential. In contrast to other biological tissues, cardiac cells have a plateau phase during which the action potential remains at about 0–10 mV. During the plateau phase, there is no potential difference between the two cells, and the ECG recording therefore registers 0 mV. This phase of the ECG is called the ST segment. At the end of the plateau, the membrane potential returns to its resting value of about −90 mV, called repolarization. Typically, the first cells to be activated in the endocardium are the last cells to repolarize. A similar sequence of events in the atria generates a deflection that represents atrial depolarization. This deflection, called the P wave, is of lower amplitude than the QRS complex and immediately precedes it. The delay between atrial and ventricular depolarization, described above, can be determined on the ECG by measuring the time between the onset of the P wave and QRS complexes, called the PR interval.

Perturbations by cardiac abnormalities in the sequence of activation or the morphology of action potentials alter the voltage relationship between the cells being recorded and therefore alter the shape of the ECG waveform. These alterations form the basis for the clinical use of the ECG to recognize disease.

Single cells or small groups of cells (such as the sinus node or the AV node) do not create sufficient current density to allow registration by pairs of extracellular electrodes. In reality, the recorded activity represents the ensemble currents of groups of cells beneath the electrodes.

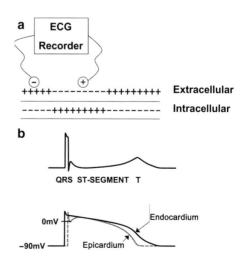

Fig. 10.2 (a) An electrocardiogram (ECG) records the potential difference between the activated (intracellularly +) and resting portion (intracellularly −) of a fiber resulting in an upward deflection beneath the electrode on the right modified from Noble D. The initiation of the heartbeat, Oxford: Oxford University Press;1979. (b) The ECG is the potential difference between two action potentials, one from the endocardium and one from the endocardium (modified from Fozzard and DasGupta[28]). The endocardial action potential occurs slightly before epicardial action potential but repolarizes earlier

10.1.2
Recording of the Heart's Electrical Activity by Electrodes on the Surface of the Skin

The conduction of the extracellular current flow generated by cardiac electrical activity to the surface of the body, where it is recorded by ECG electrodes, is complex. It has been modeled as the movement of pairs of positive and negative electrical charges, called dipoles, that arise from boundaries between positively and negatively charged areas of the heart (i.e., from the boundaries between resting and activated cells) and "travel" to the recording electrodes on the skin. They have a magnitude that depends on the voltage difference at the boundary and a direction. Thus, they can be represented as a vector that is recorded by the surface electrode.[1] Models using single and multiple dipoles have been used, as have models based on *solid angle theory* in which an infinite number of dipoles arise from the boundary at the edge of an area at a different voltage (e.g., during activation).[2] None of these models has been entirely satisfactory because of the complexity of conduction from the heart to the surface; the electrical activity arises from irregular and complexly shaped boundaries in an irregularly shaped heart that is located in a variable and asymmetrical position in the chest. The activity must then be conducted from the heart to the skin surface through irregularly shaped organs and tissues of varying resistances (e.g., air-filled lungs vs. solid organs vs. bone) and across the boundaries between them. In addition, conductivity changes with factors such as body temperature, alterations in volume, and changes in electrolyte concentration. For that reason, modeling conduction from the heart to the surface has been challenging. Though theoretically possible, the solution to the *inverse problem*…that is, reconstructing the heart's electrical activity from the surface ECG…remains elusive despite attempts to devise and test algorithms to do this.[3]

10.2
How is the ECG Organized?

Since the propagating wavefront that is initiated in the sinus node (or in the case of abnormal rhythms, at an abnormal site of impulse formation) "travels" to the ventricles and depolarizes them in a specific sequence, it has a constantly changing direction and amplitude. For ventricular activation, the sequence of depolarization is shown in Fig. 10.3.

The instantaneous direction of the wavefront as it activates the ventricle is shown as the arrows in the figure, as is the resulting QRS complex as viewed from the position of electrodes over the right and left ventricles. The individual arrows have both direction and amplitude and can be arranged on a circle as *vectors*. Initial activation occurs on the left side of the septum and depolarizes the septum from left to right (vectors 1 and 2 in Fig. 10.3). These vectors are directed toward external electrodes labeled V1 and V2 and therefore generate an upward deflection in those leads. They are moving away from V5,6 and therefore generate a downward deflection in those leads. Activation of the massive left ventricular free wall (vectors 3,4,5) generates forces toward V5,6, producing a large upward deflection, and away from V1,2, generating a large downward deflection. Activation of the right ventricular free wall is not shown in the figure. While it occurs simultaneously with that of the left ventricular free wall, it contributes relatively little to the QRS complex because of cancelation by the larger activation forces in the much more massive left ventricular free wall.

10 Electrocardiography

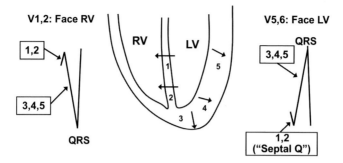

Fig. 10.3 Numbered arrows represent vectors for the activation of the ventricle and the resulting QRS waveform for exploring electrodes V1,2, facing the right ventricle (RV) and V5,6, facing the left ventricle (LV). Numbers on the QRS correspond to the vectors

The average of all of the vectors is called the axis and is a clinically useful component of ECG analysis. Axis is typically calculated for the P, QRS, and T-wave but can be calculated for any portion of the ECG waveform. In order to determine the vectors and axis, the ECG must be recorded from several points (referred to as *leads*) on a sphere surrounding the heart. Varying formats and varying numbers of leads have been used to do this. The following description applies to the most commonly used format, typically referred to as the standard ECG (note that other formats are used for different purposes such as Holter monitoring, exercise testing, and vectorcardiography). Six leads are recorded from electrodes attached to the left and right arms and the left leg, recording the so-called frontal plane. Six additional leads are recorded by placing electrodes on the chest wall, recording the horizontal plane. The arm electrodes, I, II, and III, record the potential difference between the arms and between the arms and the left leg as shown in Fig. 10.4 that shows which of the limbs is positive in relation to the other. Leads I, II, and III can be viewed as representing the limbs of an equilateral triangle that "view" the heart's electrical activity along the directions shown in Fig. 10.4.

Representing the limb leads as the sides of an equilateral triangle is arbitrary but allows clinically useful information to be calculated and deduced regarding the sequence of depolarization of the heart. It has stood the test of over a century of use.

The three leads represent a closed electrical system. The sum of the potential differences in a closed system is 0 (Kirchoff's law). Therefore, II = I + III, an equation described a century ago by Einthoven. Note that the sequence of terms in this equation is based on the arbitrary assignment of positive and negative poles: e.g., if lead II were made positive at the right arm, the equation would become I + II + III = 0). Because of this relationship, recording any two of these leads provides enough information to mathematically derive the waveform in the third lead.

The leg and two arm electrodes can be connected together through resistors to form a single, new terminal. This terminal was described by Frank Wilson in 1934 and has been called the Wilson Central Terminal (WCT). It is described by the following equation:

$$WCT = (LA + RA + LL)/3,$$

where LA = left arm, RA = right arm, and LL = left leg.

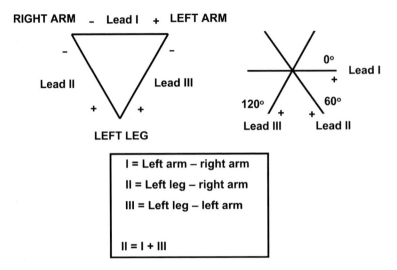

Fig. 10.4 Electrodes attached to the arms and legs, as shown, form leads that are superimposed on a circle. The positive end of each lead is shown

It is convenient (though not entirely accurate) to think of the WCT as having, by Kirchoff's law, a potential of 0. In reality, the potential may not be precisely at 0, but it varies negligibly over time and therefore provides an electrical reference terminal (cathode) that can be used to obtain the potential difference between it and any other exploring electrode (anode).[4] By using this terminal, the following three additional limb leads that have been called VR, VL, and VF can be recorded:

$$VR = RA - WCT.$$

$$VL = LA - WCT.$$

$$VF = LL - WCT.$$

These leads generate complexes that are of very small amplitude. This is not surprising, since the term for the WCT subtracts a portion of the voltage for the limb being explored (e.g., per the equations, for VR, 1/3 of the voltage for RA is subtracted). Therefore, VR, VL, and VF are no longer used. Rather, the equation for the circuit is modified by omitting in the WCT term the lead for the limb being explored, creating the so-called *augmented limb leads*, aVR, aVL, and aVF. This technique was described in 1942 by Emmanuel Goldberger[5] and the formula for the leads is

$$aVR = RA - (LA + LL) / 2.$$

$$aVL = LA - (RA + LL) / 2.$$

$$aVF = LL - (RA + LA) / 2.$$

The augmented limb leads may be thought of as viewing the heart from a second set of three reference points that are skewed 30° from the equilateral triangle that is formed by leads I, II, and III. The axes of this triangle can be superimposed on a circle to form what is known as the hexaxial reference diagram (Fig. 10.5).

By substituting and rearranging the terms for the six frontal plane leads, it can be shown that all of their information can be derived from any two of the leads I, II, III. Modern ECG machines record electrical activity from two limb leads and derive the other leads mathematically. Formats that do not contain this redundancy have been devised. However, the redundancy presents the information in a way that makes human interpretation much more convenient and therefore, the format has been retained.

In addition to the frontal plane leads, six additional leads are recorded in the horizontal plane. To obtain these leads, an exploring electrode, V_x, is compared to the WCT as follows:

$$V_X = V_X - WCT.$$

The exploring electrodes are applied at specific positions on the chest to form the pattern shown in Fig. 10.6.

Thus, a standard ECG consists of 12 leads, of which 8 (the precordial leads and two of the limb leads) provide independent information.

10.2.1
Required Accuracy and Precision

From the first recording of a human ECG by Waller in 1887 and the development of the first practical ECG recording device, the string galvanometer, by Einthoven in 1902 (an achievement for which he won the Nobel Prize), ECGs were analog recordings. Starting in the 1970s, digital processing was introduced and, while some small, portable ECG recorders still make analog recordings, the majority of ECGs obtained today are digitally

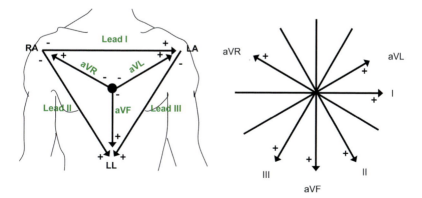

Fig. 10.5 The hexaxial reference diagram is obtained by superimposing the six limb leads (modified from Boron and Boulpaep[29])

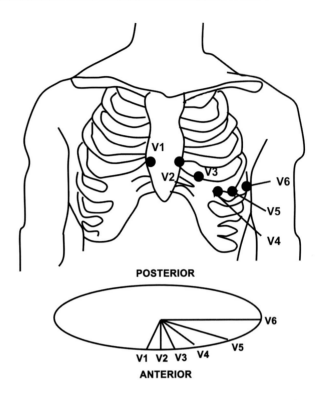

Fig. 10.6 The position of the precordial leads (modified from Thaler[30]).

processed. Fidelity in an ECG refers to how well it reproduces the heart's electrical activity as projected to the skin surface. Fidelity of a digitally processed ECG refers to the ability of the recording to faithfully reproduce the analog signal.[6] The required fidelity varies depending on whether the tracing is intended for interpretation by a human, digital interpretation by a computer, storage or transmission over a data network, with the greatest fidelity being required for computerized interpretation. Several criteria have been published for each of these purposes, and allowable distortion is often expressed as a percentage or microvolt error of the absolute or root mean square signal. Required fidelity for visual interpretation, for example, as quoted from the American Heart Association recommendations of 1990, is that the "deviation of recorded output from an exact linear representation of the input signal may not exceed 25 µV or 5%, whichever is greater."[6] Five criteria that are more stringent are listed for computerized interpretation and for digital transmission and storage in these recommendations.

10.3
High-Pass (Low-Frequency) Filtering of the Analog Signal

Since heart rates are generally not expected to be <30 beats/min, the lowest frequency event on an ECG is 0.5 Hz.[6] Fourier analysis of the ECG waveform (see Chap. 3) has shown that other ECG components have most of their energies in the 1.0 Hz range for the T-wave and up to 30 Hz for the QRS complex. Thus, most of the energy resides below 30 Hz[7] and high-pass filtering at 0.5 Hz should record all information contained in the ECG. However, high-pass filtering at 0.5 Hz leads to distortion of low-frequency components of the ECG such as the ST segment and T-wave.[8] This occurs because the degree of amplification of different frequency components of the ECG signal may vary because the response is not linear. This situation is analogous to a nonlinear music amplifier that distorts the music by, for example, emphasizing the high frequencies and muffling the bass, a situation that anyone who has adjusted the base or treble controls on a stereo system has experienced. The nonlinearity often occurs at the extremes of the frequency range and therefore affects lower frequency events such as the ST segment and the T-wave. Thus, as shown in Fig. 10.7 the current standard for analog recording calls for low-frequency filtering with a cutoff of 0.05 Hz, with a constant degree of amplification between 0.14 and 50 Hz, which incorporates the frequency range of the ECG. No more than a 30% decrease in gain is allowed at the extremes of the range.[9]

10.4
High-Pass (Low-Frequency) Filtering in Digital Systems

Filtering at 0.05 Hz, while minimizing distortion of the ECG, allows distortion of the tracing by very low-frequency signals that have a frequency of >0.05 Hz. These signals arise from events such as respiration and slowly changing voltage due to changes in resistance and capacitance at the interface between the electrolyte solution in the ECG electrode and the subject's skin. The latter change can be decreased by careful skin preparation and sometimes by simply waiting a few minutes until the electrode to skin interface reaches steady state. These sources of noise could be eliminated by choosing a higher cutoff, but that would result in distortion of

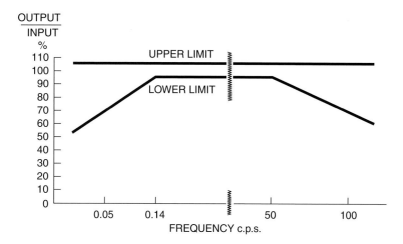

Fig. 10.7 The fidelity of the output of a direct-writing ECG machine must be between the solid lines. The ordinate shows the ratio between the input (i.e., the "true" ECG) and the output (the printed ECG) (copied with permission from Kossmann et al[9])

components of the ECG even though those components' fundamental frequencies are above the cutoff. This occurs because of another source of distortion related to high-pass filtering; electrical signals passing through a recorder are slightly delayed. This delay may vary slightly for different frequencies and may distort the ECG waveform by shifting the phase of the sine waves being recorded (see Chap. 4). It has been shown experimentally that such phase distortion may result in artifactual shifts of the ECG recording, particularly of the ST segment and may result in ST elevation that may lead to false diagnoses of myocardial injury.[7] Modern digital ECG recording systems are not dependent upon the use of electronic filters as were analog recorders. Rather, filtering can be accomplished using microprocessors. Software has been developed that uses various ways of compensating for the phase shift, for example, by filtering acquired data a second time in reverse time.[6] Other techniques, beyond the scope of this discussion, are used as well, often in combination with one another.[10] These techniques allow high-pass filtering at higher frequencies, eliminating baseline wander while faithfully preserving the content of the ECG. As a result, the standard for the low-frequency limit has been increased from 0.05 Hz, as was required for analog ECGs, to 0.67 Hz.[6]

10.5
Low Pass (High Frequency) Filtering

As noted above, *most* of the energy of the ECG resides below 30 Hz. Therefore, low pass filtering at as low as 40 Hz, eliminating or attenuating frequencies higher than that, should be adequate and should eliminate unwanted signals above the cutoff frequency, including 50 or 60 cycle artifact, muscle tremor, artifact from poor electrode contact, or electrode motion. However, the ECG contains frequencies above 30 Hz, particularly at the peaks of the Q, R, and S waves. Thus, filtering at a relatively low frequency can attenuate those signals. This may decrease the amplitude of the QRS complex, diminish or abolish Q-waves, and abolish clinically important notches in the QRS waveform. Thus, the standard for the high-frequency cutoff for analog and printed ECGs has been 100 Hz (leading to the "traditional" frequency range of 0.05–100 Hz). Since the ECG contains information at frequencies of even >100 Hz this cutoff leads to diminution of very high-frequency components of the ECG (such as small Q-waves, the peak of the R-wave, waveforms in the ECGs of infants and pacemaker artifacts) and can lead to an error in waveform amplitude of 25 μV (0.25 mm on a standard ECG recording). A 0.25 mm error is not likely to affect a visual interpretation of an ECG but may affect a computer-generated interpretation. Therefore, modern digital ECG recorders employ higher frequency cutoffs, typically 150 Hz.[6,11]

10.6
Common Mode Rejection

As described earlier in this chapter, the ECG records a wavefront whose instantaneous direction, represented by vectors, changes as it propagates through the heart. Hence, at each instant of the ECG, the vector is preferentially directed toward one of the leads in the horizontal and frontal planes. Voltages that are recorded *equally* by all of the ECG-recording electrodes are unlikely to represent the biological ECG signal. Such voltages typically arise from electrical equipment in the room and are usually much larger than the low-amplitude ECG signal. Traditionally, an ECG amplifier compares the signal between the recording electrodes and a reference electrode located on the right leg. If a signal appears at the same amplitude at each site, it is rejected. However, this traditional system rarely works perfectly, particularly for the interference produced by AC line current, which in the USA has a frequency of 60 Hz, so other strategies are used as well. For example, since common mode signals, particularly 60 Hz interference, are also picked up by the loops of wire that connect the recording electrodes to the device, most digital ECG recorders perform analog to digital conversion in a small module that is not within the ECG recorder but in a small box that is very close to the patient, thereby minimizing lead loops. In addition, filters are used to remove any remaining 60 Hz interference. In countries with power grids that use different frequencies (usually 50 Hz), machines typically can be programmed so that they filter power line interference at the correct frequency or, for some models, can automatically determine the line frequency.[12]

10.7
Analog to Digital Conversion

According to the Nyquist theorem (see Chap. 2), digital sampling must occur at a rate that is at least twice the frequency of the highest frequency component contained in the signal to prevent distortion. To preserve the higher frequency components of the ECG mentioned in the preceding paragraph, a sampling rate of at least 500 Hz, five times the traditional 100 Hz high-frequency cutoff, has been recommended, with yet a higher sampling rate of 834 Hz for ECGs from infants. Barr and Spach[13] showed, in an elegant series of experiments, that sampling at lower rates results in substantial deterioration in waveform quality. Figure 10.8 shows an example from their experiments from a subject with an anterior infarct. The sampling rate is shown on the left. Note that at 500 Hz, the tracing is faithful to the original. At lower sampling rates, the Q-wave and notches on the QRS complex, both of which are potentially clinically important, are abolished.

The current American Heart Association standard calls for a 500 Hz sampling rate, but allows lower rates if other hardware and software characteristics of the recorder allow it to meet criteria for fidelity.[6] Under some circumstances, manufacturers use a sampling rate even higher than 500 Hz: nonbiological signals such as pacemaker artifacts have a much higher frequency content than the biological signals that constitute the ECG. In early models of digital ECG recorders, pacemaker artifacts were highly distorted and often varied in shape from beat to beat because the sampling frequency was lower than that of the artifact. Thus, a pacemaker artifact with a biphasic waveform might be sampled either during its positive or negative phase, resulting in the variability in waveform. To overcome this, some modern ECG systems use a very high sampling rate of up to 15,000 Hz (which is called oversampling), although the programs that interpret the tracings often do so using signals at the standard 500 Hz.[12,14] As predicted by the Nyquist theorem, other

Fig. 10.8 The top tracing is an analog recording from a patient with an anterior MI. Tracings below are recorded at the sampling rate (samples/sec) indicated on left. Numbers on the right show the mean error (%) (copied with permission from Barr and Spach[13])

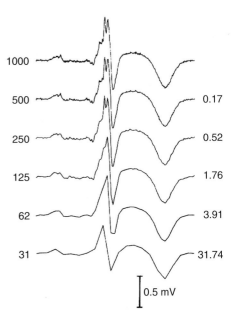

high-frequency signals, such as the peak of the QRS complex and pediatric ECG waveforms are more likely to be distorted than lower-frequency signals, such as P and T-waves, PR and T-P segments. This allows manufacturers to use variable sampling rates, oversampling for high-frequency components, and sampling at lower frequencies, sometimes <500 Hz, for low-frequency components of the waveform. These techniques preserve the fidelity of the ECG while creating smaller files.

10.8
Formation of a Template for ECG Analysis: Signal Averaging

Signal preparation by filtering and common mode rejection removes much of the noise that hampers ECG interpretation. However, factors such as patient movement, respiration, and interference from ambient electrical sources often result in residual noise that is not removed by these processes. To provide an ECG waveform that is suitable for computerized interpretation, a representation of the dominant waveform in each lead that is as free of such noise as possible must be created. This additional reduction in noise and in beat-to-beat variability is achieved by means of signal averaging (see Chap. 7), in which the average value at each data point in a time-aligned ECG waveform is used to create a template for each lead. Proper alignment of waveforms is, of course, crucial to this process, and identification of at least some portion of the waveform elements (typically the QRS, which is usually the largest and easiest to identify) must first occur. Methods whereby this is done are discussed in the next section. Since the object of creating a template of a single lead is, in part, to eliminate noise that could lead to misdiagnosis by the algorithm, some systems use the median waveform rather than the average waveform to create the template. Median waveforms are more effective than mean waveforms in eliminating large outlying values (such as noise) in an otherwise uniform waveform (like the ECG). The reason for this is illustrated in Figs. 7.9 and 7.10 in Chap. 7. Using the average or median beat has been shown to create more uniformity in interpretation, though noise may create errors in amplitude measurement, identification of fiduciary points (and therefore in waveform alignment), and of QRS labeling.[15] These errors are proportional to the amount of noise[16] and might be minimized if common standards for these measurements and for measuring and compensating for noise were adopted by manufacturers.[15,17]

Many computerized algorithms make their measurements of ECG intervals from a template that is created by superimposing waveforms from several or all leads. This method eliminates the possibility of inaccurate measurements due to isoelectric portions of the waveform. For example, if the vector representing the onset of atrial activation is perpendicular to lead II, the beginning of the P-wave in that lead will be indistinguishable from the preceding isoelectric T-P interval. The measurement of the PR interval by a human reader or an algorithm using just lead II will, therefore, be underestimated. Alternatively, a falsely long PR interval (and a falsely short QRS duration) measurement will occur if the lead being measured has a QRS complex that begins with an isoelectric segment. By measuring intervals on a template that represents an ensemble of all leads, electronic algorithms improve accuracy by eliminating errors due to segments that are isoelectric in any single lead.

10.9
Formation of a Template for ECG Analysis: Identification of Fiducial Points

Determination of the onset and offset of P, QRS, T, and U waves is crucial in order to measure standard ECG intervals and to create rational diagnostic statements. Several methods for doing this are used by manufacturers, including assessment of amplitude thresholds, changes in slope, and template matching. These techniques may be used alone but are often used in combination with one another. These techniques as well as their advantages and disadvantages are discussed in Chap. 5. Some algorithms initially identify the QRS in order to superimpose waveforms for signal averaging and then use the clean, signal-averaged global ECG to identify the other fiduciary points such as P and T wave onset and offset to avoid errors caused by an isoelectric initiation or termination of a waveform in any single lead, as discussed above. Initial QRS identification may be done by highly filtering the global QRS to eliminate low- and high-frequency "distractors" and assessing when the amplitude of this filtered signal exceeds a voltage threshold. The process of waveform detection by amplitude is illustrated in Chap. 5, Fig. 5.2. The voltage threshold may be increased briefly (full or partial blanking) after detection of a QRS to avoid detecting the T-wave and misidentifying it as a QRS complex. Further refinement is achieved by creating a template of the detected QRS waveform in each lead and comparing it with other waveforms in order to identify statistical matches. New templates are formed when the voltage threshold is met but the shape of the beat does not match that of the template of the initial waveform. These waveforms are grouped by shape and are also used for waveform matching. The template matching technique is illustrated in Chap. 5, Figs. 5.9–5.10. Using this process, the predominant QRS as well as other QRS shapes are identified and, pending further analysis, are classified as the predominant beat (usually sinus) or as non-sinus beats. Once the QRS has been identified, signal averaging is performed using either mean or medians and a global QRS is created. The global QRS is then used to identify the P, QRS, and T-wave onsets and offsets for interval measurement and further waveform analysis. This is typically done by obtaining the first derivative of the waveform to search for changes in slope as described in Chap. 5, Figs. 5.4–5.7.[12] Identification of waveform features such as the QRS complex also allows the rate to be calculated. Since cardiac rhythms are often irregular (as in sinus arrhythmias, sinus rhythms with ectopic complexes, atrial fibrillation), the rate that is presented in the interpretation typically represents an average obtained by calculating the interval between the first waveform identified as being a QRS and the last, dividing by the total number of intervals and converting the resulting interval to beats per second.

10.10
Computerized Analysis of the ECG

Since the subject of this book is signal processing, detailed discussion of interpretive algorithms is beyond its scope and will be discussed only briefly. Computerized algorithms have been in use since the 1960s and have been extensively refined, revised, and tested over the years as computer technology has improved and as new clinical information has led to revision of ECG criteria. Modern programs analyze data obtained simultaneously from the eight ECG leads that provide independent data (see Sect. 10.2). After fiducial points identifying the onset and offset of P, QRS, and T-waves are generated as described above, individual waves are identified, often by using minimal area criteria (voltage x time) to identify features such as multiple P-wave "humps," Q, R, R', S, S', T, and U waves. Detailed measurements of these waves and features (amplitude, area, deviation compared to fixed points such as the QRS onset) are obtained and used to generate a matrix of features for the computerized analysis.12 Determination of fiducial points, rate determination and wave identification allows basic measurements (PR interval, QRS duration, QT interval) to be made. Typical programs use extensive decision tree analysis in which the feature matrix is queried by a series of true/false tests that result in the generation of diagnostic statements. For example, fulfillment of QRS voltage criteria may result in a diagnostic statement such as *voltage criteria for left ventricular enlargement*, but if additional criteria are met for features such as P-wave abnormalities, widened QRS and repolarization abnormalities, the more definitive statement, *left ventricular hypertrophy* is used, often with a description of the feature (e.g., *left ventricular hypertrophy with QRS widening*).[12] The decision tree is highly complex, since it must test the measurement matrix for multiple possible abnormalities, and many branches of the test interact with other branches (e.g., meeting criteria of one test, for example left bundle branch block, may result in suppression of statements for other tests, such as left ventricular enlargement). Since criteria are age or gender dependent (e.g., voltage criteria for left ventricular enlargement), correct diagnosis is often dependent upon accurate entry of age and gender by the ECG technician. Some programs use statistical methods to incorporate probability statements (possible, probable, etc) to the interpretive statements.

10.11
Reliability of Interpretive Algorithms

Recommendations have been made for a set of standard, well-defined, and minimally ambiguous terminology for diagnostic statements.[18,19] Statements have been categorized into three types: Type A refers to statements defining specific lesions such as myocardial infarction or ventricular enlargement that can be confirmed by objective, non-electrocardiographic criteria. Type B statements refer to anatomic or functional abnormalities such as arrhythmias and conduction abnormalities. Type C statements are neither Types A or B. Type C statements include electrocardiographic features such as axis deviation and nonspecific repolarization abnormalities.19 This categorization and the use of standardized statements are useful in establishing criteria by which the validity of computerized diagnostic statements are evaluated. Type A statements can be validated by using databases that have been established using objective, validated diagnostic criteria while type B and C statements require either intracardiac electrical measurements or, particularly for type C statements, comparison with interpretations by experts. Manufacturers rely on established databases of reference ECGs for the creation of algorithms, which must be validated on different sets of reference ECGs (including technically imperfect and noisy ones) than were used in their creation.[20] Performance metrics such as sensitivities, specificities, positive and negative predictive values have been reported for many of the criteria and are used by manufacturers in assessing and reporting the performance of their algorithms.[12] While these metrics demonstrate that computerized programs perform well, differences between systems may be substantial enough to affect diagnostic conclusions. For example, a difference of up to 8 ms in Q-wave duration measurement was demonstrated in an analysis of the performance of ten ECG analysis programs.[21] While many of these studies are old and may not reflect more recent improvements in interpretive algorithms, they underscore the importance of overreading computer-interpreted tracings by an expert human. Analyses have shown that expert ECG readers often perform better than the programs. In a comparison of eight cardiologists' interpretations of tracings containing common ECG abnormalities with those of nine computer programs, the cardiologists' total accuracy was 6.6% higher than that of the computer programs and the sensitivities for many of the diagnoses was greater when interpreted by cardiologists. Nonetheless, the best programs came close to matching the performance of the cardiologists.[22] Compared to either computerized or physician interpretation alone, the combined use of a computerized algorithm with physician overreading may lead to the greatest accuracy and may cut physician time by up to 28% without increasing the false positive rate.[23,24] This may be true because the computerized ECG minimizes errors by identifying findings that the physician may have overlooked while the physician spots errors in measurements and diagnostic statements by the algorithm. Thus, the physician reader and the computerized system provide a system of checks and balances to one another. Computer-generated interpretations that contain errors may lead to significant mismanagement of patients or to the performance of unnecessary and costly diagnostic testing (e.g., when a preoperative ECG contains an erroneous statement indicating the possibility of an ischemic process). Such errors may also influence the physician overreader to make an incorrect interpretation. In a study in which second and third year internal medicine residents...who are often at the front line of patient care...interpreted tracings both with and without computer-generated interpretations, accuracy dropped when the computer's interpretation was incorrect, suggesting that the reader often agreed with the erroneous statement. Nonetheless, overall accuracy was improved by the presence of the computer interpretation.[25] Thus, current standards call for physician review of all ECGs.[14]

10.12 Potential Artifacts

One of the most common sources of ECG artifact arises from lead misplacement, most commonly when limb leads are interchanged as a result of technician carelessness. Interpretive algorithms are sometimes able to recognize lead switches but interpret the tracings as though leads were applied correctly. Lead switches can lead to major errors in interpretative statements, including spurious identification of myocardial infarction. Figure 10.9a shows an example in which the left arm and left leg electrodes were reversed. This resulted in Q-waves in leads I and aVL that suggested a high lateral wall myocardial infarction when in fact, the patient was having an acute inferior MI as shown, in Fig. 10.9b, in which leads were applied correctly. With a firm knowledge of the relationship between leads, as discussed earlier in this chapter (see Sect. 10.2), astute ECG readers can often recognize and correct for lead switches using the relabeled leads to accurately interpret the tracing.

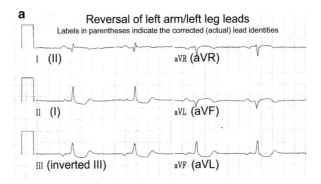

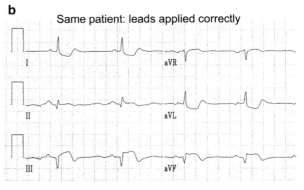

Fig. 10.9 (**a**) Left arm and left leg leads have been reversed. The lead designations in parentheses indicate the true lead identities. Failure to recognize the lead reversal might lead to an erroneous diagnosis of high lateral wall myocardial infarction because of the apparent Q-waves in the lead I and aVL positions (which are really II and aVF, respectively). (**b**) With correct placement of leads, the ECG shows an inferior wall myocardial infarction, probably recent

With the use of modern ECG electrodes and machines, artifacts resulting from poor electrode–skin interface or due to hardware component problems have become less frequent but are not uncommon. They may arise due to technical errors such as poor skin preparation, patient movement or tremor, and interference from other electrical devices. The latter may result in so-called 50 or 60-cycle noise. As noted previously, techniques to reduce noise include common mode rejection, which eliminates environmental sources of noise that appear simultaneously on more than one recording electrode. Visual displays of the ECG signal prior to its recording provide the technician the opportunity to evaluate the signal and make appropriate adjustments. However, external sources of noise may still appear. ECG artifact can be mistaken for pathological events, including ventricular tachycardia, a problem that arises both with human readers and with electronic interpretation algorithms. Usually, though, skillful readers can distinguish artifact from arrhythmias. An example of artifact, recorded with ECG telemetry, that mimics ventricular tachycardia can be seen in Chap. 18, Fig. 18.5.

10.13
Data Storage and Compression

Computerized ECG technology provides a means for long-term electronic data storage, making the large banks of filing cabinets and the attendant filing clerks that once were a hallmark of ECG departments a thing of the past. As with electronic storage of all medical records, this has eliminated the once all too common problem of lost and misfiled ECGs and has resulted in cost saving. ECGs stored on small, portable recording devices can be transmitted electronically from the clinic to the ECG server and from the server to remote sites, allowing centralized overreading by expert cardiologists of tracings obtained at satellite clinics or in the field. Stored records are used by the interpretive algorithms to generate comparison statements.

Current standards call for transmitted ECGs and ECGs retrieved from electronic storage to conform to within 10 μV of the original tracing[6,14] but the goal of data compression is to produce a "lossless" ECG, in which the tracing, when uncompressed, looks identical to the original. This could be achieved by storing all of the original data for each tracing but that has been impractical because it requires a large amount of memory since single institutions may record hundreds of ECGs daily. While the cost and physical size of storage has been decreasing, manufacturers have used data compression to improve the efficiency of storage and to speed transmission of ECG data. Greater compression of the original data has the benefit of decreasing the size of files for transmission and storage but increases the likelihood that retrieved, reconstructed ECGs will differ from the original. Data compression is feasible because an ECG contains a great deal of redundant information. In a subject with a normal, regular rhythm, waveform components such as P, QRS, T-waves, and their connectors look more or less the same for each beat on the tracing. Exceptions to this redundancy occur in pathological situations such as arrhythmias. Compression algorithms exploit this redundancy by using various techniques that allow storage of only a basic waveform, either directly or as a representation of its component sine waves, and information to indicated statistical deviations from the basic waveform. Dozens of algorithms for doing this have been described. In general, they utilize direct data compression, in which redundant and nonredundant information is obtained by analyzing the ECG signal, or transformation compression in which the spectral and energy characteristics of the signal are analyzed to find the redundancies. Direct methods use techniques such as statistically comparing a waveform sample with future samples. For example, if the preset error threshold of a sample in a waveform at point A is not exceeded until point B occurring 400 ms later, it can be assumed that points A and B are connected by a line, which can be interpolated between the two points to reconstruct the waveform. Lower preset error thresholds result in higher fidelity of the reconstructed waveform but in less compression and larger files. Some compression algorithms store data describing waveform characteristics such as their slopes, amplitudes, and inflection points. An inverse method to the compression algorithm is used to reconstruct the original ECG waveform. Details of the compression algorithms are highly mathematical. The interested reader is referred to the review of this topic by Jalaleddine.[26]

Following analog to digital conversion at 500 samples per second (see Sect. 10.7), a 10 s ECG containing information for the eight recorded leads requires about 80 kB of memory plus memory for associated data such as demographic and clinical information, matrices for interpretation, and the edited interpretation.[14] Applying compression algorithms to the same ECG can result in a file size of about 4.5 kB (depending on the compression algorithm used) vs. the 80 kB for the original data.[27] Authors of algorithms for data compression have presented data showing that compression and decompression can be achieved with very high levels of fidelity to the original tracings. For example, compression ratios (ratio of original file size to compressed file) of 24:1 have been achieved with very low levels of distortion.

References

1. Bayes de Luna AJ. *Textbook of Clinical Electrocardiography*. Dordrecht: Martinus Nijhoff; 1987.
2. Holland RP, Arnsdorf MF. Solid angle theory and the electrocardiogram: physiologic and quantitative interpretations. *Prog Cardiovasc Dis*. 1977;19(6):431–457.
3. Cheng LK, Bodley JM, Pullan AJ. Effects of experimental and modeling errors on electrocardiographic inverse formulations. *IEEE Trans Biomed Eng*. 2003;50(1):23–32.
4. Wilson FN, Johnston FD, Macleod AG, Barker PS. Electrocardiograms that represent the potential variations of a single electrode. *Am Heart J*. 1934;9(4):447–458.
5. Goldberger E. A simple, indifferent, electrocardiographic electrode of zero potential and a technique of obtaining augmented, unipolar, extremity leads. *Am Heart J*. 1942;23(4):483–492.
6. Bailey JJ, Berson AS, Garson A Jr, et al. Recommendations for standardization and specifications in automated electrocardiography: bandwidth and digital signal processing. A report for health professionals by an ad hoc writing group of the Committee on Electrocardiography and Cardiac Electrophysiology of the Council on Clinical Cardiology, American Heart Association. *Circulation*. 1990;81(2):730–739.
7. Tayler DI, Vincent R. Artefactual ST segment abnormalities due to electrocardiograph design. *Br Heart J*. 1985;54:121–128.
8. Berson AS, Pipberger HV. The low-frequency response of electrocardiographs, a frequent source of recording errors. *Am Heart J*. 1966;71(6):779–789.
9. Kossmann CE, Brody DA, Burch GE, et al. Recommendations for Standardization of Leads and of Specifications for Instruments in Electrocardiography and Vectorcardiography. *Circulation*. 1967;35(3):583–602.

10. Ahlstrom ML, Tompkins WJ. Digital filters for real-time ECG signal processing using microprocessors. *IEEE Trans Biomed Eng.* 1985;32(9):708–713.
11. Golden DP, Wolthuis RA, Hoffler GW. A spectral analysis of the normal resting electrocardiogram. *IEEE Trans Biomed Eng.* 1973;20(5):366–372.
12. GE Healthcare (2003–2006). *Marquette™ 12SL™ ECG Analysis Program: Physician's Guide; Revision D (2003–2006).* General Electric Company.
13. Barr RC, Spach MS. Sampling rates required for digital recording of intracellular and extracellular cardiac potentials. *Circulation.* 1977;55(1):40–48.
14. Kligfield P, Gettes LS, Bailey JJ, et al. Recommendations for the standardization and interpretation of the electrocardiogram: Part I: The Electrocardiogram and Its Technology: A Scientific Statement From the American Heart Association Electrocardiography and Arrhythmias Committee, Council on Clinical Cardiology; the American College of Cardiology Foundation; and the Heart Rhythm Society Endorsed by the International Society for Computerized Electrocardiology. *Circulation.* 2007;115(10):1306–1324.
15. Zywietz C, Willems JL, Arnaud P, et al.; The CSE Working Party. Stability of computer ECG amplitude measurements in the presence of noise. *Comput Biomed Res.* 1990;23(1):10–31.
16. Farrell RM, Rowlandson GI. The effects of noise on computerized electrocardiogram measurements. *J Electrocardiol.* 2006;39(4 suppl):S165–S173.
17. Willems JL, Zywietz C, Arnaud P, et al. Influence of noise on wave boundary recognition by ECG measurement programs. Recommendations for preprocessing. *Comput Biomed Res.* 1987;20(6):543–562.
18. Mason JW, Hancock EW, Gettes LS, et al. Recommendations for the Standardization and Interpretation of the Electrocardiogram: Part II: Electrocardiography Diagnostic Statement List: A Scientific Statement From the American Heart Association Electrocardiography and Arrhythmias Committee, Council on Clinical Cardiology; the American College of Cardiology Foundation; and the Heart Rhythm Society: Endorsed by the International Society for Computerized Electrocardiology. *Circulation.* 2007;115(10):1325–1332.
19. Surawicz B, Uhley H, Borun R, et al. Task force I: standardization of terminology and interpretation. *Am J Cardiol.* 1978;41:130–145
20. Willems JL, Arnaud P, van Bemmel JH, et al. A reference data base for multilead electrocardiographic computer measurement programs. *J Am Coll Cardiol.* 1987;10(6):1313–1321.
21. Willems JL, Arnaud P, van Bemmel JH, et al. Assessment of the performance of electrocardiographic computer programs with the use of a reference data base. *Circulation.* 1985;71(3):523–534.
22. Willems JL, Abreu-Lima C, Arnaud P, et al. The diagnostic performance of computer programs for the interpretation of electrocardiograms. *N Engl J Med.* 1991;325(25):1767–1773.
23. Brailer DJ, Kroch E, Pauly MV. The impact of computer-assisted test interpretation on physician decision making: the case of electrocardiograms. *Med Decis Making.* 1997;17(1):80–86.
24. Willems JL, Abreu-Lima C, Arnaud P, et al. Effect of combining electrocardiographic interpretation results on diagnostic accuracy. *Eur Heart J.* 1988;9(12):1348–1355.
25. Tsai TL, Fridsma DB, Gatti G. Computer decision support as a source of interpretation error: the case of electrocardiograms. *J Am Med Inform Assoc.* 2003;10(5):478–483.
26. Jalaleddine SM, Hutchens CG, Strattan RD, Coberly WA. ECG data compression techniques – a unified approach. *IEEE Trans Biomed Eng.* 1990;37(4):329–343.
27. Reddy BR, Christenson DW, Rowlandson GI, Zywietz C, Sheffield T, Brohet C. Data compression for storage of resting ECGs digitized at 500 samples/second. *Biomed Instrum Technol.* 1992;26(2):133–149.
28. Fozzard HA, DasGupta DS. ST-segment potentials and mapping. Theory and experiments. *Circulation.* 1976;54:533–537.
29. Boron WF, Boulpaep EL. *Textbook of Medical Physiology.* Philadelphia, PA: W.B. Saunders Company; 2002.
30. Thaler MS. *The Only EKG Book You'll Ever Need.* Philadelphia, PA: Lippincott Williams & Wilkins; 2003.

Intravascular and Intracardiac Pressure Measurement

11

Clifford R. Greyson

Intravascular pressure measurement is one of the oldest techniques employed in clinical medicine. By 1733, long before accurate external blood pressure measurement had been developed by Korotkoff, Stephen Hales had performed direct measurement of arterial blood pressure by inserting a brass tube into a horse's artery and observing the height of the resulting blood column. By 1828, Poiseuille had improved on intraarterial blood pressure measurement by using a fluid-filled catheter connected to a mercury manometer. In 1848 Ludwig invented the kymograph, a smoke-covered rotating cylinder that provided the means for graphical recording of dynamic signals for many years to come. By connecting the kymograph to a fluid-filled intraarterial catheter, the first graphical representation of the arterial pulse waveform was obtained.[1] Today, intravascular pressure measurement is performed so routinely in intensive care units, operating rooms and catheterization laboratories, that it is easy to forget that numbers and graphical representations of pressure are strongly affected by the measurement system, and indeed, can misrepresent reality. The signal processing techniques commonly used in intravascular and intraventricular pressure measurement are generally quite rudimentary and limited to simple filtering (see Chap. 4), averaging, and peak and trough detection. Less well-appreciated, but equally important, are the alterations in the raw signal introduced by the measurement system itself. In some cases, these artifacts can lead to serious errors in diagnosis. This chapter will provide an overview of how both intended and unintended signal processing affect the appearance and interpretation of data obtained using this nearly universal technique.

"Pressure" is defined as force per unit area. The SI unit for pressure, designated the *Pascal* (abbreviated Pa), is expressed in units of Newtons per square meter (N-m^{-2}). However, intravascular and intracardiac pressures are more commonly expressed in terms of millimeters of mercury (abbreviated mmHg, also known as Torr), largely due to the historical use of mercury manometers for pressure measurement. Occasionally, "centimeters of water" is used as a pressure unit (where 1.34 cm of water is roughly equivalent to 1 mmHg) because it may be directly correlated with bedside physical examination, such as observation of the jugular venous pulses. Since mercury manometers have been almost

---

C.R. Greyson
Denver Department of Veterans Affairs Medical Center, University of Colorado at Denver,
1055 Clermont Street, Denver, CO 80220, USA
e-mail: clifford.greyson@ucdenver.edu

entirely supplanted by mechanical or electrical pressure transducers, it is possible that Pascals will be adopted in the future, but this is not yet common in the medical literature.

In contrast to the smoked drum kymograph system used in the latter part of the nineteenth century and the paper-based pen recording systems used throughout the middle of the twentieth century, nearly all pressure waveform data in the twenty-first century are now acquired and stored digitally. In the clinical arena, the majority of pressure measurements are performed using a fluid-filled (saline or blood) catheter inserted into the vascular space of interest, connected to an external pressure transducer. The transducer (see Chap. 1) consists of a strain gauge connected to a bridge amplifier, which in turn is connected to the analog to digital converter or digitizer. In the research setting, miniaturized pressure transducers (micromanometers) mounted on the ends of catheters may be inserted directly into the vascular spaces of interest. Micromanometer catheters are increasingly employed in the cardiac catheterization lab to measure intracoronary pressures as well. Micromanometer catheters provide extremely high-fidelity measurements and were used to acquire the data in many of the illustrations below. These data will also be used to illustrate limitations to the fluid-filled catheter-based technique.

Pressure measurements are inherently dynamic. For clinical purposes, typical measurements derived from the pressure recording include maximum (usually systolic), minimum (usually diastolic), early diastolic, end-diastolic and mean pressures, and the first derivative of intraventricular pressure with respect to time (dP/dt). It is important to remember that intravascular and intraventricular pressures are normally referenced to atmospheric pressure; moreover, because static hydraulic pressure varies from head to toe (just as water pressure increases toward the bottom of a swimming pool), the measured pressures are generally obtained relative to a standardized position, most commonly the right atrium.

A frequent error in pressure measurement is the failure to zero the transducer with the transducer reference point placed at the level of the right atrium (for a fluid-filled catheter, the opening of a stopcock connected to the transducer is used as the reference point); micromanometer catheters do not require atmospheric zeroing.

For most text-based reporting and routine clinical care, it is rarely necessary to obtain pressure measurements with more precision than a few millimeters of mercury. However, for graphical display of dynamic waveforms, precision of 0.1 mmHg or better is desirable to avoid quantization artifacts (see Chap. 2). Figure 11.1a shows a typical ventricular waveform acquired from the left ventricle of a pig acquired using a high-fidelity micromanometer catheter (discussed further below) displayed with 0.1 mmHg precision. The panel on the left shows the full-scale tracing, while the panel on the right shows an expanded area concentrating on diastolic pressure. Figure 11.1b shows the same data displayed with 1 mmHg rather than 0.1 mmHg precision. Notice that even measurements as course as 1 mmHg precision allow reasonable estimates of left ventricular systolic, diastolic, and end-diastolic pressure, but result in the false (artifactual) appearance of abrupt changes in pressure during diastole due to quantization artifact of the true diastolic pressure waveform.

The sampling rate necessary for accurate representation of pressure waveforms is modest in comparison to sampling rates commonly used for electrical phenomenon. Figure 11.2 shows the power spectrum derived from the discrete Fourier transform (see Chap. 3) of the ventricular waveform shown in Fig. 11.1a. As can be seen for this recording, where the

11 Intravascular and Intracardiac Pressure Measurement

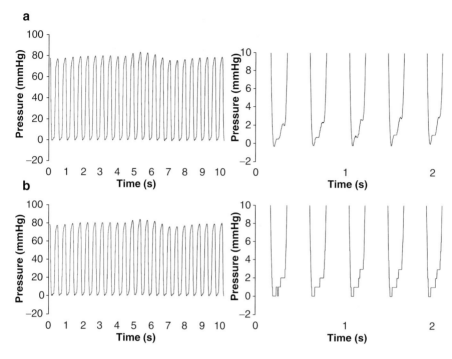

Fig. 11.1 Pressure waveform obtained using a high-fidelity micromanometer catheter from the left ventricle of a pig. (**a**) and (**b**) show the full-scale tracing on the *left* and an amplified tracing on the *right* focusing on diastolic pressures. In (**a**), the data are quantized with 0.1 mmHg precision. In (**b**), the data are quantized with 1 mmHg precision and demonstrate quantization artifact

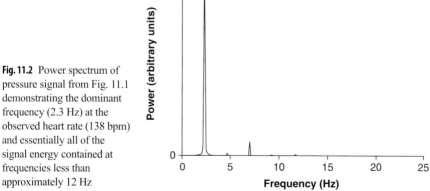

Fig. 11.2 Power spectrum of pressure signal from Fig. 11.1 demonstrating the dominant frequency (2.3 Hz) at the observed heart rate (138 bpm) and essentially all of the signal energy contained at frequencies less than approximately 12 Hz

heart rate was 138 bpm (about 2.3 Hz), the dominant frequency component was at the underlying heart rate, and the dominant harmonics were found below five times the heart rate (about 12 Hz). According to the Nyquist theorem (see Chap. 2), a sampling rate of 24 Hz would theoretically be necessary to reproduce the underlying waveform, consistent with an old rule of thumb that sampling rate for ventricular pressure should be about ten times the heart rate.

On occasion, the first derivative of pressure change with respect to time (dP/dt) is calculated as an index of contractile function. Typical values for dP/dt range from 200 to 500 mmHg/s for right ventricular pressure and 1,000–2,000 mmHg/s for left ventricular pressure. Because taking the derivative of a signal attenuates lower frequency components and amplifies higher frequency components of a signal, a higher sampling rate is necessary to reproduce the signal. For the dP/dt of the signal shown in Fig. 11.1, 99% of the signal is found below 21 Hz, requiring about a 40 Hz sampling rate. Again, this is consistent with the rule of thumb that sampling rates of 20 times the heart rate should be used when dP/dt is to be calculated.

Another way of understanding the sampling rate requirement is to calculate the time for pressure to rise from end-diastole to peak; with a left ventricular dP/dt of 1,500 mmHg/s, it takes less than 100 ms for pressure to rise from minimum to maximum; therefore, to provide a reasonable number of samples over this period of time (5 samples, for example), samples would need to be obtained no less frequently than every 20 ms, i.e., at a rate of 50 Hz.

The data in Fig. 11.1 were originally sampled at 500 Hz. Figures 11.3a–d show the ventricular pressure waveform as it appears when sampled at rates of 50, 20, 10, and 5 Hz. As discussed previously, 50 Hz (Fig. 11.3a) preserves nearly the entire signal. At 20 Hz (Fig. 11.3b), minor distortions are becoming apparent, and at 10 Hz (Fig. 11.3c), severe distortion of the waveform is occurring. At 5 Hz sampling rate (Fig. 11.3d), a sinusoidal oscillation in the recorded pressure appears. This is a result of *aliasing* (see Chap. 2), which occurs when the sampling rate is inadequate to accommodate the main frequency components present in the underlying signal. To accommodate a variety of clinical situations and to reduce the need for filtering, sampling rates of anywhere between 100 and 500 Hz are more commonly used for pressure recording.

With a sampling rate of 100 Hz and 16 bit recordings (sufficient for 0.1 mmHg precision), required data rates are very low (<1 MB/hr per channel) and rarely are a limiting factor in recording system design.

Up to this point, we have discussed the effect of the recording system on the pressure signal. However, the recorded physiologic signal can potentially be altered anywhere along the chain from the vascular space to the data storage system. To understand how the measuring system affects the resulting recorded waveforms, it is important to understand how pressure waveforms are recorded by the clinical pressure measurement system and how those waveforms are propagated and altered within the body.

We begin with the left ventricle of the heart, because this initially produces the energy that results in blood pressure development, propagation of pressure into the arterial system, and oscillating pressure waveforms. Later, we will briefly consider waveforms produced by the right ventricle of the heart, although the underlying issues are nearly identical.

We have already analyzed the frequency content of the intraventricular pressure signal as measured with a micromanometer catheter. Such catheters, sold by manufacturers such

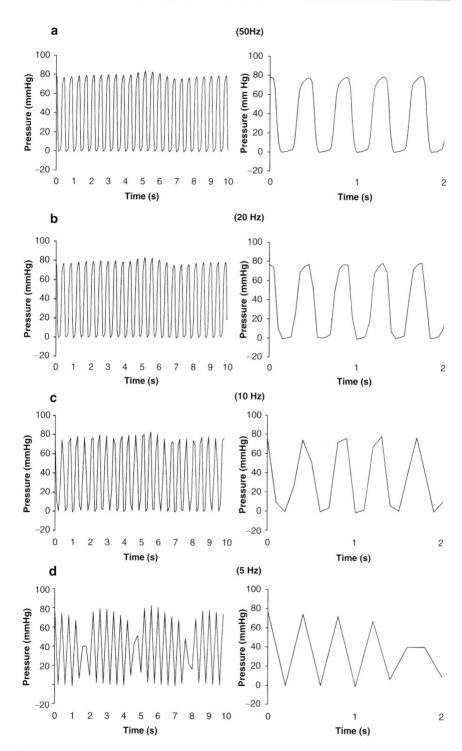

Fig. 11.3 The left ventricular pressure waveform from Fig. 11.1 is shown with sampling rates of 50 Hz (**a**), 20 Hz (**b**), 10 Hz (**c**), and 5 Hz (**d**). Each is shown for a 10 s period and with an expanded time scale of 2 s

as Millar Instruments and Scisense Corporation, consist of a miniaturized pressure transducer mounted on the end of an intravascular catheter. By placing the pressure transducer at the location of the pressure to be measured, distortion of the signal by signal components other than the analog to digital conversion system is entirely eliminated. The frequency response of such pressure transducers is typically flat between DC and 1,000 Hz, permitting high-fidelity measurement of pressure waveforms with extremely high heart rates (such as small rodents which can easily attain 800 bpm).[2] Because frequency response of the micromanometer catheter is so flat, these pressure tracings, if sampled at sufficiently high rates and with sufficient precision, can be considered for all practical purposes to be a perfect reflection of the true intraventricular pressure at the location of the transducer membrane. Nevertheless, potential errors in obtaining the measurement of interest may be introduced by the presence of debris such as protein deposits or clotted blood at the catheter tip that may damp the transmission of pressure from the vascular space to the transducer, by errors in the location of the transducer (such as placing the catheter within a coronary sinus rather than within the ventricle, or in a small arterial side branch rather than within the artery of interest itself), and by abrupt movement of the tip of the catheter such as may occur if the catheter is within a high-velocity jet of blood produced by a stenotic or regurgitant valve. Nevertheless, the pressure measured via the catheter tip is an accurate reflection of the true pressure at the tip's location even in these settings. It is always important to consider what is actually being measured.

In most clinical settings, pressures are measured with a fluid-filled catheter inserted into the vascular space of interest. This catheter is then connected to an external pressure transducer via a length of tubing. The frequency response of the external pressure transducer is also flat over the relevant range; however, the presence of the fluid-filled catheter alters the frequency response in ways that will be made clear shortly. Figure 11.4 shows an intraventricular pressure waveform as measured simultaneously using a micromanometer catheter (Fig. 11.4a) and using a large bore saline-filled catheter inserted directly into the apex of the heart and connected to a standard clinical transducer by a short clinical-grade pressure line (Fig. 11.4b). Notice that the catheter-based pressure measurement demonstrates a

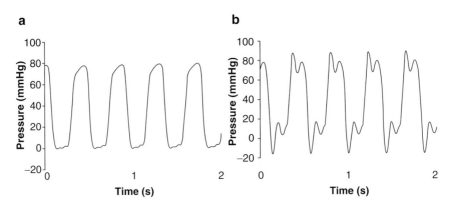

Fig. 11.4 (a) Ventricular pressure measured using a micromanometer catheter. (b) Simultaneous ventricular pressure recording using a short length of pressure tubing

peak just after its initial upstroke and a dip just after its downstroke. The power spectra of the pressure signals in Figs. 11.4a and b are shown in Figs. 11.5a and b, respectively, with magnified views of the dominant components in Fig. 11.5c and d. Notice the increased amplitude of the frequency components in the 6–15 Hz range relative to the amplitude in the 1–5 Hz range in the catheter-based measurement. These artifacts of pressure measurement are a result of resonance and amplification of higher frequency components by the catheter system. This effect is similar to the amplification of a vibrating string produced by a musical stringed instrument's sound box. This artifact is worsened considerably when the short piece of pressure tubing is replaced with a long piece of pressure tubing (Fig. 11.6). Thus the length of the pressure tubing used for the fluid-filled catheter-based technique should be minimized to improve the fidelity of the recordings.

It is possible to calculate the frequency response of the catheter-based system using Fourier analysis as described in Chap. 3 of this book. Using the Fourier transforms of the two signals, the "transfer function" of the catheter system can be determined. By examining the transfer function, which shows the relative amplification or attenuation of each frequency component of the measured signal, the response of the system to different underlying waveforms can be predicted. In particular, waveforms with a greater predominance of

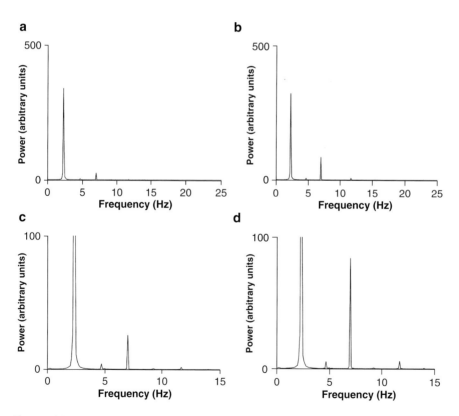

Fig. 11.5 (**a**) Power spectrum of signal shown in Fig. 11.4a. (**b**) Power spectrum of signal shown in Fig. 11.4b. (**c**) Magnified view of (**a**). (**d**) Magnified view of (**b**)

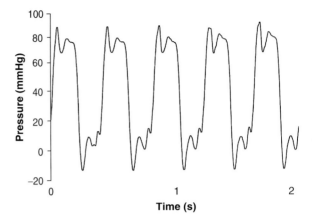

Fig. 11.6 Ventricular pressure measured using a long length of pressure tubing

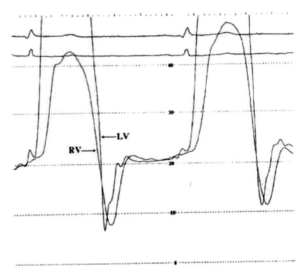

Fig. 11.7 Intraventricular pressure measurement in a patient with constrictive pericarditis

high frequency components will tend to be more distorted than waveforms dominated by lower frequency components because the transfer function amplifies high frequency components more than low frequency components.

Why should such distortions in the appearance of the waveform be important? One example is a common clinical scenario involving measurement of intraventricular pressure to determine whether constrictive pericarditis is present. An indication of constriction is the presence of the "square root sign" (Fig. 11.7, Vaitkus et al[3]), which reflects an alteration in the ventricular filling dynamics imposed by the noncompliant pericardial sack.[3] If not appreciated, the artifactual occurrence of a square root sign due to measurement system resonance, as seen in Fig. 11.6, could result in an erroneous diagnosis of constrictive pericarditis.

Just as in an electrical circuit where a signal generator, such as a time-varying voltage source, is coupled to a circuit, the ventricle is coupled to a vascular circuit. In the case of the

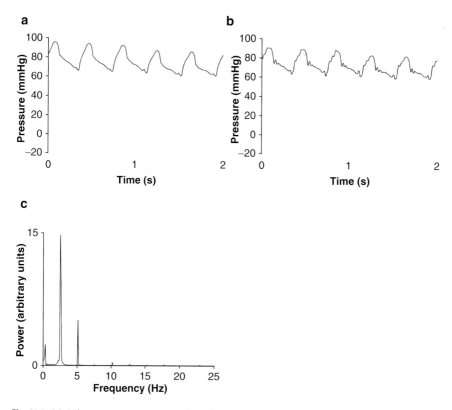

Fig. 11.8 (a) Micromanometer-measured aortic root pressure. (b) Catheter-measured aortic root pressure. (c) Power spectrum of signal in (a)

left ventricle, this is, of course, the arterial system. Arterial system compliance and resistance result in attenuation of high frequency components of the pressure signal, similar to how a resistor and capacitor in an electrical circuit function as a low-pass filter (see Chap. 4).

Figures 11.8a and b show recordings of aortic root pressure obtained with micromanometer and fluid-filled catheter systems, respectively, along with the power spectrum of the micromanometer-measured waveform (Fig. 11.8c). Notice that the waveforms are much more similar to each other than were the corresponding ventricular waveforms. The power spectra of the signals show why this is so. In contrast to the ventricular waveform, the arterial waveform has essentially no energy above 6 Hz where amplification by the catheter-based system starts to become problematic, and is thus less susceptible to distortion by the catheter-based system's transfer function.

The vascular system itself carries the potential to distort the measured signal if the measurement is not determined at the point of interest. Figure 11.9 shows recordings of arterial pressure measured with a saline-filled pigtail catheter at the level of the aortic root and from the right femoral artery. Notice that the dicrotic notches (*arrows*) seen in the aortic root tracing are absent and the pressure tracing is slightly blunted in the femoral artery tracing due to "low pass filtering" from the arterial system. In some cases, arterial

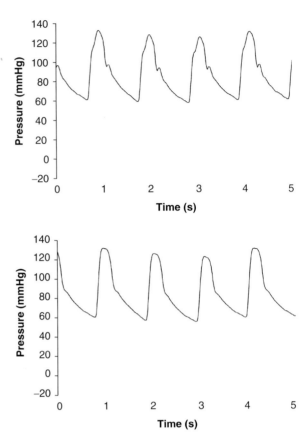

Fig. 11.9 On the top panel is arterial pressure measured at the level of the aortic root using a pigtail catheter vs. pressure measured simultaneously from an introducer sheath in the right femoral artery on the bottom panel. The *arrows* point to the dicrotic notches

stiffening due to atherosclerosis may result in amplification of certain frequency components as seen previously for pressure tubing; in such cases, systolic pressure may be increased and diastolic decreased from the values obtained at the aortic root. Although this is sometimes referred to as an artifact of "reflected waves," this, more accurately, is amplification due to resonance.

Finally, attention needs to be paid to the type of fluid filling the catheter. Figure 11.10 shows intraventricular pressure tracings obtained from a pigtail catheter filled with saline and then filled with intravenous contrast. The high-density, high-viscosity contrast agent attenuates the high frequency signals from the catheter; this would considerably reduce the value of peak dP/dt derived from this signal.

Signal processing of pressure waveforms is usually limited to minor filtering and the derivation of maximum, minimum, and mean values. While this would seem to be straightforward, a major difficulty in catheterization laboratories is standardizing the portion of the signal to be used. For example, end-diastole is commonly defined as the point corresponding to the upstroke of the QRS complex of a simultaneously recorded electrocardiogram signal. Where filtering (whether intentional or unintentional) introduces phase distortions and time delays in the pressure signal, the calculated end-diastolic pressure may be substantially altered because the ECG signal is not similarly altered and is, therefore, no longer

Fig. 11.10 Clinical recording of intraventricular pressure using a saline-filled pigtail catheter on the *top panel* and a radiocontrast filled pigtail catheter on the *bottom panel*

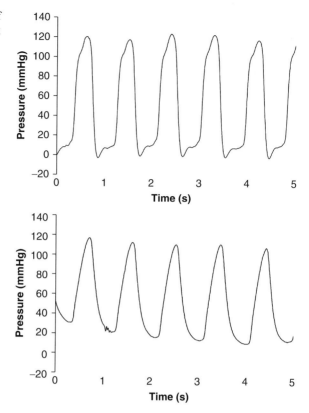

synchronous with the pressure signal. The extent to which any given clinical system filters signals and/or corrects for timing changes is difficult to determine because the signal processing algorithms are usually proprietary, so inspection of the raw hemodynamic waveforms should always be performed before accepting the automatically calculated values.

Apart from alterations of the raw signals themselves, automated derivation of values from raw hemodynamic signals is subject to the same errors that may occur in manual measurements. For example, when systolic, diastolic, or mean values of pressure waveforms are not obtained with attention to the phase of the respiratory cycle, substantially different measurements may be obtained from those made during the inspiratory phase or at end-expiration (the time used in research laboratories).

These issues become far more important when pressure measurements are being obtained from the venous and pulmonary circulation, since the magnitude of variation in pressure due to respiration is a much greater proportion of the underlying pressure variation. Figure 11.11 shows a pulmonary artery occlusive ("wedge") pressure tracing obtained from a patient where the substantial variation in intrathoracic pressure has a major impact on measurement of left atrial pressure. In this case, the computer-calculated value for pulmonary artery occlusive pressure was 15 mmHg (apparently based on averaging over the respiratory cycle), although the reference standard definition (which assumes pressure is measured at end-expiration) is closer to 20 mmHg.

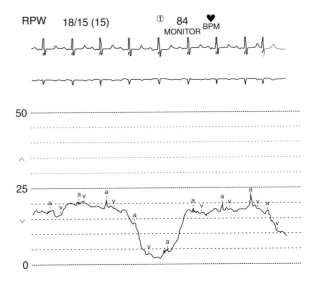

Fig. 11.11 Pulmonary occlusive pressure recording in a patient during normal respiration

Depending on how the data are sampled, summary values provided by the hemodynamic system may provide dramatically different results from what would be reported if the pressure tracing were observed directly.

In summary, while only minimal signal processing of intravascular and intracardiac pressure measurement is used explicitly in the typical clinical setting, "intrinsic signal processing" by the measurement chain may substantially alter the appearance of the measured signals, and in some cases, may even lead to erroneous conclusions and diagnoses. The most significant effects occur at the "front end" of the measurement chain, which includes the catheters and pressure transducers used. In most contemporary health care settings, the "back end" components of the signal measurement chain, such as the transducers and electronics, are unlikely to have an important effect, although inattention to the algorithms used to derive values from raw hemodynamic signals may be misleading in common clinical scenarios.

Acknowledgment Supported by the Department of Veterans Affairs, and NIH/NHLBI R01 HL068606

References

1. Booth J. A short history of blood pressure measurement. *Proc R Soc Med.* 1977;70(11): 793–799.
2. Hartley CJ, Reddy AK, Taffet GE. In-vitro evaluation of sensors and amplifiers to measure left ventricular pressure in mice. In: Engineering in Medicine and Biology Society, 2008. EMBS 2008. 30th Annual International Conference of the IEEE Engineering in Medicine and Biology Society. IEEE Engineering in Medicine and Biology Society. August 20–25 2008:965–968.
3. Vaitkus PT, Cooper KA, Shuman WP, Hardin NJ. Constrictive pericarditis. *Circulation.* 1996;93:834–835.

Blood Pressure and Pulse Oximetry

12

Grace M.N. Mirsky and Alan V. Sahakian

Oscillometry and pulse oximetry rely on signal processing for the detection of cardiogenic events (those arising from the activity of the heart) in a signal which is inherently sensitive to motion and other sources of artifact. In situations where more than one correlated physiological signal is available simultaneously (e.g., when the ECG is being acquired along with the cuff pressure in oscillometry), it is possible to use adaptive or other signal extraction techniques to enhance the desired component of the signal.

12.1
Noninvasive Blood Pressure Recordings

Arterial pressure is an important clinical indicator which must be properly monitored in the intensive care unit (ICU). Intraarterial recordings are typically treated as the gold standard; however, there are a number of noninvasive techniques that may be used to make these measurements, which include both manual and automatic techniques. Some of the major techniques will be discussed here; these include palpation and auscultation, oscillometric, ultrasonic, and tonometric methods.

12.2
Palpation and Auscultation

The methods of palpation and auscultation for blood pressure measurement are the two basic manual methods.[1] A sphygmomanometer, which includes an inflatable cuff, a rubber bulb for inflation of the cuff, and a manometer to detect pressure, is used for both manual methods. The inflatable cuff is placed around the patient's upper arm, at the level of the heart in order to avoid hydrostatic effects. The cuff is inflated until the pressure is above

---

G.M.N. Mirsky (✉)
McCormick School of Engineering, Northwestern University, Evanston, IL, USA
e-mail: gracenijm2008@u.northwestern.edu

the patient's systolic pressure; the pressure in the cuff is then slowly released. A palpable pulse in the wrist is produced as the blood spurts out from under the cuff. This pulse can be felt from a downstream artery and is used to identify the patient's systolic blood pressure.

Audible sounds, called Korotkoff sounds, can be heard through a stethoscope placed over a downstream artery, rather than feeling for the pulse as in the palpation method. The first Korotkoff sound heard indicates the systolic pressure; the transition to muffling indicates the diastolic pressure. Therefore, by the auscultation method, the clinician can identify both the systolic and diastolic pressures, whereas the palpation method is only capable of identifying the systolic pressure. Furthermore, since both methods rely on the senses of the clinician administering the technique, there are inherent limitations of each. For the palpation method, a sensitive tactile sense is necessary to properly detect the pulse at the appropriate time to give a correct blood pressure measurement. For the auscultation method, a sensitive auditory sense is necessary to properly hear the Korotkoff sounds, as well as the transition from muffling to silence. The palpation technique may be used in noisy environments, while the auscultation technique may not.

12.3
Oscillometry

Automated devices can be used for continuous monitoring, so they are frequently employed in the ICU rather than sphygmomanometer techniques.[2] The method is similar in principle to auscultation, but the small pressure oscillations in the cuff are used rather than any sounds.[1] The cuff is quickly inflated to a pressure about 30 mmHg greater than the expected systolic pressure; it is then slowly released so that the pressure can slowly decrease. When the first large increase in oscillation amplitude is observed, the systolic pressure is recorded as the pressure of the cuff. When a significant reduction in oscillation amplitude is observed, the pressure of the cuff is recorded as the diastolic pressure. At the point of maximum amplitude oscillation, the cuff pressure is recorded as the mean arterial pressure.

Oscillometric methods are capable of continuous recording, but they also have their limitations. It has been shown that the results from the oscillometric and the auscultation methods may differ significantly.[3] In the elderly age group, the differences between oscillometric and auscultation methods happen more frequently than in other age groups. Intraarterial systolic blood pressure is underestimated when using oscillometric methods, particularly in overweight critically ill patients.[1] It has recently been suggested that the high-pass filter used to extract the oscillometric pulses from the cuff pressure may change the shape of those pulses.[2] This may partially explain the measurement discrepancies observed between different patient groups.

There has been a significant amount of work dedicated to improving the oscillometric blood pressure recording method. Nelson et al. tested the accuracy of an improved algorithm for oscillometric devices, called DINAMAP SuperSTAT, which was intended to increase the speed at which blood pressure recordings were acquired for neonates, while still maintaining reasonable accuracy.[4] The algorithm works by fitting a modified Gaussian curve to the oscillometric data; the parameters of the Gaussian are selected in order to minimize the least squared error to the measured data. In addition, since the pulses are not symmetric, a skew factor is added to adjust the Gaussian curve to more accurately model the data. Systolic, diastolic, and mean arterial blood pressure measurements are determined from the fit curve. The measurements made by the oscillometric device were compared with intraarterial recordings. The study authors found that in 15 subjects, there was a 35% reduction in determination time when operating in stat mode and 55% in auto mode. Improvements in speed are especially important for this patient group, since they have a tendency to be less tolerant than other patient groups.

Due to the popularity of oscillometric devices, there has been an increased variety of these devices made by numerous manufacturers. Sims et al. studied the interdevice differences and repeatability for nineteen low-cost oscillometric blood pressure measurement devices.[5] The study authors found that results for a particular device were repeatable within a mean of 1 mmHg; however, the measurements of blood pressure between the different devices had much more variation. The mean differences between devices were 4.4 mmHg for systolic pressures and 3.6 mmHg for diastolic pressures; the mean ranges were 23 and 15 mmHg, respectively. The variations are most likely attributable to the different manufacturers' individual implementations of the oscillometric technique in their devices; the values for systolic and diastolic blood pressure are computed by the devices by using the cuff pressure at the maximum pulse height as well as the rate of change of the pulse height, but the specifics of how this is accomplished differ according to the manufacturer. The authors found that while results from the same device were accurate and sufficient for assessing clinical trends over time, the differences between the tested devices were large enough to be considered significant. The authors concluded that the clinical accuracy of measurements made by a particular device must be ultimately determined by a clinical trial, since the absolute measurements of blood pressure are not reliable. In another study, Sims et al. performed a survey of the market for automated non-invasive blood pressure measurement devices in the European Union.[6] They found that a majority of the models were not properly validated by clinical trials according to any of the acceptable protocols.

The modern oscillometer uses a microprocessor for control and signal processing as seen in Fig. 12.1. During an oscillometric blood pressure determination procedure, the cuff is inflated to above systolic pressure and then deflated either continuously or in a stepwise fashion to a pressure below diastolic. The pattern of small-amplitude oscillations in cuff pressure (i.e., the AC component of the pressure), which are coupled from the artery beneath the cuff, has a characteristic increase at systolic blood pressure, a maximum at the mean arterial blood pressure, and decrease at diastolic blood pressure. Thus it is an envelope of oscillation amplitudes taken at decreasing pressures, which is operated on to determine the systolic, mean, and diastolic pressures. This is shown in Fig. 12.2.

Motion, including both voluntary and involuntary patient movement (e.g., shivering) as well as environmental motion in the case of use in an ambulance, gives rise to artifact which must be rejected in order to make an accurate pressure determination. Some of this rejection must happen in real-time, while the cuff is inflated, in order to have useful data to work with. Some signal processing is also performed on the envelope after it has been acquired. Note that the duration of cuff inflation must be limited for patient safety, and this may make a determination very difficult or impossible in the presence of sustained motion.

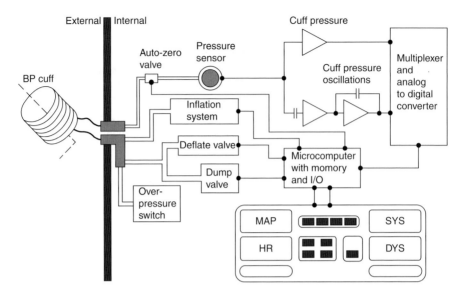

Fig. 12.1 Block diagram of the oscillometer (copied with permission from Ramsey[24])

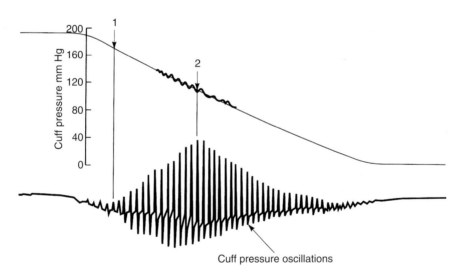

Fig. 12.2 The total cuff pressure (*upper signal*) and AC component of the cuff pressure (*lower signal*) during an oscillometric determination of blood pressure. Note the amplitude envelope pattern of the AC component as the total pressure decreases. There is a characteristic increase in AC amplitude when the total cuff pressure reaches systolic, a maximum at mean pressure, and a significant decline at diastolic (copied with permission from *Medical Instrumentation: Application and Design*)

The most common signal processing method for motion artifact rejection is based on the principle that cardiogenic events tend to happen at regular intervals and with similar shapes (morphologies). In particular, two successive events should have very similar morphologies and amplitudes and be separated by the prevailing interbeat interval. Note that using this fact may lead to difficulty in determining blood pressure in the presence of marked arrhythmia.

Morphological comparison can be accomplished using combinations of slopes (as determined by numerical differentiation signal processing algorithms) amplitudes and durations. It is also possible to use correlation methods.

12.4
Finapres and Portopres

Finapres is an oscillometric blood pressure measuring technology of notable interest. It was first introduced in the early 1980s; the name is an acronym for FINger Arterial PRESsure.[7,8] The device is comprised of an inflatable finger cuff with a built-in photoelectric plethysmograph, which is able to measure the finger arterial blood volume under the cuff. The front-end box includes a fast proportional pneumatic valve connected to a source of compressed air, an electromagnetic transducer, and the electronics for the plethysmograph. The set-point of the finger artery blood volume is determined by using a value of two thirds of the maximum, a point at which the arterial wall is considered "unloaded." The cuff pressure is continuously adjusted in order to maintain the arterial pressure at this set-point. The set-point is also periodically readjusted in order to account for variations in vasomotor tone. Using the pressure waveform, the heart rate as well as systolic, diastolic, and mean arterial pressures are determined. Portopres is a portable version of the Finapres device, which was introduced in the 1990s for 24 h ambulatory blood pressure recordings. A limitation of the Finapres and Portopres devices is that the pulse waveform is known to be distorted when it is acquired from peripheral arteries instead of central arteries. Consequently, systolic blood pressure values tend to be overestimated by these devices.

Polito et al. compared the auscultatory method and the Finapres for blood pressure measurements during resistance exercise[9] and found that there were small and systematic differences. There was high correlation of both systolic and diastolic blood pressure between the two methods.

12.5
Doppler Ultrasonic Flowmeter

Blood pressure may be measured using a Doppler sensor to detect the motion of blood vessel walls, as the amount of occlusion is varied.[1] The transmitted signal is directed toward the blood vessel wall as well as the blood. According to the Doppler shift principle, the received signal is shifted in frequency[10]; the difference in frequency between transmitted and received signals is proportional to the velocity of the blood as well as the movement of the vessel walls.[1] When the cuff pressure is between systolic and diastolic blood pressure of the patient, the blood vessel opens and closes as blood is pushed through with each heartbeat. The ultrasonic system detects the opening and closing of the vessel, and as pressure in the cuff is increased, systolic pressure is eventually reached and the opening and closing coincide. The diastolic pressure may be acquired similarly; pressure is decreased until the closing signal from one pulse coincides with the opening signal of the following pulse.

The advantages of this technique are that it may be used in noisy environments, and it may also be used in hypotensive patients.[1] It has also been shown to be more accurate than standard manual techniques for patients in shock.[10] The major disadvantage is that patient movement can result in error, since the path between the sensor and blood vessel may be altered.[10] This limitation makes the ultrasonic technique not very suitable for neonates due to frequent movement.

12.6
Arterial Tonometry

The principle behind arterial tonometry is that by flattening the anterior wall of the artery (usually radial or carotid) without occluding the vessel, tangential pressures are eliminated.[2] This allows the sensor to record the pressure within the artery. The resulting pulse waveforms recorded by tonometry are substantially similar to those recorded from intraarterial catheters. The arterial pressures recorded from the radial artery are calibrated using the pressures measured from the brachial artery. Assuming unchanged mean and diastolic blood pressure between the aorta and radial artery, a generalized transfer function is then applied to the blood pressure waveform. While the systolic aortic pressure and pulse pressure are reasonably estimated by this method, the high frequency components of the signal may suffer from distortion.

While this method has been shown to be feasible for hemodynamically stable patients, there are a number of limitations for radial artery tonometry. Carotid artery tonometry provides the advantages that blood pressure measurements are recorded close to the aortic root and the transfer function does not need to be used.[2] Nevertheless, it has not been thoroughly evaluated for its usefulness in critically ill patients.

12.7
Ambulatory Blood Pressure Monitoring

Ambulatory blood pressure monitoring is useful in many situations, particularly since it has been shown that blood pressure may vary throughout the day and in response to different physiological and psychological factors.[11] Consequently, ambulatory recordings can give clinicians a much better overall picture of a patient's blood pressure fluctuations throughout the day rather than a single, isolated measurement. This can be important for examining the distribution pattern of blood pressure and particularly if certain events trigger changes in blood pressure. For instance, white coat syndrome refers to elevated blood pressure in the clinical setting, as a result of a patient's psychological reaction to the physician. The ambulatory blood pressure monitor usually records heart rate and blood pressure every 10–20 min during waking hours and every 20–30 min during sleeping hours, typically for a total duration of 24 h.

12.8
Pulse Oximetry

12.8.1
Relevance

The amount of oxygen in arterial blood can be an important clinical indicator of how effectively gas exchange is occurring in the lungs; however, obtaining a sample of arterial blood can be difficult and painful, since arteries are usually deeper than the superficial veins used to draw blood.[12] Pulse oximetry provides the ability to quickly and painlessly measure the amount of oxygen in the blood by determining the level of oxyhemoglobin in a noninvasive, fast, and inexpensive manner. Ninety-eight percent of oxygen in the blood exists as oxyhemoglobin, in which oxygen is bound to hemoglobin, and the remaining 2% is dissolved in the plasma. Therefore, detection of oxyhemoglobin levels in the blood provides meaningful insight into the true oxygen saturation of the blood.

The pulse oximeter is currently a standard monitoring device in the ICU, where its recordings are commonly utilized as the basis of therapeutic interventions.[13] It is an especially important tool for the detection of hypoxemia. Lack of oxygen delivery to the vital organs of the body can quickly lead to severe consequences.[14] There are also a number of respiratory conditions that may result in low levels of arterial oxygen saturation in which pulse oximetry may alert the clinician. These include poor lung compliance, increased airway resistance, low pulmonary diffusion capacity, airway obstruction, ventilatory muscle weakness, increased true venous admixture, low inspired partial pressure of oxygen, and hypoventilation.

12.8.2
Principles

The pulse oximetry measurement of oxygen saturation (SpO_2) is obtained by shining light of two wavelengths, red and infrared, through a tissue bed.[14] Typically, the finger or earlobe is used so that light may pass through the tissue. Pulse oximetry is based upon two physical principles.[15,16] First, the light absorbance of oxygenated hemoglobin and reduced hemoglobin is different when using red or infrared light. Second, the oscillating component (AC) of each results from the volume change between the emitter and detector of the sensor. There is also a stable component (DC), which results from light attenuated by skin, fingernails, tissue, bone, and static blood. The reliable range of pulse oximeters is between

70 and 100% oxygen saturation; the devices are empirically calibrated by desaturating healthy subjects in this range. The oxyhemoglobin is measured at multiple stable points within the range of 70–100% oxygen saturation, and a calibration curve can be computed by obtaining absorption data for both wavelengths (red and infrared). Using the equation (12.1), the raw data become a "ratio of ratios," and the value of r may then be related to a specific value of true oxygen saturation (SaO_2) read during desaturation. This allows for estimation of the value of SaO_2 for any r, using the calibration curve.[17]

$$r = (AC_{red} / DC_{red}) / (AC_{infrared} / DC_{infrared}) \tag{12.1}$$

However, there are several assumptions for this equation to be valid. First, the hemoglobin present in the blood is only either oxyhemoglobin or reduced hemoglobin. Second, the only absorbers present in the blood are the same ones present during empirical calibration. Third, the pulsating blood is arterial blood only (not venous). These assumptions result in several limitations of this work, which will be discussed in the next section.

Most pulse oximeters also provide a photoplethysmograph, which is obtained from the same data used to compute SpO_2.[14] It may be used in the clinical setting to determine heart rate by applying signal processing techniques to the photoplethysmographic signal. The heart rate is observable from these data because during systole, the quantity of hemoglobin in the fingertip is increased, light absorption is decreased, and the opposite is true during diastole.[16] The pulse waveform from which the heart rate is determined can be derived from the infrared signal, which is primarily influenced by arterial blood. The height of the pulse component of the photoplethysmographic waveform is related to the pulse pressure, while the shape of the waveform varies from one subject to another. In addition to allowing for the estimation of heart rate, the plethysmographic pulse wave has also been shown as a potential indicator of fluid responsiveness.

12.8.3
Limitations

One limitation of pulse oximetry results from the sensitivity to ambient light.[15] Fluorescent and xenon arc surgical lamps can cause falsely low SpO_2 readings; however, this effect may be reduced by shielding the sensor with an opaque covering. A second limitation results from low perfusion. Disease states that cause low perfusion, such as low cardiac output, vasoconstriction, or hypothermia, result in difficulty in separating the true signal from the background noise because a lower perfusion level is related to a lower oscillating component of the signal.[17] Therefore, the noise caused by the motion is more significant relative to the magnitude of the true physiological signal. For example, a study found that for 20 cardiac surgery patients who were experiencing hypothermia and low perfusion, only two had measurements using the pulse oximeter, which were within ±4% of the CO oximeter value.[15] Another limitation occurs because one of the assumptions for pulse oximetry is that the hemoglobin in the blood is only either oxyhemoglobin or reduced hemoglobin. Consequently, the presence of dyshemoglobins such as carboxyhemoglobin and methemoglobin can cause inaccurate oximetry readings. These inaccuracies occur because the two wavelengths of light used for pulse oximetry are selected specifically to distinguish only oxyhemoglobin and reduced hemoglobin. In addition, some intravenous dyes that may be used in surgical procedures, including methylene blue, indocyanine green, and indigo carmine, can also cause falsely low SpO_2 readings; this effect can last up to 20 min. Also, certain colors of nail polish, including green, blue, and black, have been shown to result in inaccurate SpO_2 readings. These errors may be eliminated by orienting the oximeter probe so that it is not over the nail polish.[15]

Another limitation of pulse oximetry results from motion artifacts.[17] When a patient moves, both venous and arterial blood move, as well as other typically nonpulsatile components, which causes the AC components of the signal to be comprised of more than only the arterial blood.[17] If in addition to motion the patient also suffers from low perfusion, the venous blood contributes even further to the pulsatile component, which causes SpO_2 to be reduced even further. Motion artifacts can cause false alarms and data dropouts. In a study by Lawless, 71% of pulse oximetry alarms in a pediatric ICU were false and a mere 7% of the alarms were clinically significant.[18] Repeated false alarms can cause clinicians to become distrustful of its significance, leading to incomplete utilization of pulse oximetry as a diagnostic monitoring tool.

There are several ways to handle motion artifacts in pulse oximetry, which may help to reduce errors and the frequency of false alarms. One such method involves increasing averaging time in order to smooth the data.[19,20] Rheineck and Kalkman found that when SpO_2 values were averaged over 10 s rather than 3 s (the default value), false alarms were reduced by almost half. Data averaging reduces false alarms in two ways: by increasing the time before an initial value is reported and by smoothing changes in oxyhemoglobin saturation over time. There are bounds, however, for the duration that the signal should be averaged. The study authors found that when the data were averaged for 42 s, though the number of false alarms was reduced even further, six of the 73 true severe hypoxemic episodes were missed. Consequently, this is not an ideal solution since there is a trade-off between the number of false alarms and the number of true hypoxemic episodes that are missed.

Another method to handle motion artifacts in pulse oximetry is by read-through motion and motion-tolerant algorithms. Manufacturers do not generally disclose the details of these algorithms, but they usually involve filtering and moving averages to process the signals.[17] Masimo signal extraction technology (SET) is one such technology which implements read-through motion as well as additional signal processing techniques, resulting in significant improvements in comparison with other technologies.[19] Masimo SET uses a proprietary discrete saturation transform (DST), which uses a reference signal generator to first collect a block of red and infrared signals. Next, the reference signal for a sample saturation value is computed; the sample saturation value may begin, for instance, at 0%. The infrared signal and reference signal are then processed with an adaptive filter that eliminates frequency content common to both the signals. This procedure is repeated for the entire range of saturation values, from 0 to 100%. A power curve is built using the output from the adaptive filter, which identifies the arterial saturation and other saturation components. The value of SpO_2 is identified as the rightmost peak of the power spectrum, since arterial saturation is greater than venous saturation. Overall, pulse oximetry with read-through motion technology consistently reports fewer false alarms and data dropouts than with conventional pulse oximetry.[17]

12.8.4
Clinical Usefulness

In a study of 102 ICU patients, SpO_2 and SaO_2 (found by arterial blood gas tests) were measured and compared. The mean difference, or bias, between the SaO_2 and SpO_2 values was −0.02% and the standard deviation, or precision, was 2.1%. While the bias was within clinically acceptable limits, the precision may not be, particularly since ICU patients may tend to be hypoxemic. The study authors concluded that for ICU patients, the differences between SaO_2 and SpO_2 may be clinically significant, even though the values are within the manufacturers' reported values; they recommended that low SpO_2 targets for therapeutic decision-making should be used only with significant caution.[13]

The usefulness of pulse oximetry to record heart rate was evaluated in the neonatal ICU. Pulse oximetry sensors were used in addition to an ECG monitoring system. Thirty stable infants were included in the study; two subsets were also analyzed, which included low perfusion index and low signal quality. For the entire patient population, the mean and standard deviation difference between heart rates determined by pulse oximetry and ECG was −0.4 ± 6 beats per minute. For the low perfusion subset, the mean and standard deviation difference was −0.4 ± 7.2 beats per minute; for the low signal quality subset, the mean and standard deviation difference was 0.9 ± 14.2 beats per minute. The study authors concluded that pulse oximetry may be very useful for newborn premature infants who cannot tolerate ECG electrodes because of their very delicate skin. They also found that pulse oximetry may potentially be suitable for use in the delivery room, but this application has not yet been shown.[21]

12.9
Signal Processing in Pulse Oximetry

As described earlier, pulse oximetry is based on measuring the steady and pulsatile components of light transmission at two wavelengths through a region of tissue containing arterial blood and other components. Figure 12.3 shows a typical transmitted light intensity signal.

The transmitted light intensity decreases with increasing volume of arterial blood during the cardiac cycle. Thus the waveform is inverted from the shape of the typical arterial blood pressure waveform. There are three essential measurements to be made from the

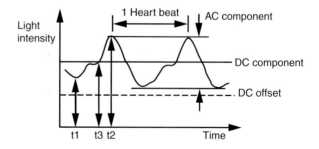

Fig. 12.3 The transmitted light intensity signal (either the red or infrared channel) (copied with permission from *Design of Pulse Oximeters*). *t1* = time of detected valley; *t2* = time of detected peak; *t3* = time at DC component

waveform using signal processing techniques. First, the DC (average)-transmitted light level is determined using low-pass filtering or integration. Second, the AC component (peak-to-peak amplitude) is determined, which involves the tasks of identifying the peaks and valleys of the waveform. This can be accomplished using slope methods or peak-pair algorithms. Finally, the interbeat intervals are measured using stable fiducial points on the waveforms. These fiducial points can be the moments of maximum slope or (as shown in the figure) peak amplitude.

12.9.1
Reducing Motion Artifact

Motion artifact can be rejected using a principle similar to that used in oscillometry. In other words, pulses that do not match others, or a mean template, can be rejected as either motion artifact or abnormal beats. However, since there are both red and infrared signals in pulse oximetry, there are other advanced methods for rejecting or even reading through motion artifact. As an example of such a method, US Patent #5,662,105, assigned to SpaceLabs, Inc.,[22] describes an adaptive signal processing technique. This signal processing algorithm employs two adaptive filters,[23] one operating on the red channel and the other on the infrared channel. The basic approach is to exploit the correlations between the two cardiogenic signals in estimating the ratio to be used in SaO2 determination.

References

1. Webster JG, ed. *Medical Instrumentation: Application and Design*. New York: Wiley; 1998.
2. Chemla D, Teboul JL, Richard C. Noninvasive assessment of arterial pressure. *Curr Opin Crit Care*. 2008;14(3):317–321.
3. Fabian V, Janouch M, Novakova L, Stepankova O. Comparative study of non-invasive blood pressure measurement methods in elderly people. *Conf Proc IEEE Eng Med Biol Soc*. 2007; 2007:612–615.
4. Nelson RM, Stebor AD, Groh CM, Timoney PM, Theobald KS, Friedman BA. Determination of accuracy in neonates for non-invasive blood pressure device using an improved algorithm. *Blood Press Monit*. 2002;7(2):123–129.
5. Sims AJ, Reay CA, Bousfield DR, Menes JA, Murray A. Low-cost oscillometric non-invasive blood pressure monitor: device repeatability and device differences. *Physiol Meas*. 2005; 26(4):441–445.
6. Sims AJ, Menes JA, Bousfield DR, Reay CA, Murray A. Automated non-invasive blood pressure devices: are they suitable for use? *Blood Press Monit*. 2005;10(5):275-281.
7. Parati G, Ongaro G, Bilo G, et al. Non-invasive beat-to-beat blood pressure monitoring: new developments. *Blood Press Monit*. 2003;8(1):31–36.
8. Imholz BPM, Wieling W, van Montfrans GA, Wesseling KH. Fifteen year experience with finger areterial pressure monitoring: assessment of the technology. *Cardiovasc Res*. 1998; 38(3):605–616.
9. Polito MD, Farinatti PT, Lira VA, Nobrega AC. Blood pressure assessment during resistance exercise: comparison between auscultation and Finapres. *Blood Press Monit*. 2007;12(2):81–86.

10. Kazamias TM, Gander MP, Franklin DL, Ross J Jr. Blood pressure measurement with Doppler ultrasonic flowmeter. *J Appl Physiol*. 1971;30(4):585–588.
11. Tseng YZ. Applications of 24-hour noninvasive ambulatory blood pressure monitoring. *J Formos Med Assoc*. 2006;105(12):955–963.
12. Silverthorn DU, ed. *Human Physiology: An Integrated Approach with Interactive Physiology*. San Francisco, CA: Pearson; 2004.
13. Van de Louw A, Cracco C, Cerf C, et al. Accuracy of pulse oximetry in the intensive care unit. *Intensive Care Med*. 2001;27(10):1606–1613.
14. Webster JG, ed. *Design of Pulse Oximeters*. Philadelphia, PA: Taylor & Francis; 1997.
15. Jubran A. Pulse oximetry. *Intensive Care Med*. 2004;30(11):2017–2020.
16. Bendjelid K. The pulse oximetry plethysmographic curve revisted. *Curr Opin Crit Care*. 2008;14(3):348–353.
17. Petterson MT, Begnoche VL, Graybeal JM. The effect of motion on pulse oximetry and its clinical significance. *Anesth Analg*. 2007;105(6 suppl):S78–S84.
18. Lawless S. Crying wolf: false alarms in a pediatric intensive care unit. *Crit Care Med*. 1994;22(6):981–985.
19. Barker SJ. "Motion-resistant" pulse oximetry: a comparison of new and old models. *Anesth Analg*. 2002;95(4):967–972.
20. Rheineck-Leyssius AT, Kalkman CJ. Influence of pulse oximeter lower alarm limit on the incidence of hypoxaemia in the recovery room. *Br J Anaesth*. 1997;79(4):460–464.
21. Singh JK, Kamlin CO, Morley CJ, O'Donnell CP, Donath SM, Davis PG. Accuracy of pulse oximetry in assessing heart rate of infants in the neonatal intensive care unit. *J Paediatr Child Heath*. 2008;44(5):273–275.
22. Tien J. US Patent #5,662,105 *System and Method for the Extractment of Physiological Signals*, Sept. 2; 1995.
23. Widrow B, Stearns D. *Adaptive Signal Processing*. Upper Saddle River, NJ, Prentice Hall; 1985.
24. Ramsey M III. Blood pressure monitoring: automated oscillometric devices. *J Clin Monit*. 1991;7:56–67.

Coronary Angiography

13

Shiuh-Yung James Chen and John D. Carroll

13.1 Introduction

Coronary angiography, the in vivo contrast study of the coronary artery tree and its lumen, is commonly used to investigate the anatomy of the coronary arteries and to assess the number, location, and severity of coronary stenoses. A minimally invasive procedure called coronary catheterization is performed where a small catheter (a thin hollow tube with a diameter of 2–3 mm) is inserted through the skin into an arterial sheath at a point where the artery is fairly superficial and easily palpable in the groin or the arm. The physician advances the catheter often leading with a soft J-shaped guidewire retrogradely with the visual guidance of fluoroscopy (a special X-ray viewing instrument), and then the catheter is manipulated in the base of the aorta immediately above the aortic valve until the catheter tip is engaged in the ostium of the coronary arteries, the blood vessels supplying blood to the heart. An injection of 5–12 mL of radiographic contrast solution containing iodine, which is easily visualized with X-ray images, visualizes the coronary tree, delineates its branching pattern, and outlines the inner diameter of a coronary artery. Both the right and left coronary artery are injected multiple times after changing the position of the X-ray system to visualize the coronary tree from different perspectives. The sequential images that are produced over the 3–6 s acquisition time are called the selective coronary angiogram, and the recorded images, if carefully and comprehensively gathered with skill, accurately reveal the extent and severity of all coronary arterial blockages.

The first human cardiac catheterization was performed in 1929, when the German physician Dr. Werner Forssmann inserted a plastic tube in his cubital vein and guided it to the right chamber of the heart. He took an X-ray to prove his success and published it on 5 Nov 1929 with the title "Über die Sondierung des rechten Herzens" (About probing of the right heart).[1] Dr. Forssmann received the Nobel Prize in Physiology or Medicine in 1959 for his pioneering contribution to the development of this widely used and often definitive diagnostic test that has dominated cardiology for decades. The selective catheterization of the

---

S.-Y. James Chen (✉)
Department of Medicine, Anschutz Medical Campus,
University of Colorado Denver, Aurora, CO, USA
e-mail: james.chen@ucdenver.edu

J.J. Goldberger and J. Ng (eds.),
Practical Signal and Image Processing in Clinical Cardiology,
DOI: 10.1007/978-1-84882-515-4_13, © Springer-Verlag London Limited 2010

coronary arteries was introduced in the late 1950s, and the first case occurred in 1958 when Dr. Sones, a pediatric cardiologist at the Cleveland Clinic, accidentally injected radiographic contrast directly into a coronary artery instead of the left ventricle. Much to his surprise the patient did not die and the image of the coronary artery was of such great detail that the clinical value was immediately clear. Afterwards, Sones and Shirey[2] developed new catheters and the technique to engage the ostia (i.e., entrance) of the two coronary arteries with subsequent selective injection of contrast dye. Coronary angiography continues today with important improvements and its use has enabled the development and refinement of coronary bypass surgery and percutaneous coronary intervention (PCI) including stent placement in millions of patients with coronary artery disease from atherosclerosis. The diagnostic procedure takes approximately 15–30 min and the patient has mild sedation and local anesthesia at the site of peripheral arterial entry.

Despite the development of other multiple imaging techniques including computed tomography (CT) and magnetic resonance imaging (MRI), selective, i.e., catheter-based, X-ray coronary angiography remains the most commonly performed method for accurate imaging of the entire coronary tree for a number of reasons.[3–5] The technology is widely available. There are many cardiologists well trained in the technique. The image interpretation and the spatial and temporal resolution are unsurpassed. Finally, the diagnostic procedure can be easily transitioned into a therapeutic procedure. In addition to specific anatomic information, angiography also has an important prognostic role in the identification of coronary artery disease and the associated risk of subsequent morbidity and mortality.[6–9] The number of diagnostic and therapeutic angiographic procedures has increased dramatically during the last several decades. Although it has been widely accepted and used, traditional angiography is limited by its two-dimensional (2-D) representation of three-dimensional (3-D) structures and the consequent imaging artifacts that impair optimal visualization. Furthermore, the techniques of image acquisition with traditional angiography are nonstandardized, subjectively chosen, and highly dependent on the 3-D visual skills of individual operators. Recognition of these limitations has resulted in the development of imaging techniques designed to specifically address the weaknesses of traditional angiographic techniques.

In this chapter, we will first describe the limitations of traditional angiography and why, in an era of complex interventions, advancements in imaging are critical for the continued improvement in patient outcomes. The technique of creation of a patient-specific 3-D coronary arterial tree from a pair of angiographic images and the basic quantitative analysis will be described. Finally, we explore the rapidly developing techniques of 3-D coronary angiography and the expanding clinical applications of this powerful new imaging tool.

13.2
Limitations of Current X-Ray Angiographic Technology in Diagnostic and Therapeutic Interventions

The soul of coronary angiography is the accurate visualization of the coronary arterial tree. Clinicians rely on traditional 2-D views or information generated from a standard X-ray imaging system to select appropriate patients for different treatments, perform catheter-based cardiovascular therapeutic or interventional procedures, and assess device-anatomy results based on the results of limited 2-D quantitative analysis as shown in Fig. 13.1. This information is subjectively processed by the operator. Subjectively selected or standard angiographic views may have no useful clinical information due to overlap or superimposed vessels (see Figs. 13.2 and 13.3). Suboptimal images may lead to mistakes, complications,

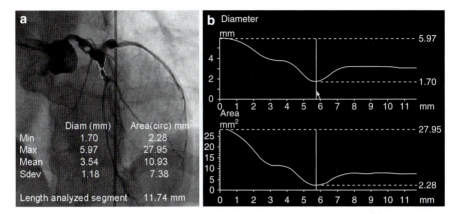

Fig. 13.1 (a) A typical example of 2-D quantitative coronary analysis results based on one selected angiogram with the interactively identified stenotic segment (outlined in *white*). (b) The plots of diameter (*upper panel*) and area (*lower panel*) profiles associated with the identified stenotic segment

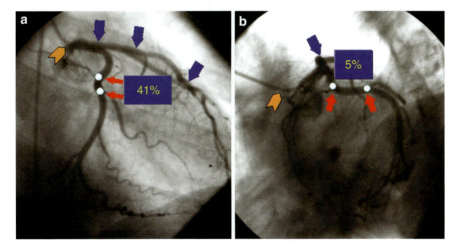

Fig. 13.2 Multiple limitations in traditional 2-D projection images are shown in this figure of the left coronary angiograms in two angiographic views. The *blue arrows* show some vessel segments that are poorly visualized due to overlap with adjacent vessels. The other vessel segment indicated by *red arrows* and *white circles* shows that the true length of a segment can be misrepresented by the phenomenon of foreshortening. The visually deceiving shortness of a segment due to severe foreshortening (41%) in (a) is better portrayed in (b) with mild foreshortening. The catheter (indicated by *orange arrows*) and target arterial segment do not lie on the same plane with respect to the angiographic views and this problem in projection images will cause an incorrect quantitative assessment due to different scaling factors

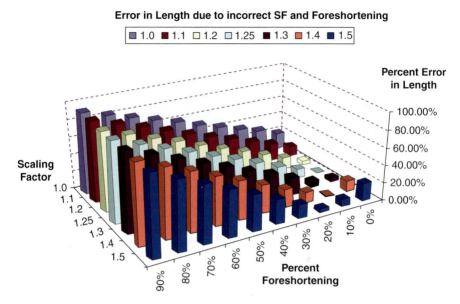

Fig. 13.3 The percent error in length estimate based on the traditional 2-D quantitative analysis on projection image resulting from the combination of various degrees of percent vessel foreshortening and incorrect scaling factors (i.e., correct scaling factor is 1.25)

and suboptimal results. Some patients with complex anatomy may need twice the number of contrast injections to adequately visualize all segments of the coronary tree. All of this occurs based on the physicians experience and skill with no computer assistance. In this case, the absence of objective signal processing techniques and the reliance on subjective evaluation may lead to variability in interpretation and outcome.

While PCI has become a more predictably successful and durable procedure due to improvements in technique, the equipment used, and stents implanted, there continues to be a sizeable proportion of patients who have procedural failure (5–8%) and in whom stent delivery is unsuccessful (2–5%).[10] In addition, even in those having successful stent deployment, it is important to consider further improvements in technology and technique that could further reduce procedure time, radiation dose, contrast volume, and wasted supplies. Challenging anatomical subsets are not rare in PCI: 16% of patients undergoing PCI have a lesion on a curved segment of >75°, 10% have lesion lengths over 20 mm, and more than 15% have lesions downstream from proximal severe tortuosity involving two to three bends of over 75°.[11] Currently, the cardiologist "eyeballs" the angiographic images that may or may not adequately display these challenging anatomical subsets. Often, the challenging nature of PCI in this group (25% of all PCI) is recognized only after the failure of initial equipment choices. The typical alterations in equipment for challenging anatomies include using larger and stiffer guiding catheters for better support, high performance hydrophilic coated guide wires with varying degrees of stiffness, initial treatment of the lesion with a variety of devices to reduce the narrowing and increase the likelihood of optimal stent deployment, and the use of specific brands of stents and multiple shorter stents to be able to deliver them to distal locations in the tortuous coronary artery tree.[11] Therefore, the goal of improvements in PCI is not only to continue to improve overall success rates, but also increase the safety, decrease the procedure time, and eliminate wasted equipment that failed with initial attempts of the trial and error approach.

Since the first percutaneous, i.e., nonsurgical, coronary intervention by Gruenzig using balloon angioplasty, extensive efforts have been made to improve this therapeutic technique and extend it to millions of patients with coronary artery disease and other vascular abnormalities. These advancements have had specific goals measured by multiple indicators of a high quality care outcome including: (1) Immediate and long-term success rates in opening narrowed vessels in a wide variety of anatomical and clinical subsets of patients; (2) safety of the procedure and freedom of the patient from complications; (3) the efficient execution and predictability of the procedure and; (4) the total cost as well as the cost effectiveness of this treatment modality. The major traditional approaches to improving these outcomes are listed below:

1. Optimal patient selection, choice of devices, appropriate pharmacotherapy, and other aspects of utilizing professional guidelines derived from high-quality scientific data especially randomized clinical trials.
2. Improved equipment and devices.
3. Improved adjunctive pharmacology.
4. Improved contrast agents.
5. Vascular access and closure techniques.
6. Improved X-ray imaging systems.
7. Adjunctive intravascular ultrasound.

Despite these major advancements, PCIs and other vascular interventions remain a group of procedures with a persistent rate of major life-threatening and disabling complications, prolonged difficult cases, unpredictable failures, and often higher than expected costs. There are several general themes that bring some understanding to this.

First, percutaneous vascular interventions often involve a vital organ (heart, brain, kidney, etc.), with mistakes, miscalculations, and unexpected events being a reality of medical practice. "Because all cardiac catheterization involve the insertion of foreign objects (i.e., cardiac catheters) into the circulatory system, it should not be surprising that a variety of adverse events (complications) can ensue."[12] These events can involve the following problems:

- Radiations burns and cumulative radiation doses of cancer-causing proportions are now of major concern for fluoroscopically guided cardiovascular therapeutic procedures.[13]
- Radiocontrast used in these procedures causes deterioration in kidney function in 13–20% of patients; especially in diabetic patients with existing renal dysfunction and is contrast volume dependent.[14]
- Improvement in coronary stents with drug-eluting properties has reduced restenosis rates but stent thrombosis, stent-fracture, and stent nondeliverability remain important issues.[15,16]

Second, patients undergoing PCI and other vascular interventions now include patients with many comorbidities, more unstable clinical states, and complex anatomy and lesion characteristics. For example in PCI, patients are older, often have an acute coronary syndrome (i.e., heart attacks), and have geometrically and biologically complex lesions involving tortuous and small coronary arteries with narrowings at ostial and bifurcation locations.

Third, the performance of these procedures is a human endeavor involving clinicians and staff with a wide range of skills and experience. New device technologies, new pharmaceutical agents, and more advanced imaging improve outcomes only if physicians and clinical teams use them effectively and conversely they are easy to use.

Improving outcomes in vascular interventions must also address core issues related to human performance. Traditional training, informal mentoring, and postgraduate medical education courses represent one approach to improve human performance. Simulator-based training and testing are emerging as exciting approaches to improving diagnostic and procedural skills, allowing objective evaluation of skills, and to decreasing the reliance on experience that has been acquired only by practicing on patients. Some of the innovative approaches currently being developed and tested to improve the outcomes of PCI and other cardiovascular interventions are listed below:

1. Advanced image processing:
   (a) 3-D reconstruction and 3-D rendering.
   (b) Automated quantitative analysis of key anatomical features.
   (c) Focused simulation of procedure tasks applied to patient-specific 3-D anatomical data sets, i.e., determination of optimal X-ray views.
2. Point-of-care information technology including medical fund of knowledge.
3. Computer-assisted decision making.
4. Simulation-based training on standard and new procedures.
5. Simulation-based testing of skill levels needed for specific procedures.
6. Robotic and other approaches to catheter manipulation.

A common theme of all these approaches is a strategy to reduce the total reliance on the clinical skills of the physician-operator and the process of skill development using patients to practice and develop experience.

An explicit breakdown is needed for all the individual tasks involved in percutaneous cardiovascular interventions and the skills required for implementing these novel approaches. The tasks involved in the performance of percutaneous vascular procedures fall into the three categories of (1) preprocedure planning, (2) procedure performance, and (3) outcome evaluation. In Fig. 13.4a, the specific tasks for the placement of an intravascular guide wire, an initial step in performing percutaneous vascular interventions are outlined. From Fig. 13.4a, b, it can be appreciated that there are multiple visual interpretative and cognitive tasks involved before the manual hand-eye coordination task of steering the guide wire. The optimal performance of each task is necessary to achieve the overall success of the procedures. Errors and mistakes in the performance of these cognitive and visual interpretive tasks can lead to bad outcomes including prolongation of the procedure, wasted equipment, and damage to the vessel wall.

Performance of each task can be understood as an interaction of the performer with the equipment used and the patient's anatomy/physiology. The interactions occur predominantly via the visual interface of X-ray imaging. The performance of these tasks, as well as

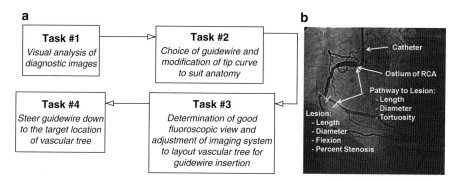

Fig. 13.4 (**a**) Sequential human task involved in placing an intracoronary guide-wire. (**b**) The required patient-specific anatomical information gathered before proceeding with the therapeutic procedure

the procedure as a whole, leads to a variety of outcomes measured as binary variables, i.e., success/failure and uncomplicated/complicated, or are continuous variables such as duration, fluoroscopic radiation dose used, contrast agents administered, and equipment cost.

13.3 Three-dimensional Modeling of Patient-Specific Coronary Arterial Tree and Quantitative Analysis based on X-Ray Angiograms

A number of techniques for estimating the 3-D structure of coronary arteries with computer assistance have been developed.[17–22] These methods are based on the known or standard X-ray geometry of projections, placement of landmarks, or the known vessel shape and iterative identification of matching structures in two or more views. Because the computation was designed for predefined views only, it is not likely to solve the modeling on the basis of two projections acquired at arbitrary and unknown relative orientations. Another method based on motion and multiple views acquired in a single-plane imaging system was proposed.[23] The motion transformations of the heart model consist only of rotation and scaling. By incorporation of the center-referenced method and initial depth coordinates and center coordinates, a 3-D skeleton of coronary arteries was obtained. However, the real heart motion during contraction and relaxation involves five specific movements: translation, rotation, wringing, accordion-like motion, and movement toward the center of the ventricular chamber. Therefore, the assumption did not correspond to the in vivo situation.

Other knowledge-based or rule-based systems were proposed for 3-D modeling of coronary arteries by the use of the model of a vascular network.[24–27] Because the rules or knowledge base were organized for certain specific conditions, it is not feasible to generalize the 3-D modeling on the basis of arbitrary projections. The advent of 3-D angiography allows improvement in the quality and potential safety of diagnostic and therapeutic endovascular procedures. Algorithms of 3-D modeling by using the cone-beam back-projection technique were proposed.[28–30] Such a technique has been successfully applied for reconstructing a nonmoving object such as brain vessels in conjunction with a rapid rotational gantry system (at more than 40° per second acquisition rate).[31-38] For a moving object such as the coronary vascular tree, the gantry system needs to be gated by the electrocardiogram (ECG) signal to synchronize the same time phase (Chap. 5). The 3-D coronary arteries were created from a set of X-ray perspective projections acquired during a rotation of the imaging gantry around the patient by the use of the technique of computerized cone-beam reconstruction.[39] Due to heart motion and the availability of only limited (four or six) projections, it was very challenging to obtain accurate reconstruction and quantitative measurement.

The basic geometric mathematics for reconstructing 3-D objects based on two views was proposed, allowing the determination of a 3-D object structure from two projection images obtained at arbitrary and unknown orientations. Iterative techniques based on nonlinear equations and optimization theory were proposed for determining the solutions that characterize two views for motion analysis.[40] The results may be suboptimal if the initial conditions are chosen beyond the proper solution space. The algorithms[41-44] require at least eight corresponding image points in the two projections for determining the 3-D position by solving a set of linear equations. In the practical situation, however, an input image error of more than one pixel (=0.03 mm) in the image intensifier (17 × 17 cm) may result in 3-D position deviations of 10 cm or more. Hence, optimal estimation has been explicitly investigated. A two-step approach was proposed[45-49] for an optimal estimation of 3-D structures based on maximum-likelihood and minimum-variance estimation. Preliminary estimates computed by the linear algorithm were used as initial estimates for the process of optimal estimation. Recently, the new C-arm imaging system is able to rapidly rotate around patients while acquiring a series of images. The 3-D coronary arterial model can then be created by the use of more than two projection views.[50-52] However, accurate segmentation of arteries in multiple images is a crucial process and time-consuming as well especially when a manual or interactive editing process is required. Among all the existing techniques, none of them has ever been applied to directly facilitate in-room clinical procedures due to the large computational cost or inadequate representation format for advanced quantitative analysis.

13.3.1
3-D Modeling Techniques

A new 3-D modeling technique was proposed to accurately reconstruct the entire coronary arterial trees based on two views acquired from routine angiograms at arbitrary orientation, without the need of calibration object, and using a single-plane imaging system.[53,54] In the proposed method, a new optimization algorithm was employed to minimize the image point and vector angle errors in both views subject to the constraints derived from the intrinsic parameters of the employed single-plane imaging system. Given five or more corresponding object points in two views, an optimal estimate of the transformation in the form of a rotational matrix R and a translational vector $\bar{t}$ can be obtained, which characterizes the position and orientation of one view relative to the other. The initial solution to the optimization process is calculated on the basis of the employed intrinsic single-plane imaging parameters. The first in-room 3-D modeling of patient-specific coronary arterial tree was performed in 1997, while the patient still lay on the table bed in the Cardiac

Catheterization Laboratory. Up to date, over 1,200 cases of coronary arterial trees have been generated in which more than 120 cases have been performed in the room during cardiac catheterization.

Either a single-plane or biplane imaging system can be employed for cardiac angiographic acquisition. The angiograms are acquired based on the selected gantry orientation in terms of left/right anterior oblique (RAO/LAO) angle, caudal/cranial (CAUD/CRAN) angle with respect to the isocenter to which the gantry arm rotates. The gantry information, accompanying the acquired images, is automatically recorded including focal *s*pot to *i*mage-intensifier *d*istance (SID), *f*ield *o*f *v*iew (FOV, e.g., 5, 7, or 9 in. mode), and gantry orientation. The proposed method of on-line 3-D modeling consists of four major steps including:

1. *Image acquisition and selection.* After routine cardiac catheterization is initiated, a standard coronary arteriogram is completed in two standard view based on two injections in a single-plane imaging system or one injection in biplane imaging systems. The table may be moved or panned during the acquisitions in a single-plane imaging system, which commonly happens during routine angiographic study in order that the projections of the whole coronary system are enclosed by the scope of image intensifier. These images are acquired at 15 or 30 frames per second in each view with an ECG signal simultaneously recorded. The acquisition time of each frame was automatically correlated with the associated ECG signal and displayed on the console to facilitate image selection and reviewing as shown in Fig. 13.5. With the acquired two angiographic sequences, a pair of cine

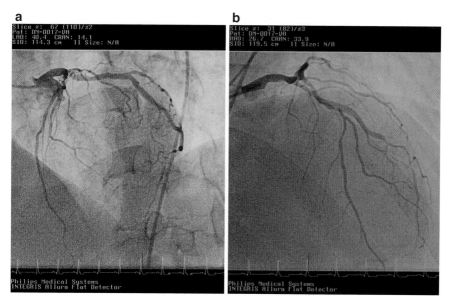

Fig. 13.5 (a) The first selected angiographic view where the first image corresponding to the seventh *R*-wave of cardiac cycle and subsequent six images at the LAO-CRAN view will be transferred. (b) The second selected angiographic view (i.e., RAO-CRAN view) where the image acquired at the third *R*-wave of different cardiac cycle along with the subsequent six images are transferred

images containing eight (at 15 frames/s acquisition rate) or 15 (at 30 frames/s acquisition rate) frames are chosen corresponding to the same or close acquisition time (e.g., end-diastole) in the cardiac cycle. They are transferred to the computer workstation through a fiber optic link for subsequent 3-D modeling and quantitative analysis.

2. *Segmentation of 2-D arterial tree and vessel feature extraction.* A semiautomatic segmentation system by the use of a curve-based deformation technique is adopted to identify the 2-D arterial tree on the pair of angiographic images. The required user interaction in the identification process involves the indication of a series of points inside the lumen of each artery in the angiogram. Afterwards, a parametric curve is formed based on the selected points, which serves as the initial estimate of the vessel centerline, as shown in Fig. 13.6a. This user-generated centerline is then refined by a deformation process. The first part of this deformation process involves applying a filter to the image (see Fig. 13.6b) for the identification of those pixels with the minimum local intensity inside the lumen. These points define the actual vessel centerline points (but not the continuous centerline itself). The final continuous centerline is generated by deforming the initially identified user-generated centerline toward the filter-derived centerline points. Our method (see Appendix A) for this deformation process is based on the algorithms reported by Kass et al and Williams et al[55,56] By the use of a deformation model, the identified "valley" pixels serve as the external force to act on the initial vessel centerline curve, so that it is gradually deformed (see Fig. 13.6c) and finally aligned with the actual vessel centerline (see Fig. 13.6d). Vessel features including bifurcation points, directional vectors at individual bifurcations, diameters and centerline points of each artery are extracted from the employed pair of angiograms to facilitate the calculation of transformation and subsequent modeling process as shown in Fig. 13.6e, f. An interactive editing tool is available to change the identified vessel centerline points and associated vessel cross-sectional diameters if the resultant vessel features are not calculated correctly due to noisy background or overlapped vessels.

3. *Calculation of the transformation defining relative location and orientation of the two views.* The spatial relationship between any two views can be characterized by a transformation in the forms of a rotation matrix and a translation vector with the 3-D coordinate system defined in the X-ray source or focal spot as shown in Fig. 13.7a. By the use of the corresponding bifurcation points and vessel directional vectors identified from the pair of images, the transformation can be calculated to define the relative location and orientation of gantry systems associated with the two angiographic views[54] as shown in Fig. 13.7b, c.

4. *Calculation of the skeleton of the coronary arterial tree.* The calculated transformation is used to establish the point correspondences between each pair of 2-D vessel centerlines based on the epi-polar theory (see Fig. 13.8a, b). Afterwards, a refinement process by the use of the minimization algorithm for segment-to-segment matching is performed as shown in Fig. 13.9a, b. By the use of the correspondence relationship and transformation, the 3-D morphologic structures of the coronary arterial tree can be computed. The resultant vessel lumen of the 3-D arterial tree is modeled as a series of cross-sectional contours with the surfaces filled between every two consecutive contours calculated from the identified 2-D diameters at the second step for rendering of the approximated morphology of artery as shown in Fig. 13.9c, d, respectively.

13 Coronary Angiography

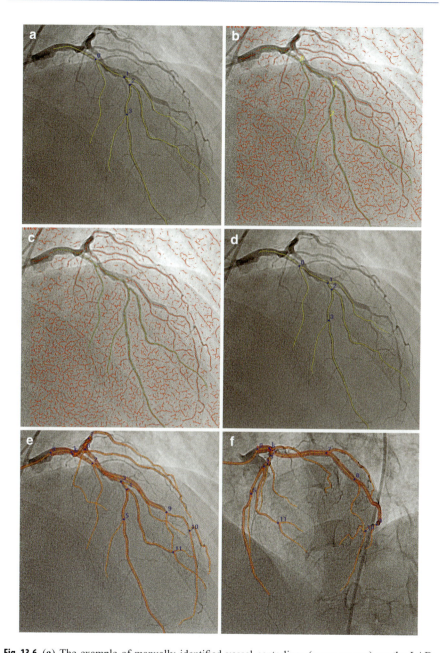

Fig. 13.6 (a) The example of manually identified vessel centerlines (*green curves*) on the LAD artery and three side-branches served as initial vessel centerlines. (b) The image forces in terms of "valley" points (*red dots*) with initially identified vessel centerlines superimposed on the image. (c) The initial vessel centerlines interacted with the image forces and are pushed or pulled toward the actual median lines of artery. (d) The resultant vessel centerlines aligned with the actual median lines of artery overlaid on the images. (e, f) The vessel features including the vessel centerline lines (*yellow curve*), bifurcation points (*blue dots*), and diameters (*short red segments*) are extracted on the pair of angiograms

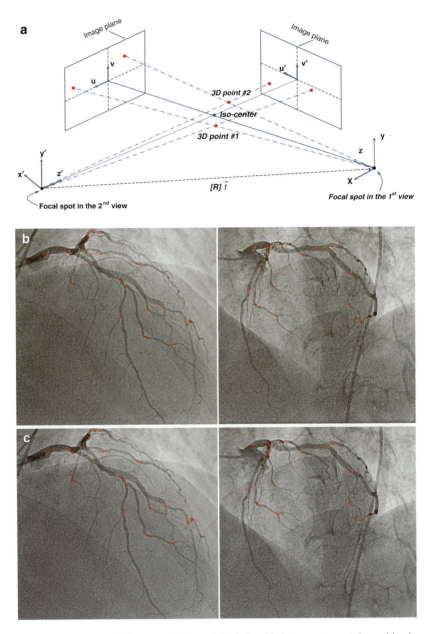

Fig. 13.7 (a) The schematic diagram of 3-D spatial relationship between two angiographic views, showing two 3-D points defined by respective x,y,z (i.e., the first view) and x',y',z' (i.e., the second view) coordinate systems and their projections in respective image planes characterized by u,v and u',v' coordinate systems. (b) The 3-D bifurcation points and associated directional vectors (*blue*) projected to the same angiographic views as used for extraction of the 2-D bifurcation points and associated directional vectors (*red*) based on the initial transformation derived from the two viewing angles. (c) The final transformation is determined after minimization of the distances between the projected 3-D and extracted 2-D bifurcation points and the angles between the projected 3-D and 2-D directional vectors in both views

13 Coronary Angiography

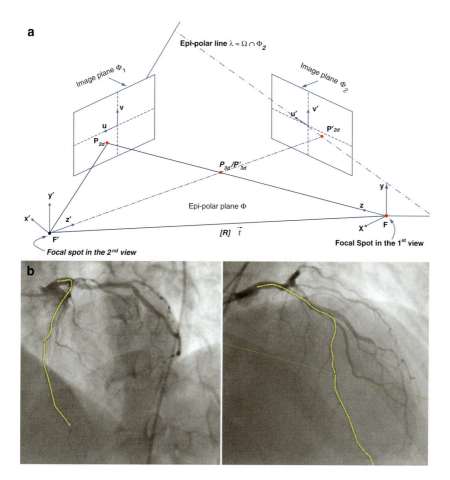

Fig. 13.8 (**a**) The schematic diagram of epi-polar theory: the epi-polar plane Ω, which is defined by the two focal spots (i.e., F in the first view and F' in the second view) and the point P_{2d} on image plane Φ_2 projected from the 3-D point P_{3d}, should contain the point P'_{2d} on the other image plane Φ_1 projected from the same 3-D point P_{3d}. Besides, the epi-polar line λ resulting from the intersection between the image plane Φ_1 and epi-polar plane Ω should pass through the projection point P'_{2d}. (**b**) The initial correspondence of a vessel centerline point (a *red dot*) in the first view (*left*) is established by calculating the intersection between the epi-polar line (a *green straight line*) and the 2-D vessel centerline curve in the second view (*right*)

13.3.2
Basic 3-D Quantitative Coronary Analysis

Coronary arteries possess a curvilinear shape as observed in all vascular trees and are unique because they also undergo a cyclical deformation due to their attachment to the myocardium. It is necessary to obtain a patient-specific 3-D vascular structure so that the dynamic curvilinear nature of the human coronary artery can be best described and quantified. The skeleton of a reconstructed 3-D artery can be mathematically defined as a curve function $p(s) = (x(s), y(s), z(s))$ connecting all the 3-D centerline points with associated cross-sectional

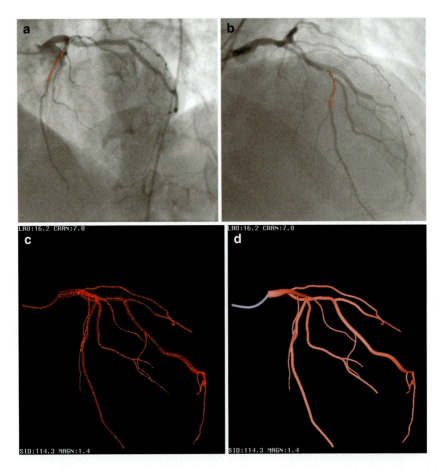

Fig. 13.9 (**a**, **b**) The typical example of segment-to-segment matching on the pair of arterial segments to refine the vessel centerline point-to-point correspondences based on a minimization process. (**c**) The calculated skeleton structure of left coronary arterial (LCA) tree in the forms of 3-D vessel centerlines and associated cross sections. (**d**) The surface-based graphic rendering technique to display the 3-D LCA tree (*pink*) and the catheter (*light blue*)

contours (e.g., circular disks perpendicular to the directional vector at each vessel centerline point) where variable s denotes the arc length along the vessel centerline as shown in Fig. 13.8e. The function that defines a vessel centerline curve is detailed in Appendix B.

13.3.2.1
Evaluation of the Length of Arterial Segment, Take-Off Angle of Side-Branch, and Volume-Based Percent Stenosis

The 3-D vessel centerline is characterized by a parametric curve function in terms of an ordered sequence of 3-D data points as described previously. With the reconstructed

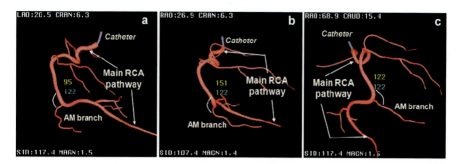

Fig. 13.10 The typical example of true 3-D take-off angle (122°) of side-branch (pointed by *arrow*) vs. its 2-D take-off angles estimated in various projection views in a right coronary arterial tree that may cause (**a**) an underestimated angle (95°), (**b**) an overestimated angle (151°), or (**c**) a correct estimated angle

coronary arterial tree, a segment of the artery, the entire artery, or a pathway consisting of multiple arteries can be selected as the region-of-interest (ROI). The length of the ROI can be calculated by the summation of the interdistance of every pair of consecutive vessel centerline points or by numerical integral of the parametric function $\rho(s)$.

Based on the generated patient-specific coronary arterial tree, the true 3-D take-off angle of a branch vessel can be estimated by calculating the angle between the two tangent vectors originating from the bifurcation; i.e., one toward the direction of precedent vessel and the other toward the direction of branching vessel. The view-dependent 2-D take-off angle of a branch vessel can be computed by first computing the branch vessel and proceeding vessel centerlines projected onto the imaging plane based on the gantry orientation followed by calculating the angle of the 2-D tangent vectors associated with the projected 3-D vessel centerlines. When the projected 2-D take-off angle is identical or very close to the true 3-D take-off angle for a specific side-branch, the corresponding gantry orientation in terms of LAO/RAO and CAUD/CRAN can be adopted as the "fluoscopic working view," minimizing vessel foreshortening for subsequent digital image acquisition or continuous fluoroscopy reviewing to facilitate the diagnostic or therapeutic procedure as shown in Fig. 13.10a–c.

By the use of 3-D modeling of the artery characterized by n vessel centerline points and associated cross-sectional diameters a_i and b_i calculated from two angiographic views, the percent luminal volume narrowing $V^{vol}_{\%narrowing}$ can be calculated, so that the resultant estimate will be more accurate than that calculated from the conventional approach based on a single 2-D image only; especially when the lesion shape is eccentric. The estimate of volume narrowing is computed based on the equation as described in Appendix C.

13.3.2.2
Evaluation of the Tortuosity of Artery

By the use of such a spline-based curve modeling technique, we are able to apply the theory of differential geometry such as Frenet-Serret apparatus (F-S theory)[57] or its variation to study the geometrical nature of the 3-D coronary artery at any time frame in the cardiac cycle. A technique based on the F-S theory of differential geometry has been developed to

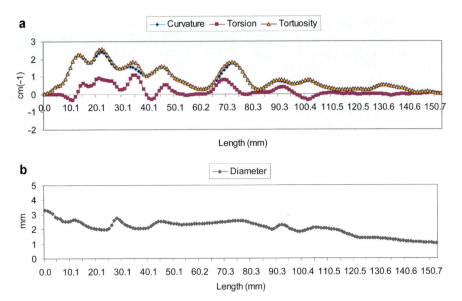

Fig. 13.11 (a) The estimates of curvature, torsion, and tortuosity associated with the pathway of the main right coronary artery as indicated in Fig. 13.10. (b) The averaged cross-sectional diameter profile of the main right coronary arterial pathway

study the geometrical nature or tortuosity of the 3-D coronary artery shape at any time frame in the cardiac cycle.[58,59] The F-S theory consists of five components: three vector fields along the given curve (the tangent $T(s)$, the normal $N(s)$, and the bi-normal $B(s)$ vectors) and two scalar valued functions (the curvature $\kappa(s)$ and the torsion $\tau(s)$), where (s) denotes the parametric variable defining the location of the point on the curve function $\rho(s)$. The curvature $\kappa(s_i)$ measures the rate of change of the angle defined by the two neighboring tangents $T(s_i)$ and $T(s_i + \delta)$ associated with the two points, $\rho(s_i)$ and $\rho(s_i + \delta)$. In other words, it characterizes the degree of bending pertinent to a local curve segment in the neighborhood between s_i and $(s_i + \delta)$ (i.e., how rapidly the curve pulls away from the plane perpendicular to the tangent vector at $T(s_i)$. Similarly, the torsion $\tau(s_i)$ measures the rate of change (or twisting) at a point $\rho(s_i)$ and how its trajectory twists out of the plane perpendicular to the normal vector $B(s_i)$. The curvature and torsion at every vessel centerline point $\rho(s_i)$ can be calculated by the use of the equations as described in Appendix D. Generally, these estimates $(T(s), N(s), B(s), \kappa(s), \tau(s))$ define a microscopic approach to look in very small neighborhoods of points. Therefore, they are regarded as primitives for assessing the local geometrical property of a vessel centerline curve (see Fig. 13.11).

13.3.2.3
Evaluation of the Discrete Flexion Point of Artery Throughout a Cardiac Cycle

Coronary arteries demonstrate significant *dynamic* shape change; i.e., vessel curvature changes with respect to time. This phasic change has been shown in cell culture models to impact endothelial function. Endothelial cells subjected to oscillating stretch demonstrate altered gene expression for endothelin, growth factors, and regulators of fibrinogen.[60] Moreover, clinical events such as restenosis appear to be accelerated at areas of cyclic curvature change, the so-called flexion areas.[61] Thus, geometric description of human coronary arteries represents a potentially useful method for understanding both the natural and treated history of coronary artery disease.

The analysis is performed by comparing the coronary trees reconstructed at two different time points (e.g., end diastole and end systole). The "enclosed angle" (θ) is defined as the angle formed by two chords that extend from a point along the centerline to the next local curvature maxima (inflection point) in each direction. The enclosed angle is calculated for end diastole (θ_{ED}) and end systole (θ_{ES}) for every point of the centerline as shown in Fig. 13.12a. The "flexion angle," defined as the difference between θ_{ED} and θ_{ES}, is calculated for every point along the centerline ($\Theta_{FP} = \theta_{ED} - \theta_{ES}$). Local maxima of acute bending are named "flexion points." If the value of Θ_{FP} is a local minimum and greater than 15°, that vessel centerline point is counted as a flexion point. In Fig. 13.12b, the right coronary arterial trees created at end diastole and end systole time points are used as an example to demonstrate the aforementioned estimates. The enclosed angles of vessel centerlines at end diastole and end systole are shown in Figure 13.12c and there are six flexion points along the main RCA pathway that are identified as shown in Figure 13.12d, respectively.

13.4
Clinical Application of 3-D Angiography

With the development of 3-D modeling techniques and basic quantitative analysis, the limitations of traditional use of 2-D angiography can be minimized. The 3-D imaging is capable of quantifying vessel curvature, measuring vessel segment length, and identifying the amount of radiographic foreshortening and vessel overlap in any simulated angiographic projection.

The 3-D modeling and optimal view selection protocol to assist on-line PCI procedure involves the following steps:

1. Routine cardiac catheterization is initiated and standard coronary angiographic acquisitions are completed in two views based on two injections using a single plane imaging system.
2. A pair of image sequences consisting of 8 (15 frames/s rate) or 15 images (30 frames/s rate) at each view are chosen and transferred to a computer workstation.
3. The 2-D coronary arterial trees are identified in the selected pair of angiograms (e.g., images corresponding to end-diastole) and the vessel features are extracted including vessel centerlines, diameters, bifurcation points, directional vectors of bifurcations, and hierarchy.
4. The processing of 3-D modeling is completed by the use of information from identified vessel features and results in a 3-D patient-specific coronary arterial tree model.
5. Manual indication of a vessel segment(s) of interest (e.g., region of a coronary stenosis) on the projection from the generated 3-D coronary model is performed by marking the proximal and distal points of the desired arterial segment(s) or bifurcation.

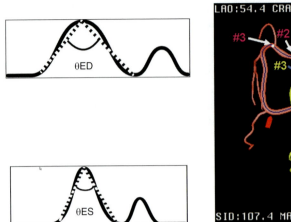
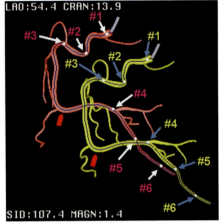
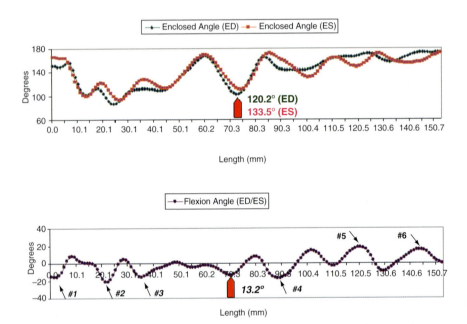

Fig. 13.12 (a) The schematic diagrams illustrating the enclosed angles of arterial centerline point at end diastole (*upper panel*) and end systole (*lower panel*). (b) The generated 3-D right coronary arterial trees at end diastole (*pink*) and end systole (*yellow*) where the pathway of the main right coronary artery is selected for 3-D quantitative analysis. (c) The enclosed angles at every vessel centerline points associated with the pathways at end diastolic and end systolic time points where the two prominent angles at end diastole (120.2°) and end systole (133.5°) are indicated by *red arrows*. (d) The plot of flexion angles calculated from the differences of enclosed angles shows six flexion points (>15°). Although the corresponding enclosed angles are prominent, the flexion angle is only 13.2° as indicated by *red arrows*

6. The processing of geometry and tortuosity analysis on the selected vessel segment/bifurcation of interest and the pathway from the ostium to the targeting segment is completed and the 3-D based quantitative estimates are reported and displayed.
7. The processing of optimal views is completed that minimize the foresortening and overlapping of the selected vessel segment(s) and results in a sequence of projections associated with the gantry orientations.

The cardiologist incorporates the created 3-D coronary model predictions of which views, in terms of gantry angles, will have minimal vessel overlap and foreshortening associated with the coronary arterial segment or bifurcation to acquire additional images for detailed diagnosis or adopt them as fluoscopic working view(s) to guide therapeutic procedure. The results of quantitative analyses will be used to optimize the selection of adequate intracoronary devices such as guide-wire, guiding catheter, and stent. The tortuosity of the pathway through which the intracoronary devices are traversed and delivered can be evaluated and quantified based on the methods described in the previous section. Generally speaking, more flexible guide-wire and catheters will be used for pathways with highly tortuous shapes or containing side-branches with acute take-off angles.

Stents are tiny flexible wire mesh tubes that prop open blocked arteries in the heart. Drug-eluting stents are coated with slowly released drugs that help prevent cell regrowth that can renarrow the artery. Implanted stents may result in a permanent modification of the curvilinearity of the artery. Although the benefits of stent implantation have been widely appreciated and yielded an explosion in the number of stents implanted around the world, the impact of arterial straightening by the stent has not been well studied. It has been hypothesized that the frequently observed straightening effect of stents implies an uneven distribution of forces within the arterial wall, potentially augmenting the injury reaction of the vessel wall and thereby increasing the rate of restenosis. The impact of stent-induced arterial straightening during cardiac contraction is also unknown, but is clearly greater at ES when arteries are normally more tortuous, shortened, and flexed.

In Fig. 13.13a, b, the proximal lesion is shown on the right coronary angiograms acquired at end diastole and end systole, respectively, and the dramatic change in shape within the stenotic region during the cardiac cycle is apparent. The first 3.5 × 18 mm CYPHER drug-eluting stent was deployed to cover the stenotic region and a significant hinge point occurred at the proximal end as shown in Fig. 13.13c. The second 3.5 × 11 mm drug-eluting stent was placed to overlap the proximal end of the first stent in an attempt to minimize the hinge point. However, a new hinge point was created from its previous location shifting it to the proximal end of the second stent as shown in Fig. 13.13d. At the end, a more flexible traditional (non drug-eluting) 4.0 × 12 mm Driver stent was implanted and overlapped with the proximal end of the second stent. At this time, it was evident that a new hinge point at the distal end of the first CYPHER stent occurred with another minor hinge point at the proximal end of the third stent as shown in Fig. 13.13e. "Hinge points" may also occur if the edge of a stiffer stent is placed close to a cyclic flexion point.

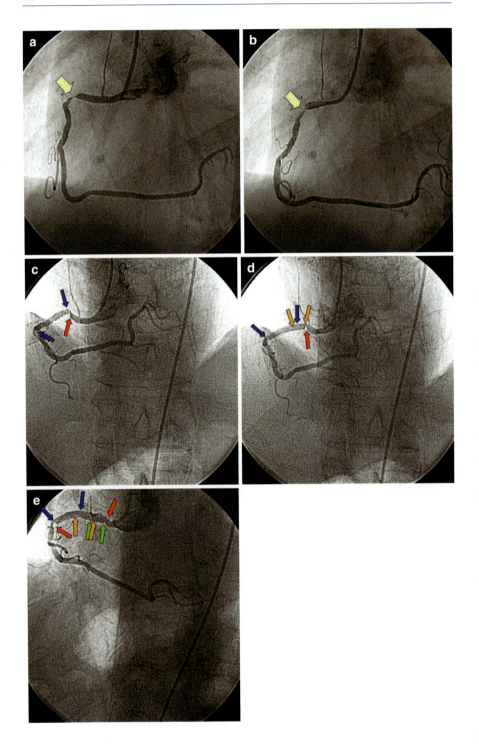

The vessel centerline point is defined as a flexion if: (a) its curvature (or enclosed angle) is a local maximum (or minimum) and greater than 1.2 cm^{-1} (or smaller than 150°) at end diastole or end systole, or (b) its curvature difference (or flexion angle) between the end diastole and end systole is greater than 0.6 cm^{-1} (or greater than 15°). By the use of the tortuosity analysis, the location of flexion point will be highlighted. If multiple flexion points appear on the arterial segment, the length between every two adjacent flexion points will also be reported to facilitate selection of the adequate size stent and determination of appropriate location for stent placement.

The typical example of a patient's left coronary arterial (LCA) tree is used to demonstrate how the 3-D quantitative coronary analysis can be utilized to assist PCI. The two pairs of routine angiograms acquired at end-diastole and end-systole are shown in Fig. 13.14a–d, where the two stenotic lesions occur at the mid left circumflex and ostium of the obtuse marginal artery. The 3-D patient-specific coronary arterial trees at end diastole and end systole are created and the stenotic segments at the obtuse marginal artery are identified for quantitative analysis as shown in Fig. 13.14e, f, respectively.

By the use of the selected vessel segments on the obtuse marginal artery, the results of advanced 3-D quantitative analyses[58,59] including curvatures, take-off angles, and dimensions of lesion size are shown in Fig. 13.15a, b, and the quantitative tortuosity and flexion points are shown in Fig. 13.15c, d, respectively. There are two flexion points identified in the area of the target lesion. The first flexion point with a large flexion angle (>30°) suggests a stent length shorter than 15 mm to avoid severe arterial straightening and cyclic bending force that may potentially cause stent fracture. Because the stenotic lesion is located near the ostium of obtuse marginal branch, the fluoscopic view requires the bifurcation region to be visualized with minimal vessel foreshortening and overlapping for PCI.[62,63] The bifurcation region in terms of two vessel segments is manually selected on the projection of the 3-D coronary tree in Fig. 13.16a. Afterwards, the optimal view map is derived that defines the combined percentage of vessel foreshortening and overlap of the selected obtuse marginal bifurcation with respect to the gantry orientation in terms of LAO/RAO and CRAN/CAUD angles as shown in Fig. 13.16b, where three viewing angles as indicated on the grey color regions on the map are suggested. The computer-predicted projections of the patient's LCA tree based on the suggested viewing angles are illustrated in Fig. 13.16c–e such that the interventionist can use them as fluoscopic working views for subsequent therapeutic intervention.

Fig. 13.13 The baseline right coronary angiograms acquired at an end diastolic time point (**a**) and a end systolic time point (**b**) show the lesion by a *yellow arrow*. (**c**) After a 3.5 × 18-mm CYPHER drug-eluting stent was placed as indicated by a pair of *blue arrows*, the narrowing was effectively eliminated, but a hinge point was created (*red arrow*). (**d**) The second 3.5 × 11 mm CYPHER drug-eluting stent ($3,000 cost) was then placed to overlap the proximal end and its portion is indicated by a pair of *orange arrows*. Note that the new hinge point was shifted to the proximal end of the new stent as indicated by the *red arrow*. (**e**) Two hinge points appeared as indicated by the individual two *red arrows* after the third 4.0 × 12 mm Driver (more flexible, nondrug-eluting stent, cost $1,000) was implanted to overlap the proximal end of the second CYPHER stent as indicated by a pair of *green arrows*

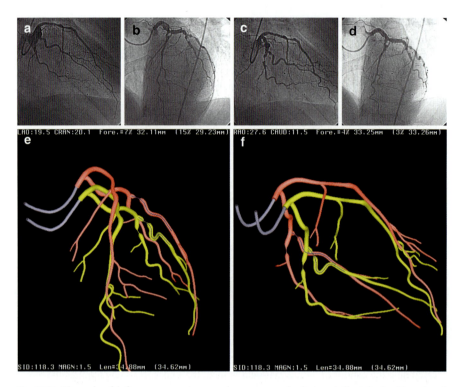

Fig. 13.14 The pair of left coronary artery angiograms acquired at end diastole (**a**, **b**) and end systole (**c**, **d**), where the two stenotic lesions are located near the bifurcation between the mid left circumflex artery and obtuse marginal side-branch. (**e**, **f**) The 3-D models of the LCA tree at end diastole (*pink*) and end systole (*yellow*) generated by the use of the two pairs of angiograms, where the stentoic segments at the obtuse marginal artery are selected for 3-D quantitative analysis

13.5 Summary

Many advances in coronary artery imaging are now being driven by the ability to process the digital images. There is clinical value in the first step of transforming 2-D projection images into a 3-D model of the patient's arterial tree. There is further value in performing a quantitative analysis of key geometric features from this 3-D tree. Finally, decision-making support can provide assistance to the physician in solving imaging tasks such as the determination of an optimal projection view of a coronary artery lesion needing treatment. Each of these three important processes must occur in the clinical environment where actions must be made within minutes of image acquisition. Furthermore, the information must be presented to the physician using graphics that are intuitive and useful. This chapter has outlined the amazing advances in coronary imaging that have come from the labor of imaging scientists and physicians working together.

13 Coronary Angiography

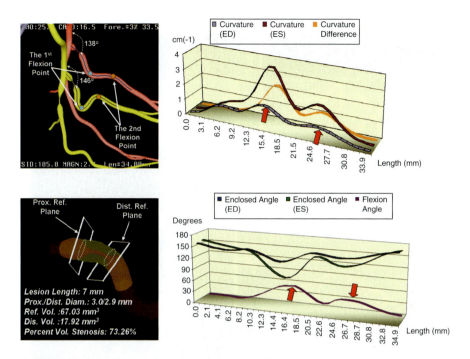

Fig. 13.15 (**a**) The arterial segments with stenosis at end diastole (*pink*) and end systole (*yellow*) are selected for advanced 3-D quantitative analysis to facilitate the selection of adequate stent size for stent implantation, where the 3-D take-off angles (i.e., 138° and 146°) of obtuse marginal branch are calculated and two flexion points (*green* and *orange circles*) are identified. (**b**) The results of advanced 3-D quantitative coronary angiography calculated at end diastole for lesion size (i.e., 7 mm length and proximal/distal cross sections diameters 3.0/2.9 mm) and percent volume stenosis 73.26%. (**c**) The individual curvatures of the stenotic segments at end diastole and end systole and the curvature differences. (**d**) The estimates of enclosed angles and identified flexion points associated with the stenotic arterial segments

13.6 Appendix A

In our implementation of the deformation algorithm, the internal energy E_{int} and image force E_{image} in energy functional E^*_{snake} are adopted as follows.

$$E^*_{snake} = \int_0^1 E_{int}(v(s)) + E_{image}(v(s))\, ds, \quad (13.1)$$

where the initial curves drawn by the operator is parameterized by $v(s) = (x(s), y(s)), s = 0,\cdots 1$. The internal energy function was further defined by a first-order term $|v_s(s)|$ and a second-order term $|v_{ss}(s)|$ in the following:

$$E_{int}(v(s)) = (\alpha(s)|v_s(s)|^2 + \beta(s)|v_{ss}(s)|^2)/2, \quad (13.2)$$

where $\alpha(s)$ and $\beta(s)$ are the weighting function. The image force term $E_{image}(v(s))$ is governed by the inverted grey level of "valley points" (e.g., the maximal grey level

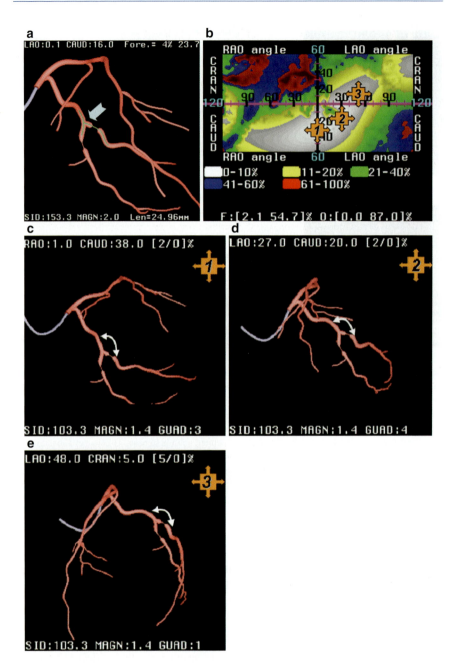

Fig. 13.16 (**a**) The bifurcation region indicated by two *green curves* is selected for optimal view analysis. (**b**) The calculated optimal view map defining the gantry angles with respect to the combined measurements of vessel foreshortening and overlap where three angiographic views are suggested (i.e., the combined vessel foreshortening and overlap <10% in *grey* color region). (**c–e**) The projections of the 3-D LCA tree based on the suggested angiographic views that shows minimal vessel overlap and foreshortening associated with the obtuse marginal bifurcation as indicated by the *double arrows*

256 − $g_{(i,j)}$) where the associated pixel have the minimal grey level $g_{(i,j)}$ within a $k \times k$ window (where k is selected as the average 2-D cross-sectional width of the artery) centered at the pixel location (i,j). If the grey level of a pixel is not the local minimum within the $k \times k$ window, the corresponding image force at that location is suppressed.

13.7
Appendix B

The skeleton of a 3-D artery can be defined as a curve function $p(s) = (x(s), y(s), z(s))$ connecting all the 3-D centerline points with associated cross-sectional contours, where $0 \leq s \leq 1$ is the parametric variable in the form of normalized arc length of vessel centerline. The employed parametric function is a *Bézier* curve $p(s)$ that is formed as the Cartesian product of *Bézier* blending functions $B_{j,m}(s)$:

$$p(s) = \sum_{(j=0)}^{m} p_j B_{j,m}(s), 0 \leq s \leq 1 \quad (13.3)$$

subject to the constraints

$$p(s_i) = (x(s_i), y(s_i), z(s_i)), \quad 0 \leq s_i \leq 1, i = 0, 1, \cdots n_s,$$

where $p(s_i), i = 0, 1, \cdots, n_s$, with $(n_s + 1) \leq 4$, denotes the individual vessel centerline points, and $p_j, j = 0, \cdots m$, denotes the $(m+1)$ control points with $n_s \geq m \geq 3$. The employed constraints ensure that the derived curve function will pass through the vessel centerline points. $B_{j,m}(s)$ is a polynomial function of degree one less than the number of control points used (i.e., at least a third order derivative function) and is defined as

$$B_{j,m(s)} = C(m, j) s^j (1-s)^{m-j}$$

and $C(m, j)$ represent the binomial coefficients

$$C(m, j) = \frac{m!}{j!(m-j)!}.$$

13.8
Appendix C

By the use of the 3-D modeling of an artery characterized by n vessel centerline points and associated cross-sectional diameters a_i and b_i calculated from two angiographic views, the percent luminal volume narrowing $V^{vol}_{\%\,narrowing}$ can be calculated as follows:

$$V^{vol}_{\%\,narrowing} = \frac{V_H - V_D}{V_H} * 100\%,$$

$$V_D = \sum_{i-1}^{n-1} \frac{(\pi a_i b_i + \pi a_{i+1} b_{i+1})}{2} l_i^{i+1},$$

$$V_H = \sum_{i-1}^{j-1} \frac{(\pi a_i b_i + \pi a_{i+1} b_{i+1})}{2} l_i^{i+1} + \frac{(\pi a_j b_j + \pi a_k b_k)}{2} l_j^k + \sum_{i=k+1}^{n-1} \frac{(\pi a_i b_i + \pi a_{i+1} b_{i+1})}{2} l_i^{i+1}, \quad (13.4)$$

where V_H and V_D denote the reference (or healthy) and diseased luminal volume of arterial segments, l_r^s represents the curve length between the rth and sth vessel centerline points, and j and k denote the jth and the kth centerline points of reference cross sections with normal lumen, respectively.

13.9 Appendix D

The calculation of curvature and torsion at every vessel centerline point $\rho(s_i)$ is characterized by the following equations:

$$T(s_i) = \frac{\rho^{(1)}(s_i)}{|\rho^{(1)}(s_i)|},$$

$$B(s_i) = \frac{\rho^{(1)}(s_i) \times \rho^{(2)}(s_i)}{|\rho^{(1)}(s_i) \times \rho^{(2)}(s_i)|},$$

$$N(s_i) = B(s_i) \times T(s_i),$$

$$\kappa(s_i) = \frac{|\rho^{(1)}(s_i) \times \rho^{(2)}(s_i)|}{|\rho^{(1)}(s_i)|^3},$$

$$\tau(s_i) = \frac{(\rho^{(1)}(s_i) \times \rho^{(2)}(s_i)) \circ \rho^{(3)}(s_i)}{|\rho^{(1)}(s_i) \times \rho^{(2)}(s_i)|^2} \quad (13.5)$$

where $\rho^{(k)}(s_i)$ denotes the kth derivative with respect to s_i. With (13.5), a single value measurement "tortuosity index" $\upsilon(s_i)$ is derived using the following equation:

$$\upsilon(s_i) = \sqrt{\kappa(s_i)^2 + \tau(s_i)^2}. \quad (13.6)$$

Generally, (13.5) and (13.6) define a microscopic approach to look in very small neighborhoods of points.

References

1. Radner S. Attempt at roentgenologic visualization of coronary blood vessels in man. *Acta Radiol.* 1945;26:497–502.
2. Sones FM Jr, Shirey EK. Cine coronary arteriography. *Mod Concepts Cardiovasc Dis.* 1962; 31:735–738.
3. Kim WY, Danias PG, Stuber M, et al. Coronary magnetic resonance angiography for the detection of coronary stenoses. *N Engl J Med.* 2001;345:1863–1869.
4. Achenbach S, Giesler T, Ropers D, et al. Detection of coronary artery stenoses by contrast-enhanced, retrospectively electrocardiographically gated, multislice spiral computed tomography. *Circulation.* 2001;103:2535–2538.
5. Achenbach S, Moshage W, Ropers D, Nossen J, Daniel WG. Value of electronbeam computed tomography for the noninvasive detection of high-grade coronary artery stenoses and occlusions. *N Engl J Med.* 1998;339:1964–1971.

6. Friesinger GC, Page EE, Ross RS. Prognostic significance of coronary arteriography. *Trans Assoc Am Physicians*. 1970;83:78–92.
7. Oberman A, Jones WB, Riley CP, Reeves TJ, Sheffield LT, Turner ME. Natural history of coronary artery disease. *N Y Acad Med*. 1972;48:1109–1125.
8. Bruschke AV, Proudfit WL, Sones FM FM. Progress study of 590 consecutive non-surgical cases of coronary disease followed for 5 to 9 years. I: arterographic correlations. *Circulation*. 1973;47:1147–1153.
9. Scanlon PJ, Faxon DP, Audet AM, et al. ACC/AHA guidelines for coronary angiography: a report of the American College Curr Probl Cardiol, March 2004 137 of Cardiology/American Heart Association task force on practice guidelines (committee on coronary angiography). *J Am Coll Cardiol*. 1999;33:1756–1824.
10. Poma J, Kuntz R, Bain D. Percutaneous coronary and valvular interventions. In: Zipes D, Libby P, Bonow R, Braunwald G, eds. *Braunwald's Heart Disease. Textbook of Cardiovascular Medicine*. 7th ed. Philadelphia PA: Elsevier Saunders; 2005:1367–1402.
11. Popma J. Coronary angiography and intravascular ultrasound. In: Zipes D, Libby P, Bonow R, Braunwald G, eds. *Braunwald's Heart Disease, Textbook of Cardiovascular Medicine*. 7th ed. Philadelphia PA: Elsevier Saunders; 2005:423–455.
12. Baim DS, Grossman W, eds. *Grossman's Cardiac Catheterization, Angiography and Intervention*. 6th ed. Philadelphia: Lippincott Williams & Wilkins; 2000.
13. Hirshfeld JW Jr et al. ACCF/AHA/HRS/SCAI Fluoroscopy Clinical Competence Statement. *JACC*. 2004;44(11):2259–2282.
14. Solomon R. Radiocontrast-induced nephropathy. *Semin Nephrol*. 1998;18:551–574.
15. Kereiakes D, Choo J, Young J, Broderick T. Thrombosis and drug-eluting stents. *Rev Cardiovasc Med*. 2004;5(1):9–14.
16. Sianos G, Hofma S, Ligthart J, et al. Stent fracture and restenosis in the drug-eluting stent era. *Cath Cardiovas Interven*. 2004;61:111–116.
17. Kim HC, Min BG, Lee TS, et al. 3-D digital subtraction angiography. *IEEE Trans Med Imaging*. 1982;MI-1:152–158.
18. Potel MJ, Rubin JM, Mackay SA, et al. Methods for evaluating cardiac wall motion in 3-d using bifurcation points of the coronary arterial tree. *Invest Radiol*. 1983;18:47–56.
19. Parker KL, Pope KL, van Bree R, et al. 3-D reconstruction of moving arterial beds from digital subtraction angiography. *Comput Biomed Res*. 1987;20:166–185.
20. Kitamura K, Tobis JM, Sklansky J. Estimating the 3-D skeletons and transverse areas of coronary arteries from biplane angiograms. *IEEE Trans Med Imaging*. 1988;MI-7:173–187.
21. Pellot CP, Herment A, Sigelle M, Horain P, Maitre H, Peronneau P. A 3-D reconstruction of vascular structures from two x-ray angiograms using an adapted simulated annealing algorithm. *IEEE Trans Med Imaging*. 1994;13(1):49–60.
22. Dumay ACM, Reiber JHC, Gerbrands JJ. Determination of optimal angiographic viewing angles: basic principles and evaluation study. *IEEE Trans Med Imaging*. 1994;13(1):13–24.
23. Nguyen TV, Sklansky J. Reconstructing the 3-D medial axes of coronary arteries in single-view cineangiograms. *IEEE Trans Med Imaging*. 1994;13(1):48–60.
24. Stansfield S. ANGI: a rule based expert system for automatic segmentation of coronary vessels from digital subtracted angiograms. *IEEE Trans PAMI*. 1986;8(2):188–199.
25. Garreau M, Coatrieux JL, Collorec R, Chardenon C. A knowledge-based approach for 3-D reconstruction and labeling of vascular networks from biplane angiographic projections. *IEEE Trans Med Imaging*. 1991;10(2):122–131.
26. Fessler JA, Macovski A. Object-based 3-D reconstruction of arterial trees from magnetic resonance angiograms. *IEEE Trans Med Imaging*. 1991;10(1):25–39.
27. Liu I, Sun Y. Fully automated reconstruction of 3-D vascular tree structures from two orthogonal views using computational algorithms and production rules. *Opt Eng*. 1992;31(10): 2197–2207.

28. Smith BD. Cone-beam tomography: recent advances and a tutorial review. *Opt Eng J.* 1990;29: 524–534.
29. Tuy HK. An inversion formula for cone-beam reconstruction. *SIAM J Appl Math.* 1983;43: 546–552.
30. Smith BD. Image reconstruction from cone-beam projections: necessary and sufficient conditions and reconstruction methods. *IEEE Trans Med Imaging.* 1985;MI-4:14–25.
31. Saint-Felix D, Picard C, Ponchut C, Romeas R, Rougee A, Trousset Y. *Three dimensional X-ray angiography: first in vivo results with a new system. SPIE: Medical Imaging: Image capture, formatting, and display.* Newport Beach, California; 1993, 1897:90–98.
32. Anxionat R, Bracard S, Macho J, et al. 3D angiography: clinical interest – first applications in interventional neuroradiology. *J Neuroradiol.* 1998;25:251–262.
33. Grass M, Koppe R, Klotz E, et al. Three-dimensional reconstruction of high contrast objects using C-arm image intensifier projection data. *Comput Med Imaging Graph.* 1999;23(6):311–321.
34. Moret J et al. 3D rotational angiography: clinical value in endovascular treatment. *Medica Mundi.* 1998;42(3):8–14.
35. Koppe R, Klotz E, Op de Beek J, Aerts H. *3D Vessel Reconstruction Based on Rotational Angiography. Proceedings CAR '95.* Berlin, June 21–24; 1995:101–107.
36. Koppe R, Klotz E, Op de Beek J, Aerts H. *Digital Stereotaxy/Stereotactic Procedures with C-Arm Based Rotational Angiography. Proceedings CAR '96.* Paris; 1996:17–22.
37. Koppe R, Klotz E, Op de Beek J, Aerts H, Kemkers R. *3D Reconstruction of Cerebral Vessel Malformations Based on Rotational Angiography (RA). Proceedings CAR '97.* Berlin; 1997: 145–151.
38. Kemkers R, Op de Beek J, Aerts H, Koppe R, Klotz E, Grass M, Moret J. *3D-Rotational Angiography: First Clinical Application with use of a Standard Philips C-Arm System. Proceedings CAR '98.* Tokyo; 1998:182–187.
39. Rougee A, Picard C, Sanit-Felix D, et al. 3-D coronary arteriography. *Int J Card Imaging.* 1994;10:67–70.
40. Roach JW, Aggarwal JK. Determining the movement of objects from a sequence of images. *IEEE Trans PAMI.* 1980;2:554–562.
41. Longuet-Higgins HC. A computer algorithm for reconstructing a scene from two projections. *Nature.* 1981;293(5828):133–135.
42. Tsai RY, Huang TS. Uniqueness and estimation of 3D motion parameters of rigid objects with curved surfaces. *IEEE Trans PAMI.* 1984;6(1):13–27.
43. Metz CE, Fencil LE. Determination of three-dimensional structure in biplane radiography without prior knowledge of the relationship between the two views: theory. *Med Phys.* 1989; 16(1):45–51.
44. Hoffmann KR, Metz CE, Chen Y. Determination of 3D imaging geometry and object configurations from two biplane views: an enhancement of the Metz-Fencil technique. *Med Phys.* 1995;22:1219–1217.
45. Weng J, Huang TS, Ahuja N. *A two-step approach to optimal motion and structure estimation. Proceeding IEEE Workshop Computer Vision.* 1987:355–357.
46. Weng J, Ahuja N, Huang T. *Closed-form solution and maximum likelihood: a robust approach to motion and structure estimation. Proceeding IEEE Conference Computer Vision and Pattern Recognition.* 1988:381–386.
47. Weng J, Huang TS, Ahuja N. Motion and structure from two perspective view: algorithms, error analysis and error estimation. *IEEE Trans PAMI.* 1989;11:451–476.
48. Weng J, Ahuja N, Huang TS. Optimal motion and structure estimation. *IEEE Trans PAMI.* 1993; 15(9):864–884.
49. Chen S-YJ, Metz CE. Improved determination of biplane imaging geometry from two projection images and its application to 3-D reconstruction of coronary arterial trees. *Med Phys.* 1997; 24(5):633–654.

50. Sprague K, Drangova M, Lehmann G, et al. Coronary X-ray angiographic reconstruction and image orientation. *Med Phys*. 2006;33(3):707–718.
51. Movassaghi B, Rasche V, Grass M, Viegever M, Nissen W. A quantitative analysis of 3-D coronary modeling from two or more projection images. *IEEE Trans Med Imaging*. 2004; 23(12):1517–1531.
52. Blondel C, Malandain G, Vaillant R, Ayache N. Reconstruction of coronary arteries from a single rotational X-Ray projection sequence. *IEEE Trans Med Imaging*. 2006;25(5):653–663.
53. Chen S-YJ, Carroll JD. On-line 3-D reconstruction of coronary arterial tree based on a single-plane imaging system. *Circulation*. 1997;96(8):1–308.
54. Chen S-YJ, Carroll JD. On-line 3D reconstruction of coronary arterial tree for optimization of visualization strategy using a single-plane imaging system. *IEEE Trans Med Imaging*. 2000; 19(4):318–336.
55. Kass M, Witkin A, Terzopoulos D. Snakes: active contour models. *Int J Comput Vis*. 1988;1: 321–331.
56. Williams DJ, Shah M. A fast algorithm for active contours. *Int J Comput Vis*. 1992;55:14–21.
57. Millman RS, Parker GD. *Elements of Differential Geometry*. Prentice-NJ: Hall, Englewood Cliffs; 1977:13–48.
58. Chen S-YJ, John Carroll D, Messenger JC. Quantitative analysis of reconstructed 3-D coronary arterial tree and intracoronary devices. *IEEE Trans Med Imaging*. 2002;21(7):724–740.
59. Chen S-YJ, Carroll JD. Kinematic and deformation analysis of 4-D coronary arterial trees reconstructed from cine angiograms. *IEEE Trans Med Imaging*. 2003;22(6):710–721.
60. Davies PF, Tripathi SC. Mechanical stress mechanisms and the cell. *Circ Res*. 1993;72:239–245.
61. Stein PD, Hamid MS, Shivkumar K, et al. Effects of cyclic flexion of coronary arteries on progression of atherosclerosis. *Am J Cardiol*. 1994;73:431–437.
62. Green NE NE, Chen S-YJ, Hansgen AR, Messenger JC, Groves BM, Carroll JD. Angiographic views used for percutaneous coronary interventions: a tree-dimensional analysis of physician-determined versus computer-generated views. *Catheter Cardiovasc Interv*. 2005;64:451–459.
63. Garcia JA, Chen S-YJ, Hansgen A, Wink O, Movassaghi B, Messenger JC. Rotational angiography (RA) and three-dimensional imaging (3-DRA): an available clinical tool. *Int J Cardiovasc Imaging*. 2007;23(1):9–13.

Echocardiography

14

John Edward Abellera Blair and Vera H. Rigolin

14.1
Introduction to Ultrasound Imaging – The Physiologic Signal

Echocardiography is an imaging modality that takes advantages of the physical properties of sound. In echocardiography, *sound pulses* generated by a *transducer* travel through the thoracic cavity, reflect off structures around and in the heart, and return to the transducer, and are processed into images. This is similar to the way sound behaves in a canyon – as sound travels through the canyon, it is reflected off the walls of the canyon and returns to the original source as an echo. The sound pulses used in echocardiography are in the ultrasound range, or greater than 20,000 cycles per second (20 KHz), and are higher than the sound audible to humans, which is in the 20–20,000 Hz range. Several mammalian species use ultrasound to locate other animals and prey, including bats, dolphins, whales, and some fish. They take advantage of the following properties of ultrasound: it can be directed and focused, travels at different speeds through different media allowing for the discrimination of types of objects, and follows the laws of reflection and refraction. Similarly, ultrasound beams can be used in medical imaging and echocardiography.

Ultrasound, like all sound waves, is a *longitudinal wave* that carries *energy* in a straight line from one point to another. In a longitudinal wave, particles in a given medium move in the same direction of the wave propagation (Fig. 14.1). As particles are compressed and decompressed along the axis of the beam, areas of *compression* or *rarefaction* are formed. This may be represented as a sine wave, where peaks represent the areas of compression and troughs represent the areas of rarefaction, both expressed in units of pressure (Fig. 14.2). A *cycle* is composed of one compression and one rarefaction, while a *wavelength* is the distance the cycle travels, and the *frequency* is the number of wavelengths per unit of time. The *velocity* an ultrasound wave travels can thus be expressed as:

$$v = f \times \lambda$$

J.E.A. Blair (✉)
Department of Medicine, Division of Cardiology,
Wilford Hall Medical Center; Lackland, AFB, TX and
Uniformed Services University of the Health Sciences, Bethesda, MD
e-mail: jblair1@gmail.com

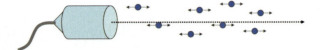

Fig. 14.1 Schematic representation of a longitudinal wave. Ultrasound produced by a transducer is directed away from the transducer (*black dotted line*) and the particles (*blue dots*) in the wave move back and forth in the same direction of the wave

where v is the velocity, f is the frequency, and λ is the wavelength. The velocity of sound, expressed in meters/second, is determined only by the medium through which the sound is traveling. Even waves with different frequencies travel through a given medium at the same velocity. In general, the velocity of sound is slowest in gasses such as air, fastest in solids such as bone, and intermediate in fluids such as blood. The velocity of sound is directly related to the stiffness of the material and inversely related to the density. Velocities of sound in various materials are reported in Table 14.1. The frequency of sound produced in echocardiography is expressed in cycles per second, or Hertz (Hz), and ranges from 2,000,000 to 45,000,000 Hz (2.0 to 45.0 MHz). Wavelength, expressed in meters (m) is therefore determined by both the ultrasound source and the medium, and is an important determinant of the resolution of an image. Another important quality of ultrasound waves

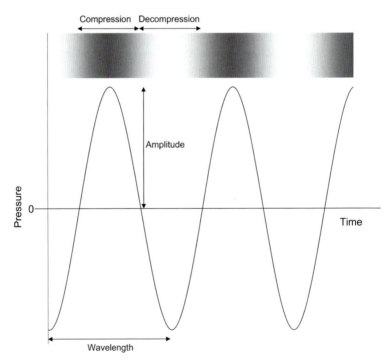

Fig. 14.2 Longitudinal wave depicted as a sine wave. Areas of compression are represented as a peak and decompression (rarefaction) as a trough. The *x*-axis is time and the *y*-axis is power. Wavelength is the distance (in units of time) from one peak to the next, while amplitude is the height (in units of pressure) from baseline to peak

14 Echocardiography

Table 14.1 Velocity of sound in various media

Medium	Velocity (m/s)
Air	330
Lung	500
Fat	1,450
Water	1,480
Soft tissue	1,540
Liver, kidney	1,560
Blood	1,570
Muscle	1,600
Tendon	1,700
Bone	3,500

is the *amplitude*, or strength of the wave, which is the difference in pressure between either the peak or trough and the average pressure of the wave. Amplitude is usually expressed in *decibels* (dB), a unit on a logarithmic scale relative to a standardized baseline value. Amplitude can be controlled by the ultrasound source. The squared amplitude is proportional to *power*, usually expressed in watts (W), and represents the rate of energy transfer of the ultrasound. *Intensity* is the ultrasound's power per unit area and is usually expressed in W/cm^2.

Since ultrasound waves carry energy, as waves enter the body, their energy is transmitted to objects within the body. As a result, the ultrasound waves weaken as they propagate – a process known as *attenuation*. Attenuation is directly proportional to the distance an ultrasound wave travels and to the frequency of the ultrasound wave. In addition, attenuation occurs in three forms: reflection, scattering, and absorption (Fig. 14.3). The above properties of ultrasound can be used for medical imaging. As ultrasound strikes an object, a portion of the wave's energy bounces, or reflects back to the sound source. *Reflection* occurs in two varieties – specular and diffuse. *Specular reflection* occurs at predictable angles from the source when the object is smooth, while *diffuse reflection* (or backscatter) occurs at multiple angles from the source when the object surface is irregular, as in most surfaces in the body. *Scattering* of ultrasound is the erratic and random motion of waves after encountering particles smaller than the source wavelength. Finally, *absorption* is the direct conversion of ultrasound energy into another form of energy such as heat, and is the most significant contributor to attenuation. Generally, transthoracic echocardiography uses transducer frequencies of 2.0–5.0 MHz. At 2 MHz, structures in the heart distant to the transducer can be imaged with minimal attenuation, at the expense of image accuracy and resolution. However, if higher frequencies were used, the ultrasound signal would become attenuated, especially at greater depths, but the image accuracy and resolution is better in the depths that are not attenuated. The goal of ultrasound imaging, therefore, is to maximize the frequency to attain adequate imaging, without losing the ability to image deep structures because of attenuation.

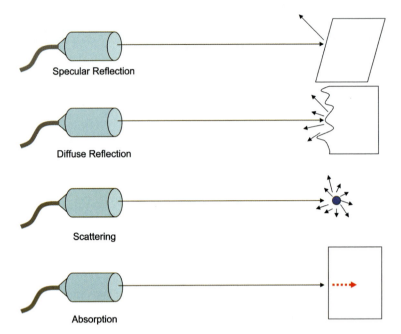

Fig. 14.3 Types of attenuation. Specular reflection occurs when ultrasound encounters a smooth surface and is reflected. Diffuse reflection occurs when ultrasound is reflected in many directions after the beam encounters an irregular surface. Scattering occurs when ultrasound of higher wavelength than an object is diffusely scattered by the object. In all cases, energy is absorbed by the object and accounts for the majority of the attenuation

14.2 Creating and Receiving the Signal – The Transducer

The ultrasound transducer is a critical element to ultrasound instrumentation. All forms of transducers convert one form of energy to another. The ultrasound transducer both *transmits* ultrasound energy converted from electrical energy and *receives* ultrasound energy and converts it into electrical energy for signal processing. The critical component of the ultrasound transducer is the *piezoelectric crystal*. Piezoelectric crystals are substances that rapidly vibrate when an electric current is applied, creating sound waves through the vibration of the material. These crystals also create electric signals when deformed by reflected sound waves. The ultrasound transducer is composed of many such crystals coupled to electrodes that connect to the ultrasound system. These crystals are arranged in two dimensions and interconnected electronically to form a *phased-array transducer*, the most common type of transducer used in cardiac ultrasound.

In order to send and receive ultrasound signals, short bursts, or *pulses* of acoustic energy are produced, alternating with periods of time where ultrasound waves are not created, or *dead time* (Fig. 14.4). Each pulse contains many cycles of ultrasound energy. The *pulse duration* is the amount of time required for the pulse to start and finish, while the *pulse length* is

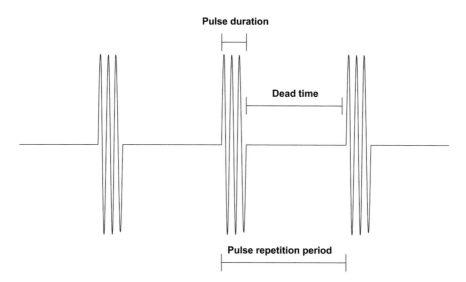

Fig. 14.4 Sending and receiving the signal. A pulse is a collection of several short bursts of ultrasound. The pulse duration is the time required for the pulse to start and finish. Dead time is the amount of time between pulses when the transducer is available to receive signals. PRP is the total amount of time from the beginning of one pulse to the end of the dead time. PRF is the number of pulses in 1 s and can be calculated using 1/PRP

the wavelength of each cycle multiplied by the number of cycles per pulse. The pulse duration and length are fixed and determined by the manufacturer of the ultrasound instrumentation, since the wavelength, frequency, and number of cycles per pulse is determined primarily by transducer design. The *pulse repetition period (PRP)* is the time from the beginning of one pulse to another, and includes the time when no ultrasound is created. *Pulse repetition frequency (PRF)* is the number of pulses transmitted each second. It is during the dead time that the transducer does not send pulses and is able to receive ultrasound energy. The PRF can be adjusted by the operator. Higher PRFs lead to less dead time and therefore less time to receive ultrasound energy, allowing reflection from more shallow structures to be imaged. Lower PRFs lead to more dead time and therefore more time to receive ultrasound energy, allowing reflection from deeper structures to be imaged. While higher PRFs result in a better ability to image a moving object, they cannot image deeper structures as well as lower PRFs. The PRF should be optimized to maximize imaging depth while capturing the moving object.

14.3
Manipulating and Embellishing the Signal

The ultrasound signal can be optimized using the components of the instrumentation and the basic principles of sound. This section will provide several examples on how the signal is manipulated or embellished in order to optimize the image.

14.3.1
Adjusting the Ultrasound Beam

The beam leaving the transducer is generally hour glass-shaped. Initially, the beam width is the same as the diameter of the active element in the transducer, narrows until it reaches its smallest diameter, then widens. The *focal point* is the point where the beam diameter is the narrowest, and is half the diameter of the active element in the transducer. The *near field* is the distance from the transducer to the focal point, while the *far field* is the portion beyond the focal point. The *focal zone* is the region on either side of the focal point, where reflections are most accurate (Fig. 14.5). The distance to the *focal point* is the *focal depth* (l), and is described in the following equation:

$$l = r^2 / \lambda$$

where *r* is the transducer radius and λ is the wavelength.

The focal depth can be increased by *increasing the transducer size* and/or reducing the wavelength (*increasing the frequency*). Since the transducer size is fixed, focal depth is controlled by adjusting the frequency, which is limited by the fact that higher frequencies result in greater attenuation and less penetration of ultrasound energy, as discussed above. In addition, the width of the far field section of the ultrasound beam, or *divergence*, depends on the diameter of the active element in the transducer, and frequency of the ultrasound (Fig. 14.6). Smaller active transducer elements produce more divergent waves, while larger active transducer elements produce less divergent waves. In addition, higher frequency ultrasound reduces divergence, while lower frequency ultrasound increases divergence.

14.3.2
Improving Resolution

Resolution is the ability to distinguish between two objects, and is one of the most important variables in echocardiography. There are four types of resolution in echocardiography:

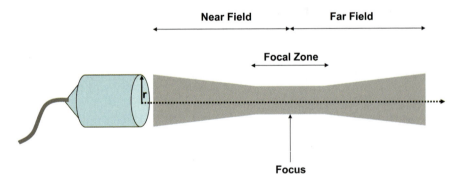

Fig. 14.5 Details of a sound beam. The focal point is the narrowest part of the beam, while the near field and the far field straddle the focal point. Imaging is optimal in the focal zone. The length to the focal point from the transducer is the focal depth, which is equal to the square of the radius of the active transducer element (r) divided by the wavelength of the ultrasound

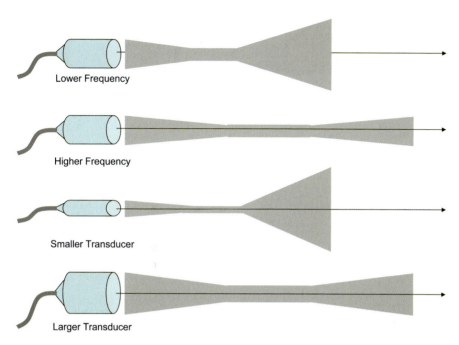

Fig. 14.6 Optimizing focal length and divergence. Lower frequencies shorten focal length and increase dispersion, while higher frequencies increase focal length and reduce dispersion. Smaller active transducer elements reduce focal length and increase dispersion, while larger active transducer elements increase focal length and reduce dispersion

axial, lateral, contrast, and temporal resolution (Fig. 14.7). *Axial resolution* is the ability to distinguish between structures parallel to the sound beam. *Lateral resolution* is the ability to distinguish between structures perpendicular to the sound beam. *Contrast resolution* is the ability to distinguish different shades of gray within the image. *Temporal resolution* is the ability to accurately track moving targets over time.

Axial resolution is directly proportional to the pulse length of the emitted ultrasound wave, and is represented in the following equation:

$$\text{Axial resolution (mm)} = \text{pulse length (mm)}/2.$$

Since pulse length is equal to the wavelength × the number of cycles per pulse, axial resolution is directly proportional to the wavelength and cycles per pulse, and inversely proportional to the frequency. To optimize axial resolution (lower number), a shorter wavelength (higher frequency) or smaller number of cycles is needed. Axial resolution is fixed and determined by the manufacturer of the ultrasound instrumentation.

Lateral resolution is best at the beam focal point, and is equal to the beam diameter. Similar to axial resolution, lateral resolution is expressed as distance, and is best when smallest. Also, lateral resolution improves with higher frequency, but for different reasons: higher frequency causes less divergence and therefore a narrower beam and better lateral resolution. In addition, the size of the active transducer element optimizes the lateral resolution because this can reduce divergence as well. Transducer design is therefore critical to the optimization of both types of resolution.

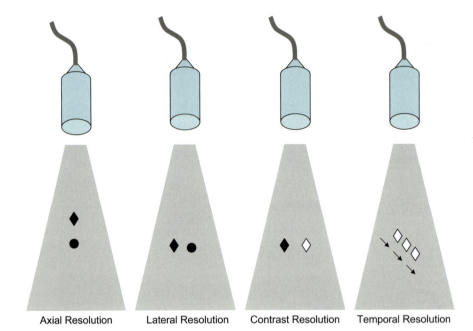

Fig. 14.7 Types of resolution. Axial resolution distinguishes between structures parallel to the sound beam and is dependent on the pulse length and frequency. Lateral resolution distinguishes between structures perpendicular to the sound beam and is dependent on the frequency and depth. Contrast resolution distinguishes different shades of gray within the image and is dependent on the processing of the image and image size. Temporal resolution tracks moving objects over time and is dependent on depth, PRF, angle, and line density

Adequate *contrast resolution* helps accurately display borders of structures and textures within structures for diagnostic purposes. Data received by the transducer are processed into grayscale images during pre- and postprocessing of the data. In addition, larger structures have better contrast resolution than smaller structures.

Temporal resolution depends on the number of images the ultrasound system can obtain over a period of time, which in turn depends on the depth of the image and the PRF. The deeper the imaged structure, the longer it takes for the sound to reach, which requires lower PRFs. Therefore, deeper structures have less temporal resolution than others. In addition, the number of echoes within a frame increases the temporal resolution, because it allows for more information to be stored in fewer frames.

14.4 Displaying the Signal

The *pulser* creates the *electrical signals* that stimulate the piezoelectric crystals on the transducer. Changes in pulser *voltage* increase the *intensity* of the ultrasound signal. The *beam former* is a sophisticated piece of equipment, often controlled by a microprocessor that converts an electrical signal from the pulser to the individual *piezoelectric crystals*. The beam former contains an electrical *switch* that sends high voltages from the ultrasound system to stimulate the crystals during transmission, and relays the low voltages from the crystals to the ultrasound system during the reception (Fig. 14.8). Received electrical signals are processed by the *receiver*, which prepares the information for display on a monitor.

An image is created when ultrasound is transmitted, reflected, received, and converted into a radiofrequency (RF) signal, and then displayed. There are several different ways this signal can be displayed. The most basic display modes are *A-mode* (amplitude), *B-mode* (brightness), and *M-mode* (motion), while modern systems can display cardiac structures in *two dimensions* and *three dimensions*.

The three basic modes operate on similar principles (Fig. 14.9). After a pulse is emitted from the transducer, it reflects upon a cardiac structure and returns to the transducer. The *A-mode* display plots the amplitude of each pulse versus the depth the pulse was reflected. The *B-mode* codes the various amplitudes as different intensities of gray and is plotted against depth. The *M-mode* displays the motion of cardiac structures over time across a single area of the heart. The reflected pulses are coded in different intensities of gray based on amplitude and are plotted as depth over time. Multiple B-mode scans taken simultaneously by a phased array system create a two-dimensional image and form the basis of two-dimensional imaging. The M-mode has the best temporal resolution, although structures orthogonal to the sound pulse are not displayed.

In order to create a two-dimensional image, multiple pulses are produced in an organized manner in order to receive reflected signals over a range of space (Fig. 14.10). Along

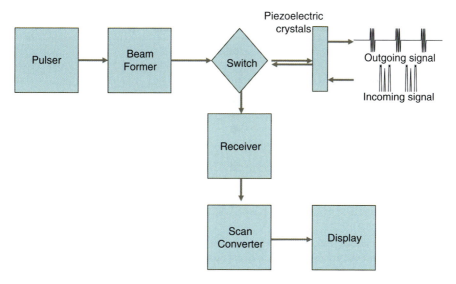

Fig. 14.8 Creating and displaying the signal. The pulser creates electrical signals and is modified by the beam former. An electrical switch sends high voltages to stimulate the piezoelectric crystal during transmission (outgoing signal), and relays low voltages from the crystals to the receiver during reception (incoming signal). The scan converter converts the data into a two-dimensional image seen on the display

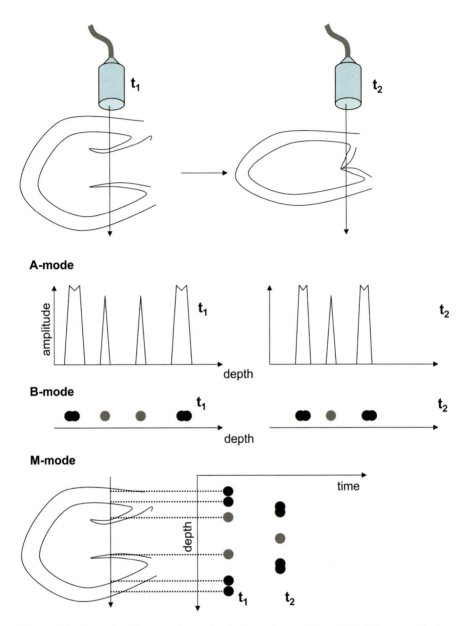

Fig. 14.9 Display modes. Time at various points in the cardiac cycle (t_1 and t_2), different amplitudes of reflected ultrasound are measured at different depths and are displayed using A-mode (amplitude vs. depth), B-mode (amplitude [brightness] in grayscale versus depth), and M-mode (amplitude in grayscale plotted as depth vs. time)

each pulse, sound is reflected back to the transducer and converted into an electrical signal that corresponds to that pulse. The signal from each pulse is stored and converted into an image, as described below.

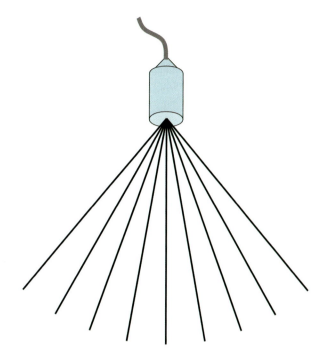

Fig. 14.10 Creation of a two-dimensional image. Multiple ultrasound pulses arranged spatially are created and received by an ultrasound transducer

As mentioned, the most common type of transducer for cardiac ultrasonography is the *phased array transducer*. Each pulse in a phased array transducer is created by 100–300 individual piezoelectric elements arranged next to each other, individually connected to its own electric circuitry. The ultrasound signal can be manipulated by changing the timing of activation of each element, resulting in steering or beam focusing, or by changing the number of activated elements, resulting in aperture narrowing (Fig. 14.11). The signals the transducer receives from each element contain several intensities of reflected waves along each element path. The information is then recreated into a two-dimensional image when all the signals from each path at any given point in time are arranged together. A three-dimensional image is created similar to a two-dimensional image, with an additional axis through which pulses are created. This process is described in more detail in Sect. 14.8.

Displays are the final output from the information gathered by the ultrasound system and are the basis for image visualization and interpretation. A *scan converter* changes the format of the data from the pulses received by the transducer arranged in a "fan" or "spoke" configuration into a horizontal "line" configuration on the monitor. Modern day echocardiography systems have *digital scan converters*, but older systems were analog.

After ultrasound signals are sent and received by the transducer, a variety of signals from increasing depths will need to be processed. Because of attenuation, deeper structures correspond to weaker returned signals. An important aspect of image processing is amplifying echoes from greater depths using a method called *time gain compensation*. This method creates an image of uniform brightness (Fig. 14.12).

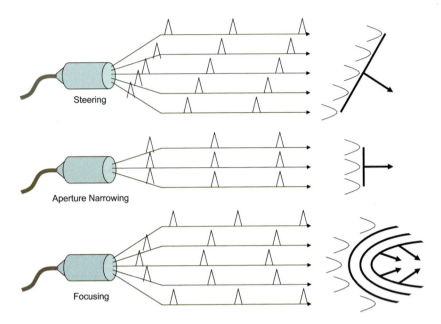

Fig. 14.11 Manipulation of the ultrasound beam with a phased array transducer. The transducer can adjust the timing of the pulses of each piezoelectric element to steer, change aperture, and focus

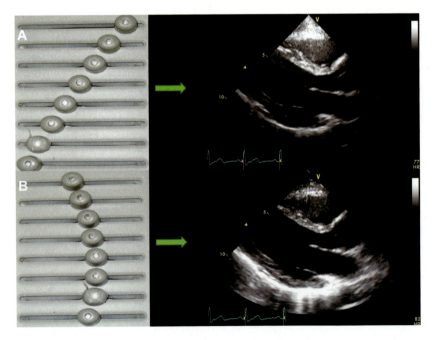

Fig. 14.12 Time gain compensation. (**a**) Amplifies echoes closer to the transducer while attenuating echoes further from the transducer, resulting in an image that does not have uniform brightness. (**b**) Adjusts the amplification of all echoes so that the final image has a uniform brightness

14.5
Doppler Echocardiography

The principles of Doppler describe the behavior of sound when it encounters moving objects. When sound encounters objects moving towards the sound source, the reflected sound returns to the source at a higher frequency, whereas when it encounters objects moving away from the source, reflected sound returns at a lower frequency. This principle was described by Christian Doppler in 1842, ultimately in the form of the following equation:

$$\Delta F = 2f_0 v / c \times \cos\theta.$$

where ΔF is the change in frequency, f_0 is the transmitted frequency, v is the velocity of the target, c is the speed of sound, and θ is the angle between the sound source and the flow. In echocardiography, Doppler is used to determine the velocities of blood and cardiac structures by interrogating them with sound. In ultrasonography, the transducer transmits the f_0 and the ΔF is measured through Fourier transformation of the actual transmitted and received waveforms. The result is a spectral display of all the resulting velocities, v over a given period of time, using the above equation to solve for v, (Fig. 14.13) where:

$$v = (\Delta F \times c) / (2f_0 \times \cos\theta).$$

An important aspect to this equation is the angle θ. The Doppler shift is maximized when the moving object is parallel to the Doppler signal (cos $0° = 1$), whereas it is zero when the moving object is perpendicular to the Doppler signal (cos $90° = 0$). For all ranges in between, the signal will be multiplied by a factor between 0 and 1. Therefore, to optimize the signal and find the maximum velocity of the moving object of interest (usually blood), the transducer would have to be exactly parallel with the blood flow. There are three basic types of Doppler used in Echocardiography: pulsed wave, continuous wave, color flow (Fig. 14.14).

Pulsed wave Doppler is similar to echocardiographic imaging – intermittent bursts of sound are transmitted and interrupted by periods when sound is received. The PRF defines

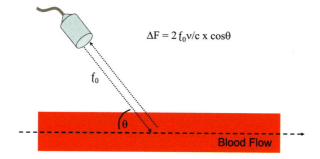

Fig. 14.13 Determination of blood and tissue velocities (v) using Doppler Echocardiography. The change in Doppler frequency (ΔF) is twice the transmitted frequency multiplied by the velocity of the target (v) divided by the speed of sound (c). If the angle of measurement (θ) is not parallel to the direction of the target, the result is multiplied by cosθ. The equation can be solved for v to determine the velocity of a given object

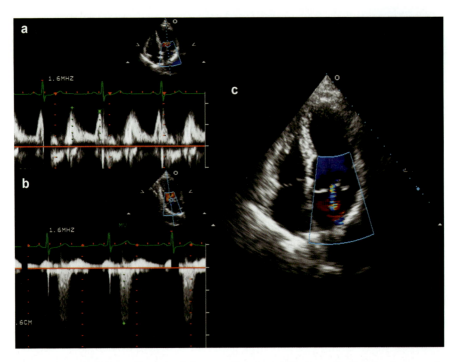

Fig. 14.14 Doppler Echocardiography. Pulse wave Doppler (**a**) displays velocities at a given sample volume, while Continuous wave Doppler (**b**) displays velocities across the entire line of interrogation. Color flow Doppler is similar to Pulse wave Doppler, but the velocities are color-coded across multiple sample volumes (**c**)

the number of alternating transmission and reception periods per second, while the PRP is the period of time between transmission or reception periods. The advantage of pulsed wave Doppler is that since the PRF can be adjusted, the instrument "listens" during a fixed time interval after ultrasound is sent, allowing velocity information at a specific depth to be analyzed at a window called the *sample volume*. Other signals outside of this volume are not measured, allowing for range resolution and absence of range ambiguity. A major disadvantage to pulsed wave Doppler is *aliasing* (see Chapter 2 for the description of aliasing). Since the transmitted signal has to travel to and from the sample volume for a signal to be measured, the Doppler shift frequency (and therefore speed) of any moving object can be measured as long as the PRF is twice that frequency. If the moving object has a Doppler shift frequency faster than twice the PRF, aliasing will occur, which will register as traveling in the opposite direction on the spectral display (Fig. 14.15). The frequency at which aliasing occurs is called the Nyquist limit, and is one-half the PRF. Sample volumes close to the transducer require less time for a transmitted signal to return, and therefore have high PRFs and Nyquist limits and are therefore less likely to have aliasing. Conversely, sample volumes far from the transducer require low PRFs and Nyquist limits, and are more likely to have aliasing. By design, pulsed-wave Doppler has good range resolution, but is limited by aliasing.

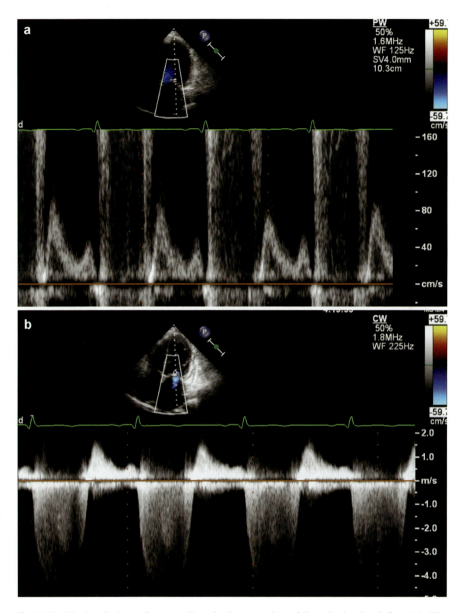

Fig. 14.15 Aliasing during pulse-wave Doppler interrogation of the mitral valve inflow (**a**). The high-velocity mitral regurgitation directed away from the probe is cut off and displayed as flow toward the probe starting at the maximum recorded velocity of 160 cm/s. Continuous wave Doppler in the same patient (**b**) displays the entire spectral array of velocities through the line of interrogation without aliasing

Continuous wave Doppler simultaneously sends and receives Doppler signals. Because there is no PRP, aliasing does not occur, making it ideal for measuring high velocity signals. However, range resolution is poor, and range ambiguity is present since all signals across the line of interrogation are represented. The combination of continuous and pulse wave Doppler imaging is a powerful tool for clinicians.

Color flow Doppler uses multiple sample volumes along multiple lines of interrogation to record Doppler shift using principles of pulsed wave Doppler. There are multiple regions of interest where flow characteristics are measured. The area over which the regions of interest exist can be controlled by the operator. Within each region of interest, the mean frequency shifts and variance are calculated. The direction and velocity are then encoded in color, and a color flow map is created for each time point in a cineloop. This information is overlayed on top of the two-dimensional or M-mode tracing. Typically, red is used to display blood flow going toward the transducer and blue is used to display flow going away from the transducer, brightness of these colors indicates higher velocity, and green or mosaic coloring is used when blood flow becomes turbulent. Similar to pulse wave Doppler, color flow Doppler has the advantage of range resolution or range specificity, but is subject to aliasing.

14.6
Factors Influencing Signal Quality

14.6.1
Noise

As with any diagnostic system, the goal is to optimize the signal to noise ratio, which is limited by the physical principles of sound, practical limitations of instrumentation design, and safety to the patient. *Noise*, or random disturbances that disrupt the signal, is generally constant, and increasing the pulser voltages increases the signal-to-noise ratio. Pulser voltages are described by many different names, such as output gain, acoustic power, pulser power, energy output, transmitter output, power, or gain. Modern ultrasound systems use the terms *thermal index* (TI) or *mechanical index* (MI) to describe power voltages. Although increases in TI or MI improve image quality, they are limited by the biological effects on the patient. Biological effects of ultrasound come in the form of thermal effects and cavitation. Briefly, thermal effects result if the TI is high enough to cause an increase in the temperature of the organ scanned. Cavitation is the interaction of sound with microscopic gas bubbles in the tissues. Cavitation takes the form of oscillating bubbles, and shear stresses at lower MIs, and transient bubble-bursting which causes very high localized temperatures and shock waves at higher MIs. Diagnostic ultrasound systems are designed to produce TIs and MIs far below the levels that could cause harmful biological effects.

Tissue harmonic imaging is another method of improving signal-to-noise ratio. One unique aspect of the interaction of sound with tissue is that sound travels faster through compressions and slower through rarefactions. This nonlinear interaction with matter creates an uneven shape of the sound beam. As the wave propagates through tissue, the peaks and troughs become slightly distorted. These minor distortions at the peaks and trough create very low-amplitude signals, which when summed together are harmonics, or signals occurring in frequencies that are multiples of the original frequency (Fig. 14.16). Tissue harmonics have two qualities that make it useful for imaging. First, as the fundamental frequency propagates through tissue, the distortion at the peaks and troughs increases, resulting in higher-amplitude harmonics at deeper depths compared to shallower depths. At the same time, the fundamental frequency weakens as it propagates through tissue, due to attenuation (Fig. 14.17). Second, higher-amplitude fundamental signals result in higher-amplitude harmonic signals, while lower-amplitude fundamental signals may not produce measurable harmonic signals. To take advantage of these two qualities, harmonic imaging suppresses or eliminates the fundamental signals, which allows for better visualization of deeper structures, and reduces the chances of artifacts resulting from the low-amplitude refracted or reflected signals created by the fundamental signal (Fig. 14.18).

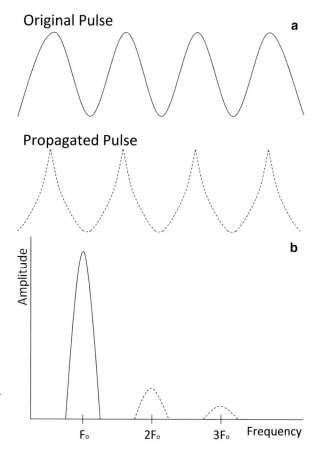

Fig. 14.16 Tissue harmonic imaging. (**a**) The nonlinear interaction of sound with matter creates distortion of the original wave, such that the propagated wave has acceleration at the peaks and deceleration at the troughs. (**b**) These distortions create low-amplitude signals, or harmonics, at multiples of the original frequency

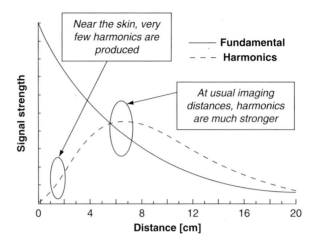

Fig. 14.17 Tissue harmonic imaging. At distances close to the surface, the fundamental frequency is stronger than the harmonic frequency. At increasing depths, fundamental frequencies are subject to artifacts such as reverberation and lobe artifacts, but the harmonic frequency increases in strength. Adapted from Thomas and Rubin[5]

14.6.2
Artifacts

An *artifact* is simply an error in imaging. Artifacts take on different forms, but include reflections of sound waves that are either not real, not seen on the image, not of correct shape or size, not in the correct position, or not of correct brightness. Artifacts result from violations of assumptions or from the physics of ultrasound.

There are six assumptions that are fundamental to the design of all ultrasound systems: (1) sound travels in a straight line, (2) sound travels directly to a reflector and back, (3) sound travels in soft tissue at exactly 15,400 m/s, (4) reflections arise only from structures positioned in the beam's axis, (5) the imaging plane is thin, (6) the strength of a reflection is related to the characteristics of the reflecting tissue. Most artifacts can be explained by identifying which of the assumptions were violated. The following are examples of common artifacts.

Reverberation artifacts are reflections caused by the bouncing of sound waves between two strong reflectors parallel to the ultrasound beam. These artifacts appear in multiples, are equally spaced, located parallel to the sound beam's main axis and at increasing depths, and are caused by violating assumption #2 (Fig. 14.19). *Comet tail* artifacts are reflections of two strong reflectors spaced closely together parallel to the ultrasound beam, and appear as single long streaks parallel to the sound beam's main axis, are similar to reverberation artifacts, and are also caused by violating assumption #2 (Fig. 14.20). *Shadowing* is a hypoechoic or anechoic region that extends beneath the structures with unusually high attenuation. Shadows are usually of the same color as the background and obscure the image, and are caused by violating assumption #6 (Fig. 14.21). *Enhancement* is the opposite of shadowing: it is a hyperechoic region and located beneath the structure with unusually low attenuation, and is also caused by violating assumption #7. *Focal*

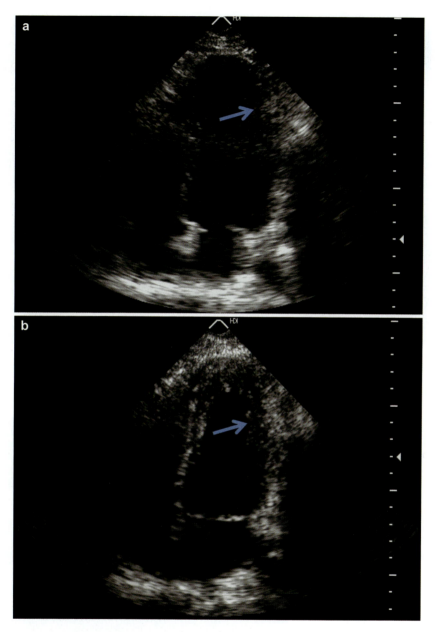

Fig. 14.18 The lateral wall of the left ventricle (*arrows*) is poorly visualized with fundamental imaging (**a**) compared to tissue harmonic imaging (**b**)

enhancement is the enhancement that is caused by highly focused beams and occurs as a bright band at the focal zone. Both shadowing and enhancement artifacts can be clinically useful by providing information that characterizes the tissue causing the artifact. *Mirror*

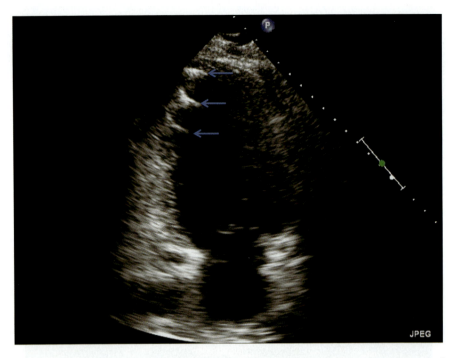

Fig. 14.19 Reverberation. A metal cannula of a left ventricular assist device is present at the apex of the left ventricle, which causes reverberation and multiples of the same image (*blue arrows*)

Fig. 14.20 Comet tail artifact (*orange arrow*) caused by a mechanical prosthetic mitral valve. Also note the lobe artifact (*blue arrow*) caused by the same structure

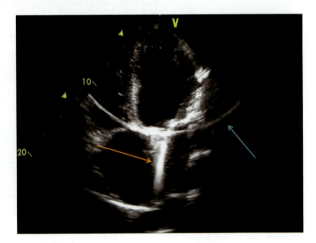

image artifacts occur when sound reflects off a strong reflector towards a second structure, which creates a replica of the structure. The artifact is an identical copy of the object that appears deeper than the real structure, while the mirror is located along a straight line

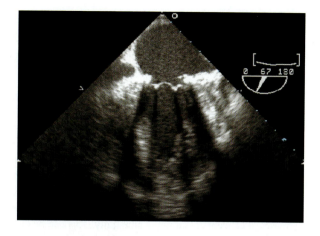

Fig. 14.21 Shadowing artifact created by a mitral valve annular ring. The ring creates enough attenuation to obscure structures behind it

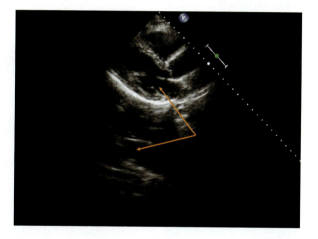

Fig. 14.22 Mirror image artifact created by the reflection of ultrasound from a calcified pericardium

between the transducer and artifact. Assumptions #1 and #2 are violated with mirror image artifacts (Fig. 14.22). *Refraction* artifacts occur when ultrasound encounters tissue with different propagation velocities, causing bending of the sound wave and a copy of a reflector that appears beside the real structure, and result from violation of assumption #1. *Speed error* artifacts occur when the speed of propagation is different than that of soft tissue, causing reflectors that are displaced and appear at incorrect depths, appearing split or cut, violating assumption #3. Occasionally, additional beams of ultrasound can appear at depths beyond the focal zone off-axis from the main ultrasound beam. If these beams or lobes are sufficient in energy to create a reflection, *lobe artifacts* are created, which results from violation of assumption #2 (Fig. 14.20). Lobe artifacts can be reduced by *apodization*, or reduction in voltage in the elements making up the periphery of the main beam, or by obtaining complementary images from alternate locations.

There are a variety of potential artifacts that can occur with Doppler imaging. The most common artifact to pulsed wave and color flow Doppler is *aliasing*, which occurs when blood flows faster than the Nyquist limit. When the Nyquist limit is too high in color flow Doppler imaging, a jet can inappropriately be enlarged as low velocity signals at the periphery of the jet are registered. Therefore, it is important to set the appropriate Nyquist limit for any given depth. In addition, high power and instrument gain can also exaggerate the jet width for the same reasons. When strong reflectors are present, occasionally large regions of color are created, which transiently obscure the true Doppler signal in a phenomenon called *ghosting*. For continuous wave Doppler, a common artifact is *mirror imaging*, which is the appearance of a mirror Doppler signal on the opposite side of the baseline, usually due to excessively high power output. *Beam width artifacts* occur when imaging deeper structures with pulse wave Doppler. As the sample volume increases in size, the deeper the structure interrogated, the likelihood of measuring adjacent signals increases, a concept called range ambiguity. This can be clinically useful, for example, in measuring the aortic outflow and mitral inflow simultaneously to measure the isovolumic relaxation time (Fig. 14.23).

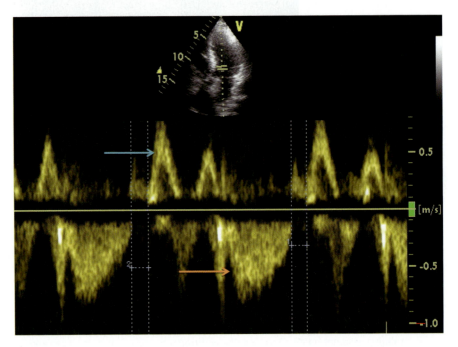

Fig. 14.23 Beam width artifact using pulse wave Doppler. The mitral inflow signal (*blue arrow*) is measured in the same sample volume as the aortic outflow signal (*orange arrow*) due to the widening of the beam at increasing depths

14.7
Storing of Data

14.7.1
Data Conversion and Storage

The transducer receives a wide range of signals, which need to be converted into a manageable scale of gray shades. Using an operation called *preprocessing*, the ultrasound instrumentation reduces the range of voltage signals into a range called the *dynamic range*, after rejecting the undesired weak echoes (noise) and filtering the strong echoes that can saturate the image. The dynamic range should be as large as possible to ensure that all clinically important signals are represented in the image. With preprocessing, the *scan converter* stores digital information as a string of 0s and 1s. Within the dynamic range, the electrical signals are converted into very small pixels that are assigned a level ranging from absolute white to absolute black, typically divided into 128 or 256 levels of gray. This step, which remaps the digital information into the range of grayscale used in video display is known as *postprocessing*. Postprocessing also includes adjustments to brightness, filtering, and other manipulations used to enhance image interpretation.

Digital information is stored either as a bitmap, or a large rectangular matrix of pixels, where the brightness or color at each position is represented by a digital value, or as a cineloop, which is a series of bitmap images that typically plays at a frame rate of 20–200 images per second. For display on a monitor, older echocardiography systems would convert the digital information into an analog video signal. However, most modern equipment is totally digital and supports the storage and communication of digital images and cineloops. The advantage of digital images is that they do not degrade when copied, transmitted, or stored, can be copied onto multiple formats, can be transmitted over large networks, can be stored in large databases, and can have patient information associated with them. One major disadvantage that remains is the amount of space required to store all data.

14.7.2
Data Selection and Compression

Image selection allows for selected "clips" of cineloops to be saved and allows for storage of the data that are selected by the sonographer. Other images observed during the echocardiography examination are not retained. Image selection reduces the amount of storage space and focuses the echocardiographic examination. However, some potentially relevant data may be lost. Once data are selected, they can be compressed into different digital formats.

The current method for digital image storage is the Digital Imaging and Communications in Medicine (DICOM) format. DICOM is also a communications standard that defines the method that medical imaging devices, picture archiving and communications systems (PACS) servers, and printers communicate in order to transport, store, or retrieve images and the associated patient information. DICOM is a standard that crosses multiple imaging modalities including ultrasound, nuclear medicine, radiology, and angiography and covers every detail of image handling, and is therefore a complex system that involves storage of the images as well as patient information without compression of the data.

Several echocardiography manufacturers have their own proprietary formats similar to DICOM. These systems allow for complex off-line analysis and manipulation of images, but complicate exchange of data between other departments, PACS, and other offline analysis systems.

Image compression can be used to reduce data storage requirements. Compression can be in two forms: lossless and lossy image compression. Lossless compression allows for perfect copying of the original image upon decompression, but results in compression by a factor of only 2–5. Lossy compression can compress images by a factor of 20–100, at the expense of image degradation. Generally, lossy compressions up to 20 times create diagnostically non-significant degradation, but may interfere with postprocessing and analysis. DICOM currently supports RLE, JPEG (lossless and lossy), JPEG2000, and MPEG2 compression formats.

14.8
Advanced Applications of Echocardiographic Imaging

14.8.1
Contrast Echocardiography

Contrast echocardiography was first described in 1968, when hand-agitated saline injected into a vein created a gas-blood interface for echocardiographic enhancement of blood within the heart. The major limitation of this method was that the bubbles created by agitating saline would be destroyed in the pulmonary capillaries and therefore would not traverse the lungs to the left ventricle. Therefore, contrast was limited to studying the right-sided structures and the presence of interatrial communications. Over time, contrast agents, or *microbubbles*, were designed to cross the pulmonary capillary beds into the left ventricle to allow for left ventricular contrast enhancement and the study of left ventricular microcirculation. Microbubbles, created by either modifying albumin or creating lipid spheres, must meet the following requirements for use as a contrast agent: it must be safely administered intravenously, metabolically inert, long lasting, small enough to pass through pulmonary capillaries (≤ 8 µm), and strong reflectors of ultrasound.

The interaction of sound and microbubbles uses the concept of harmonics, similar to tissue harmonics discussed earlier. When a microbubble is struck by ultrasound, the high pressure component of the sound wave compresses the microbubble, while the low pressure component allows for expansion of the microbubble. Since microbubbles expand to a greater extent than they shrink, the microbubbles change shape unevenly, resulting in the conversion of a small amount of energy from the fundamental frequency to the harmonic frequency. Both the fundamental and harmonic frequencies are returned back to the transducer, and echocardiography instrumentation can selectively receive the harmonic frequencies (Fig. 14.24). The extent of the harmonic resonance depends on the MI of the ultrasound beam. At low MI, (<0.1) there is no significant harmonic resonance, while at intermediate mechanical indices (0.1–1.0) moderate harmonic resonance is created. Beams with high mechanical indices (>1.0) cause destruction of the microbubbles and very strong harmonic reflections.

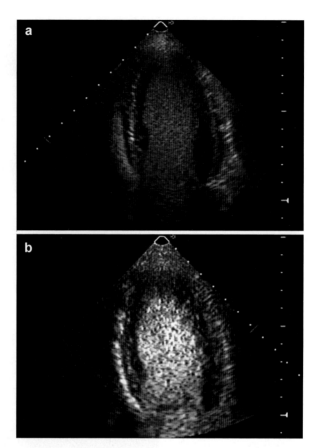

Fig. 14.24 Use of harmonic imaging with contrast echocardiography. Echo contrast is less well visualized with fundamental imaging (**a**) compared to harmonic imaging (*arrow*) (**b**)

Approved clinical uses of contrast harmonics include opacification of the left ventricle for better image enhancement (Fig. 14.25), enhancement of Doppler signals, identification of intracardiac structures, evaluation for ischemia, and elimination of lobe artifacts. Contrast for myocardial perfusion is currently under investigation.

14.8.2
Three-Dimensional Echocardiography

In order to understand three-dimensional structures of the heart, multiple two-dimensional images need to be acquired, and reconstructed mentally by the echocardiographer. Technology has advanced such that a three-dimensional image can be created either as a series of two-dimensional images reconstructed into a three-dimensional image (reconstruction technique), or as a real-time three-dimensional volume of ultrasound data (volumetric technique).

The reconstruction technique is older and requires off-line reconstruction of images. With transthoracic echocardiography, two-dimensional images can be obtained using

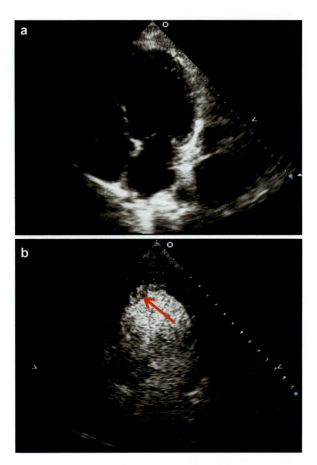

Fig. 14.25 Use of microbubbles for contrast in a patient with a poorly defined apex without microbubbles (**a**). After the injection of microbubbles, a left ventricular thrombus can be found at the apex (*red arrow*) (**b**)

freehand scanning with specialized equipment to locate the transducer in space or by mechanically rotating the probe over 180°. In both situations, the final three-dimensional image is reconstructed from the two-dimensional images, and cineloops are created by gating the images according to the cardiac and respiratory cycles.

The volumetric technique is now the technique of choice for 3D echo imaging. This technology demands advanced transducers that contain 3,000–4,000 piezoelectric elements. A pyramid-shaped three-dimensional volume of about 30–60° can be acquired and displayed in real time. Initially, only the outer surface of the entire 3-dimenstional volume is displayed on the echocardiographic machine or workstation. In order to visualize important cardiac structures, layers of the three-dimensional volume must be removed, through a process called cropping. Through cropping and slicing of the three-dimensional space, the structures of interest and the relationship with other structures can be examined (Fig. 14.26).

Three-dimensional echocardiography is a relatively new clinical field, and applications of this technique are growing as the technology improves and becomes more accessible. The ability to accurately define left and right ventricular geometry, define valvular

14 Echocardiography

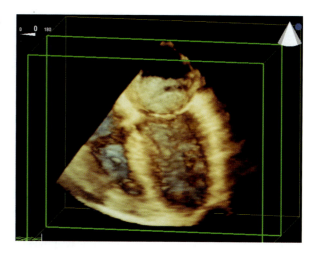

Fig. 14.26 Three-dimensional echocardiography. A three-dimensional volume is cropped, revealing the left ventricle and mitral valve for close examination

pathology, and evaluate congenital heart disease is one of the current applications. 3D echo color Doppler imaging is also available, although frame rates are slower than 2D echo color Doppler imaging. Pulsed-wave and continuous Doppler are not yet available for three-dimensional imaging.

14.8.3
Intravascular Ultrasound

Intravascular ultrasound (IVUS) is a catheter-based technique that uses a miniaturized transducer that is inserted into arteries for in vivo visualization of vascular anatomy. It allows for detailed visualization of all arterial layers in a particular length of artery. The instrumentation includes a specially adapted ultrasound machine dedicated to catheter-based imaging, an IVUS catheter, motorized pullback system, and an interface that ensures sterility of the catheter. The catheter is placed in the vessel of interest using conventional catheter techniques, and the motorized pullback system pulls the catheter back at a set rate (usually 0.5–1.0 mm/sec) while the transducer sends and receives ultrasound. The pullback system allows for calculation of lesion length, provides frame of reference based on anatomic landmarks, and allows for comparison of other IVUS studies within the same vessel.

The transducer sits on the end of the catheter and can be either a *mechanical* or *phased array* system. The mechanical transducer consists of piezoelectric elements arranged perpendicular to the catheter that rotate at 1,800 rotations per minute about the axis of the catheter. Fast rotation of the transducer can be accomplished because the imaging depth is very shallow (approximately 1–5 mm), and therefore the PRF can be very high, and the required information at a given point in the rotation can be gathered quickly. The resulting image is a circular map of the artery from the perspective of the catheter. Mechanical transducers have the advantage of high spatial resolution, but have the disadvantage of limited catheter flexibility due to the mechanical drive shaft required to rotate the transducer. As a result, in a tortuous vessel, the drive shaft may be constricted, resulting in uneven rotation, creating artifact called *nonuniform rotational distortion* (NURD). Phased array transducers have multiple piezoelectric transducer elements along the circumference of the catheter tip. Each element sends and receives signals from a small sector, and the final image is a summation of all signals from all sectors, resulting in an image similar to that created by a mechanical transducer. Phased array transducers are more flexible than mechanical transducers, can move through tortuous vessels more easily, and do not create NURD. However, these transducers require complex programming to add sectors together and have lower spatial resolution due to the finite number of elements that can be used, and lower temporal resolution due to computational speed. However, as element miniaturization and processor technology are improving, phased array transducer images are approaching those created by mechanical transducers.

IVUS provides images of the inside of an artery. In order to create an image, ultrasound reflects off the structures of the artery. Arteries contain three major layers: intima, media, and adventitia. The intima is a thin layer of endothelial cells that line each vessel. In vessels with atherosclerosis, the intima thickens due to deposition of lipids and inflammatory cells. The media is a layer of smooth muscle that surrounds the intima. Finally, the adventitia is the outermost layer of the vessel that primarily consists of connective tissue and provides structural support for the vessel. Each of these three layers has different densities and consistencies, such that when ultrasound interacts with each layer, a unique acoustic signal is reflected. When ultrasound leaves the transducer, it interacts with blood, which appears as a dark signal. It then encounters the intima, which is reflected back to the transducer as a bright ring. Unless the intima is heavily calcified, ultrasound is able to penetrate the media, which consists of homogenous smooth muscle cells and returns as a hypoechoic (black) region, until ultrasound interacts with the adventitia, which reflects ultrasound and appears as a bright region. Therefore, all the three layers can be visualized as different shades of gray based on their relative densities and consistencies (Fig. 14.27).

IVUS can be used for studying various vascular structures, including coronary arteries, to assess the degree of atherosclerosis and to guide stent deployment, and peripheral arteries, to assess peripheral arterial disease severity. Since the structures measured are within millimeters of the ultrasound probe, rather than centimeters in transthoracic echocardiography, higher frequencies (up to 45 MHz) can be used. The attenuation that occurs at higher depth is not clinically useful and therefore not included in the final display. IVUS takes advantage of the accuracy and resolution of higher-frequency signals due to the limited range of depths needed for a clinically important image.

14.8.4
Intracardiac Echocardiography

Intracardiac echocardiography is a technique used to image cardiac structures in great detail, using a small probe inserted into the right cardiac chambers through a central vein. Because the structures imaged are closer to the probe, higher frequency transducers (up to 10 MHz) can be used without losing signal intensity; for the same reasons IVUS can use higher-frequency signals. This technique can be used to guide interventional and electrophysiological procedures.

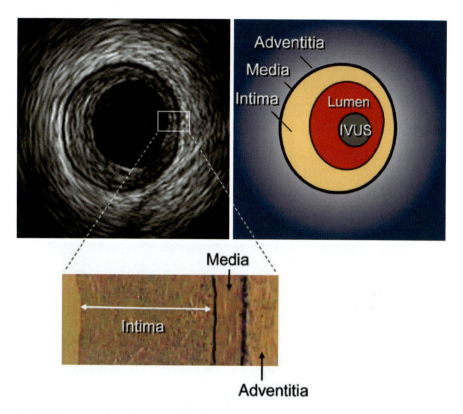

Fig. 14.27 Intravascular ultrasound. The layers of the vessel can be differentiated based on their densities and echocardiographic properties (see text). Reproduced, with permission from[4]

14.8.5
Tissue Doppler Imaging

Tissue Doppler imaging (TDI) is a Doppler technique used to measure velocities of myocardial tissue in real-time. The basic physical principles of Doppler imaging of blood flow apply to TDI for myocardial motion, with different processing of the received signal to obtain the necessary information. Two major differences in blood and tissue signals are used to discriminate between the two: blood flow velocities are fast (usually 100 cm/s, up to 600 cm/s) but low-amplitude, while tissue velocities are slow (usually 10–20 cm/s) and higher-amplitude. When pulsed wave Doppler is used to assess blood flow, low-velocity, high-amplitude myocardial signals are considered noise and are eliminated using a filter (high-pass filter). With TDI, the filtering should be performed in the opposite way, where high-velocity, low-amplitude, blood flow signals are eliminated using a filter (low-pass filter) (Fig. 14.28). Tissue Doppler is currently being used to assess systolic and diastolic function of the left ventricle.

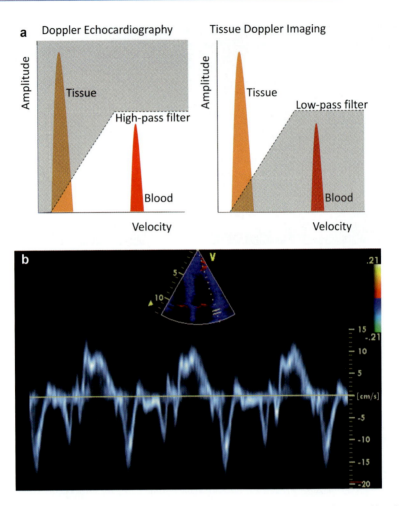

Fig. 14.28 (a) Tissue Doppler Imaging (TDI). High-amplitude, low-velocity signals created by ultrasound reflections off tissues are filtered out using a high-pass filter in conventional Doppler (*rejected area in gray*). Low-amplitude, high-velocity signals of blood are filtered out using a low-pass filter in TDI (*rejected area in gray*). (b) TDI signal is displayed as a spectral Doppler signal similar to conventional Doppler. Note that the velocities are much lower than conventional Doppler

14.9 Conclusion

Echocardiography is a technique based on basic physics of sound. Sound in the ultrasonic range can be transmitted and received, and the signal can be converted into a digitized image for clinical use. Various techniques such as two-dimensional echo, three-dimensional echo, intravascular echo, intracardiac echo, and Doppler echocardiography have been developed, and the techniques have become ubiquitous in clinical practice.

References

1. Edelman SK. *Understanding Ultrasound Physics*. 3rd ed. Woodlands, TX: ESP Publishers; 2005.
2. Feigenbaum H, Armstrong WF, Ryan T, eds. *Feigenbaum's Echocardiography*. 6th ed. Baltimore: Lippincott Williams and Wilkins; 2004.
3. Otto CM, ed. *The practice of Clinical Echocardiography*. 3rd ed. Philadelphia, PA: Saunders; 2007.
4. Baim DS, ed. *Grossman's Cardiac Catheterization, Angiography, and Intervention*. 7th ed. Philadelphia, PA: Lippincott Williams and Wilkins; 2005.
5. Thomas JD, Rubin DN. Tissue harmonic imaging: Why does it work? *J Am Soc Echocardiogr*. 1998;11:803–808.
6. Garcia-Fernandez MA, Zamorano J, Azevedo J, eds. *Doppler Tissue Imaging Echocardiography*. Madrid: McGraw-Hill; 1998.

Nuclear Cardiology: SPECT and PET

15

Nils P. Johnson, Scott M. Leonard and K. Lance Gould

15.1 Introduction

Nuclear cardiology utilizes radioactive tracers to image primarily physiology as opposed to anatomy. Its two key imaging techniques, single photon emission computed tomography (SPECT) and positron emission tomography (PET), offer tradeoffs in terms of availability, cost, artifacts, quantification, and complexity. This chapter discusses the physiologic signals of interest in nuclear cardiology, from their acquisition to processing to reproducibility and noise.

15.2 Physiologic Signals

Two primary physiologic signals can be sampled by nuclear cardiology. The first is flow via the coronary arterial tree through the left ventricular myocardium. The second is metabolic pathways within the left ventricular myocardial cells. Signals of cardiac chamber size and contractile function by radionuclide angiography and ECG-gated SPECT or PET are not discussed here since these signals are better imaged by other techniques. Emerging signals such as myocardial innervation are not yet mature or wide-spread enough for inclusion at this time.

15.2.1 Flow

The coronary arteries originate from the aortic root and branch over the epicardial surface of the heart. Via this network, blood reaches the myocardial tissue to supply nutrients and

---

N.P. Johnson (✉)
Department of Medicine, Division of Cardiology,
Northwestern University, Feinberg School of Medicine, Chicago, IL, USA
e-mail: n-johnson4@md.northwestern.edu

J.J. Goldberger and J. Ng (eds.),
Practical Signal and Image Processing in Clinical Cardiology,
DOI: 10.1007/978-1-84882-515-4_15, © Springer-Verlag London Limited 2010

remove the waste products of metabolism. Radionuclide tracers introduced into the blood stream are taken up by metabolically active and structurally intact myocardial cells. The exact mechanism and characteristics of the uptake and washout depend on the tracer.

Figure 15.1 shows a generalized curve representing tracer concentration within the myocardial tissue following its systemic injection. While both tracer uptake and washout occur continuously, the first part of the curve is dominated by uptake, due to high tracer concentration in the blood stream, and the second part of the curve can be dominated by either washout, due to the high tracer concentration in the myocardial cells, or decay, in the case of retained tracers. Compartmental models identifying intravascular, interstitial, and intracellular components contribute to the overall blood tracer curve.

Radioactive tracer decay produces counts detected by a scanner, as detailed below. Thus tracer concentration itself is not measured directly. Static imaging (acquiring one image with a long temporal duration) effectively integrates the area under the curve in Fig. 15.1 over the duration of the scan, as shown in its subfigure. During this time the overall tracer concentration decays from its initial value, depending on the specific half-life of the agent, as described in more detail below. If the scan time is long compared to the half-life of the tracer (as is typical in PET imaging), then such changes in the net balance of the tracer concentration become important considerations in static imaging. If the scan time is short compared to the specific half-life of the tracer (as is typical in SPECT imaging), then such changes in overall tracer concentration have less impact. As counts are integrated over a long period, static imaging offers a high signal-to-noise ratio.

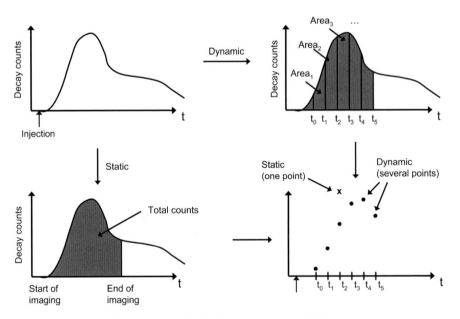

Fig. 15.1 Theoretical radiotracer dynamics for flow after injection. Subfigures show the integrative effects of static and dynamic imaging, which reduce a continuous curve into discrete sample(s). In the bottom right curve, the datum (single point) obtained by static imaging is shown by the "x" and the multiple points obtained by dynamic imaging are depicted by circles

Dynamic imaging consists of acquiring sequential images each with a short temporal duration. It is effectively serial static imaging where the duration of each static image is small compared with the overall duration of the scan, as demonstrated in the subfigure of Fig. 15.1. The short temporal images of dynamic imaging reduce the signal-to-noise ratio when compared to static imaging. However it offers the ability to model the curve in Fig. 15.1 at a higher temporal resolution needed for studying radionuclide kinetics into and out of the different myocardial spaces.

The physiologic range of flows spans an order of magnitude. Resting myocardial flow is typically on the order of 1 mL/g/min. Hyperemia produces flows up to 5 mL/g/min. Flow to hypoperfused myocardial tissue is roughly 0.5 mL/g/min, while flow to infarcted tissue is essentially 0.1 mL/min/g. Clinically these ranges of flow need to be distinguished from each other and, within the range of diminished and hyperemic flow, differences of 0.5 mL/g/min have clinical impact.

Ideally, flow quantification would provide absolute flow values over the entire dynamic range from 0 to 5 mL/g/min with a precision of less than 0.5 mL/g/min. Currently however, quantitative flow models are not yet routinely used clinically due to their complexity. An analysis of published quantitative results using PET tracers shows a variability of roughly 25–30% (standard deviation divided by the mean flow), as discussed later. This works out to approximately 0.2 mL/g/min under resting conditions and 0.8 mL/g/min during hyperemia. Thus quantitative flow has the potential accuracy and precision to meet clinical, diagnostic needs.

Current practice, however, employs relative radionuclide uptake as a measure of relative myocardial flow whereby radionuclide uptake throughout the left ventricle is normalized to the maximal observed radionuclide uptake. Relative radionuclide uptake indicating relative myocardial perfusion has the drawback that global flow reductions are not identified and the degree of hyperemia among scans performed on different occasions cannot be directly compared. The area of maximal radionuclide uptake may have severely reduced absolute flow due to diffuse disease that remains undetected. However relative imaging simplifies acquisition and processing protocols.

The spatial resolution of the flow signal acquired depends on the tracer and modality used, as detailed in the next section. Typically this resolution is on the order of voxels sized 4–6 cm^3 for PET and 6–8 cm^3 for SPECT suitable for identifying abnormal flow patterns due to coronary artery stenosis. However, myocardial perfusion may vary on very fine spatial levels, as shown by microsphere work.[1] It is unlikely that these fine heterogeneities of flow can be observed with current nuclear imaging techniques but are not currently of clinical importance.

15.2.2
Metabolism

Myocardial blood flow must deliver nutrients to the myocardial cells to meet their metabolic needs and remove waste products. Under normal conditions, the heart primarily utilizes fatty acids for metabolic fuel. However, under conditions of relative hypoperfusion or frank ischemia, cellular metabolism switches to glucose for anaerobic glycolysis. Thus, imaging these metabolic pathways can alter clinical decisions regarding the need for mechanical revascularization or the presence of primary metabolic derangements in the myocardium itself (termed a cardiomyopathy).

Two general types of tracers exist for metabolic imaging, those that participate in the fatty acid pathways and those that participate in the glucose pathways. The next section of this chapter discusses technical properties of these tracers. Conceptually, however, their signal reflects the relative utilization of their associated metabolic substrate. Models to quantify metabolic pathways have been limited by their complexity and unclear validity when simplified into a handful of parameterized constants.[2] Generally the practice has been to study simple relative uptake of these metabolically-active tracers.

Much like Fig. 15.1, an analogous curve exists for the concentration of metabolically active tracers after intravenous injection. Often, however, the time course achieves a relatively stable steady-state as changes in metabolic utilization have a longer time course than the duration of the nuclear scan. For example, Fig. 15.2. shows the conceptualized counts obtained after injection of a fatty acid-analog nuclear tracer. Static imaging of integrated counts from its decay produces a map of relative uptake, similar to the subfigures of Fig. 15.1. Dynamic models do exist for fatty acid and glucose metabolism[3]; however, these are infrequently used and current guidelines argue against their use due to the wide variation of normal values.[4]

Unlike flow, for which invasive measurements have validated noninvasive quantitative models, metabolic imaging does not have such well-established correlates. Thus, the accuracy and precision have not been well studied. Data do exist on using metabolic imaging to predict if surgical revascularization will result in a return of contractile function.[5] In general, these studies show a reasonable accuracy (sensitivity of approximately 90% and specificity of approximately 65%) for the binary outcome of improved contractile function. However, these data do not define accuracy of metabolic imaging for quantifying in vivo metabolism.

Reproducibility of metabolic imaging by nuclear tracers is limited. Absolute rates of glucose uptake in the myocardium can only be estimated via tracer methods under steady-state conditions.[2] Intersubject variability of absolute glucose uptake is large, varies physiologically with diet, and normalization to maximum relative uptake is necessary for intersubject comparison.[6] An analysis of published results shows a 30% variability (standard deviation divided by the mean flow), as discussed later.

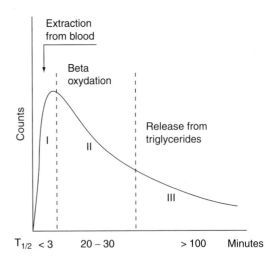

Fig. 15.2 Theoretical radiotracer dynamics for metabolism after injection[53] (copied with permission from *Noninvasive Imaging of Cardiac Metabolism*, page 42)

Spatial resolution for metabolic imaging again depends on the tracer and imaging modality used, as detailed in the next section. The resolution is similar when compared to flow imaging.

15.3
Basic Description of the Techniques

15.3.1
Photon Detection

Regardless of the nuclear tracer utilized, the useful result of its decay pathway is the production of one or more photons. The energy level and number of photons produced vary. PET and SPECT scanners can be categorized generally as position-sensitive radiation detector systems that utilize crystals to absorb the energy of incident photons (scintillation detectors). Once absorbed in the crystal, a portion of a photon's energy is released as visible light, the magnitude of which is proportional to the energy of the incident photon. The scintillation light is detected by light sensitive devices, usually photomultiplier tubes (PMT), which produce electronic pulses proportional to the light detected. In modern systems, these electronic pulses are digitized directly at the PMT. Down-stream electronics discriminate out photon events that may have undergone a loss of energy via a scattering interaction (see below) or background radiation, as well as coincidence determination in PET systems.

The type of crystal is based on expense, ease of fabrication, relative light output per unit of photon energy absorbed, and the rate at which light is generated and decays from the crystal. In general, SPECT systems utilize large single plates of thallium doped sodium iodide, NaI(Tl) coupled to an array (9–64+) of PMTs. NaI(Tl) is relatively inexpensive to manufacture and produces a relatively high light yield per unit of absorbed photon energy. But its relatively low effective atomic number and density are not well suited to absorbing (stopping) the higher energy 511 keV photons of PET tracers.

PET systems, in contrast, typically utilize multiple rings of small crystal blocks, coupled to four PMTs. Most PET scanner crystals are made of bismuth germinates (BGO) or lutetium oxyorthosilicate (LSO). Both materials have higher effective atomic numbers and density than NaI(Tl), making them more efficient absorbers of PET tracer photons with the disadvantage of lower light yield. LSO produces more light than BGO and also emits its light more than 2–3 times faster than BGO, increasing the sensitivity and maximum count rate for LSO-based scanners.

In general, then, a photon emitted from the patient at the end of the decay pathway interacts with a crystal on the face of the camera. The photon interaction with the crystal releases electrons, which are directed into a photomultiplier that amplifies the electrical signal before converting it into a digital signal by an analog-to-digital converter. The incoming photon produces a signal in proportion to its energy level. When the magnitude of this signal falls within a specified zone, the camera registers a "count," equivalent to the detection of the incoming photon whose energy is within the expected range for the utilized tracer.

15.3.2
Attenuation

Photons exiting the body have the potential to interact with its tissue before reaching the scanner. Such interactions can reduce the energy of the photon, alter its direction (scatter), or absorb it completely. Figure 15.3 demonstrates that attenuation modifies the nonattenuated energy spectrum by producing a leftward smear and resulting tail. A photon that is absorbed by the body will not be detected by the camera. Scatter changes the direction of the photon. This scatter can result in the photon's not being detected at all (if its direction is changed away from the camera) or seeming to come from a different location within the body. Finally, energy discrimination is used to "filter out" and reject photons whose energy is reduced below a certain limit. Photon attenuation will cause some photons to fall below the lower cutoff and thereby not be counted. Attenuation correction techniques will be discussed later.

15.3.3
Single Photon Emission Computed Tomography (SPECT)

Tracers that can be imaged by SPECT systems decay and produce single (that is "unpaired") photons via nuclear and electron transitions (although an isotope may have several possible

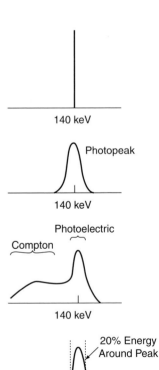

Fig. 15.3 Effect of scatter and attenuation on the photon energy signal from an ideal tracer to that measured in practice[52] (copied with permission from *Nuclear Cardiac Imaging: Principles and Applications*, page 43). Photoelectric effect and Compton scatter cause the smearing of the original sharp signal

transitions, each with a characteristic energy). Two common flow isotopes and one common metabolic isotope are typically employed. Table 15.1 lists the physical properties for these tracers. Note the long half-life for all of them, when compared to the acquisition protocol, as described below. The long half-lives allow the tracers to be produced centrally and transported to imaging facilities.

For each SPECT acquisition, typically a dual-head camera with two faces approximately 90° apart steps through a 180° orbit about the patient. At each step (typically 64 steps, each for 25 s) counts are acquired as they exit the patient. Collimator covers over the camera face allow localization of each count to a narrow volume defined by the collimator septations, as shown in Fig. 15.4.

Table 15.1 Common SPECT tracer properties

Isotope	Compound	Half-life	Photon energy (keV)	Physiologic signal
Tl-201	N/A (acts as potassium analog)	74 h	60–80	Flow
Tc-99m	SestaMIBI, teboroxime, tetrofosmin	6 h	140	Flow
I-123	BMIPP	13 h	159	Metabolism

BMIPP β-methyl-*p*-iodephenyl-pentadecanoic acid (free fatty acid); *I* iodine; *MIBI* methoxyisobutyl-isonitrile; *Tc* technetium; *Tl* thallium

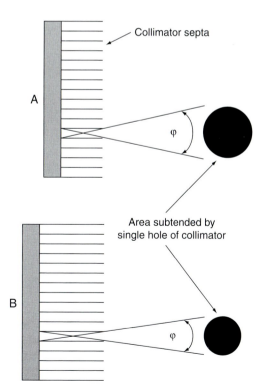

Fig. 15.4 Effect of collimator septa on image localization in SPECT[54] (copied with permission from *Nuclear Medicine and PET/CT: Technology and Techniques*, page 275). Note that increased length of the collimator septa (longer in B compared to A) narrows the volume subtended for imaging

Different techniques exist for attenuation correction of SPECT images. However only recently has true correction become more widely available through commercial vendors. The details of several frequently used attenuation correction techniques will be discussed in the next section of this chapter.

In an effort to identify the effects of attenuation, a patient may be reimaged in the prone position. This technique alters the tissue composition between the heart and the camera. A change in the signal between supine and prone conditions suggests that the variation is due to tissue attenuation as opposed to the underlying physiologic state. As such, prone imaging seeks to identify the existence of attenuation artifacts as opposed to truly correcting the signal for their effect.

Figure 15.5 shows common clinical protocols for SPECT imaging of the heart, both for flow and metabolism. Total protocol times run approximately 4 h. Note that this is relatively short when compared with the tracer half-lives as given in Table 15.1.

15.3.4
Positron Emission Tomography (PET)

Tracers that can be imaged by PET systems decay via the beta pathway, converting a proton in the nucleus into a neutron and emitting a positron (a positive electron) with a range of kinetic energies. The positron travels some distance in the tissue (described by a characteristic average distance for each tracer, termed the effective positron range) then combines with an electron to annihilate both and produce two 511 keV photons 180° apart. Thus two higher-energy photons are emitted and detected by the camera, compared to one lower-energy photon in SPECT. The most common isotopes for flow and metabolism are listed in Table 15.2 along with their physical properties. Note the short half-life for all of them, when compared to the acquisition protocol and when compared to SPECT tracers. The short half-lives, apart from F-18, demand that the tracers be produced at the imaging site immediately at the time of the study.

For each PET acquisition, a stationary series of 360° detector rings surround the patient. If two photons are detected almost simultaneously at detectors located 180° apart, then these simultaneously detected counts are assumed to represent a positron annihilation along the path connecting the two detectors, as demonstrated in Fig. 15.6. Note, that the near simultaneous detections can be due to true annihilations or random coincidences, as demonstrated in Fig. 15.7.

Several factors limit the resolution of PET systems. First, the positron always travels some distance before annihilation occurs. Second, the two photons are emitted apart slightly less than 180° due to residual positron momentum, which degrades image resolution by about 1–2 mm. Third, the spatial resolution of the detection system itself varies with the size of the detector and the distance of the annihilation from the detector. These factors combine to place a lower limit on the detection resolution of the radioactive decays, even before these counts have been processed into an image.

Corrections need to be applied to PET images for variable detector efficiency, random coincidences, tracer decay, and the dead time of the detectors, in addition to scatter and attenuation. The details of attenuation correction will be discussed in the next section. The other corrections are technical and will be not discussed here but can be found in standard

15 Nuclear Cardiology: SPECT and PET

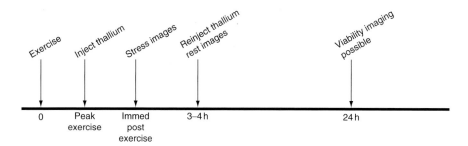

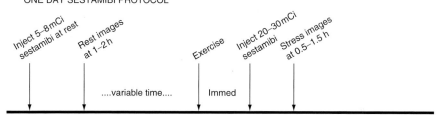

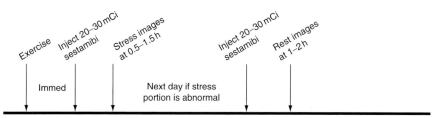

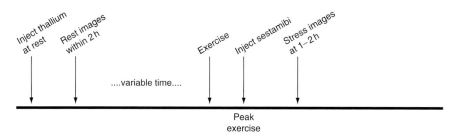

Fig. 15.5 Typical SPECT clinical protocols for viability and flow[51] (copied with permission from *Essentials of Nuclear Medicine Imaging*, pages 108–110)

texts on nuclear imaging.[7] Two different techniques have been employed for attenuation correction of PET images: computed tomography (CT) and a rotating rod technique. Historically a rotating germanium (Ge-68) rod has been used, although current commercial scanners favor a built-in CT system.

Table 15.2 Common PET tracer properties

Isotope	Compound	Half-life	Mean positron range (mm)	Physiologic signal
Rb-82	N/A (acts as potassium analog)	75 s	2.6	Flow
N-13	Ammonia	10 min	0.6	Flow
F-18	FDG	110 min	0.2	Metabolism

F fluoride; *FDG* fluorodeoxyglucose (glucose analog); *N* nitrogen; *Rb* rubidium

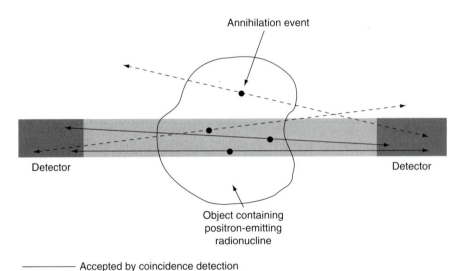

Fig. 15.6 PET tracer decay produces a positron which annihilates with an electron to produce two photons which are seen by detectors 180° apart[7] (copied with permission from *Physics in Nuclear Medicine*, page 326)

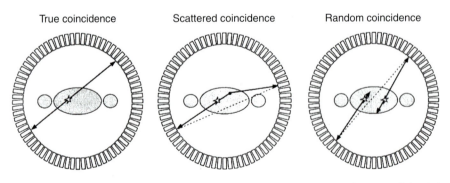

Fig. 15.7 In addition to true coincident detections, random and scatter detections occur[7] (copied with the permission from *Physics in Nuclear Medicine*, page 341)

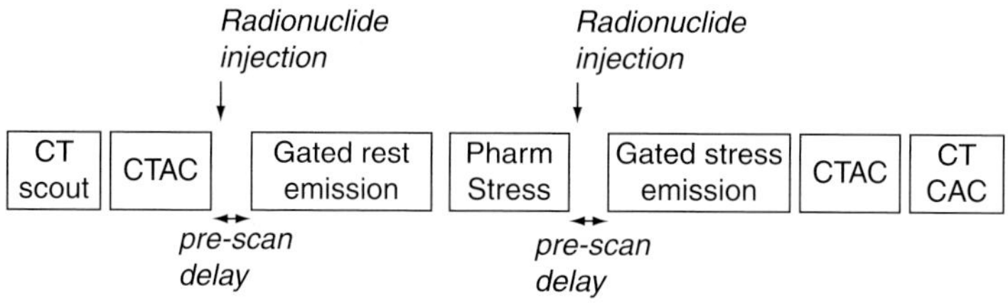

15 Nuclear Cardiology: SPECT and PET

```
      Radionuclide                    Radionuclide
       injection                       injection
           ↓                               ↓
 ┌────┐┌──────┐┌──────────┐┌───────┐┌────────────┐┌──────┐┌────┐
 │ CT ││      ││Gated rest││ Pharm ││Gated stress││      ││ CT │
 │scout││ CTAC ││ emission ││ Stress││  emission  ││ CTAC ││ CAC│
 └────┘└──────┘└──────────┘└───────┘└────────────┘└──────┘└────┘
            ←──pre-scan──→          ←──pre-scan──→
                delay                    delay
```

Fig. 15.8 Typical PET clinical protocol for flow[52] (copied with permission from *Nuclear Cardiac Imaging: Principles and Applications*, page 561). *CT* computed tomography; *CTAC* CT-based attenuation correction; *CAC* coronary arterial calcium

Figure 15.8 shows common clinical protocols for PET imaging of the heart, both for flow and metabolism. Total protocol times run approximately 30 min. Note that this is relatively long when compared to the tracer half-lives as given in Table 15.2 and much shorter than SPECT protocol times.

15.4 Key Signal Processing Techniques Used

Both SPECT and PET acquisitions offer raw data of a similar nature: counts produced by nuclear decays that can be isolated to a portion of the field-of-view. Image reconstruction seeks to use this localized count information to recreate the original distribution of radioactive material inside the patient. After the tracer distribution has been recreated, it in turn must be processed for display. Often this consists of rotating and reslicing the data into planes aligned with the axes of the heart, as opposed to the axes of the human body.

15.4.1 Forward Projection and Simple Backprojection

Figure 15.9 shows a point source of radioactive tracer whose activity has been recorded by a detection camera at various angles about a 180° rotation. The data set compiled by combining all the projections is called a sinogram, as shown in Fig. 15.9. The process of converting the distribution of radioactive material into a sinogram is termed "forward projection" or a "Radon transformation" and occurs during SPECT or PET acquisition. The goal of image reconstruction is to undo this process (or find its inverse transformation).

The most elementary image reconstruction technique is termed simple backprojection, as it undoes forward projection. Figure 15.10 demonstrates how each projection is spread evenly over the reconstruction image along the path which created the projection. By utilizing ever more projection angles, the final image appears similar to the original distribution of material. However, note that the sharply defined object has been blurred and the originally empty

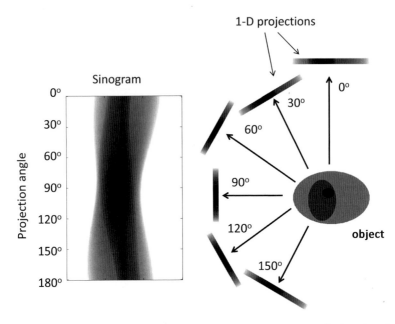

Fig. 15.9 Forward projection of an object creates a sinogram. The sinogram displays the 1-D projections of the 2-D cross-section of the object at incrementing angles as the detector revolves around the source

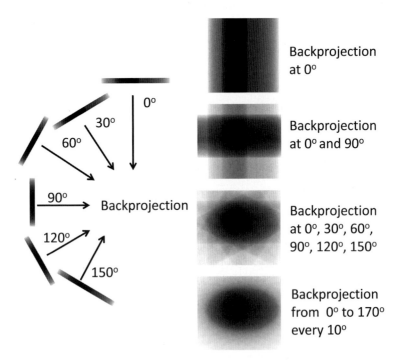

Fig. 15.10 Simple backprojection produces a blurred image and suffers from count diffusion into the background

background now has diffuse activity. Such blurring and count diffusion are inherent problems with simple backprojection which more sophisticated techniques seek to overcome.

15.4.2
Filtered Backprojection (FBP)

By applying a filter to the projection data before performing backprojection, some of the problems with image blurring and diffusion of counts into the background can be reduced. Such filters are generally applied in the frequency domain instead of the spatial domain. First, the projection data at each angle is transformed to the frequency domain. Next, the transformed data is multiplied by the chosen filter. After transforming the filtered frequency projection data back into the spatial domain, the backprojection algorithm described earlier is applied.

Figure 15.11 demonstrates the same radioactive object as in Fig. 15.9, but now its projection data have been filtered. Compared to the simple backprojection of Fig. 15.10, the filtering has reduced both the blur and the background noise. Various types of frequency filters can be chosen, and Fig. 15.12 shows typically employed filters. These offer different tradeoffs between image resolution and artifacts. Figure 15.13 demonstrates the same image reconstructed using filtered backprojection with various filters applied to identical projections with introduced noise.

15.4.3
Iterative Reconstruction

A different and more computationally intensive method for image reconstruction takes an initial "guess" for the distribution of radioactive tracer and improves this in a

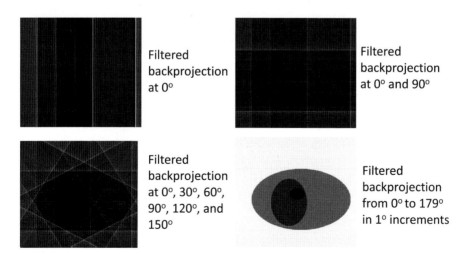

Fig. 15.11 Filtered backprojection helps reduce the problems associated with simple backprojection in Fig. 15.10. The blurring with simple backprojection is reduced by attenuating the low frequency components of the projections

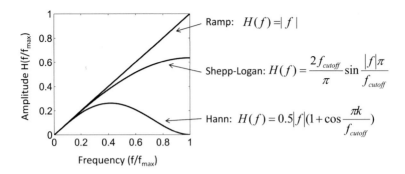

Fig. 15.12 Various filters that can be used with filtered backprojection

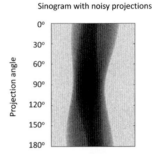

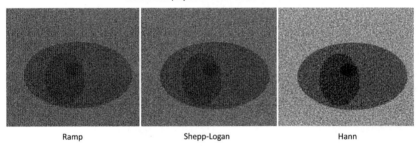

Fig. 15.13 An image reconstructed filtered backprojection from a noisy sinogram using three different filters

cyclic fashion. At each step of the cycle, the current estimate for the image is forward projected to produce a sinogram, as in Fig. 15.9. This sinogram is compared to the one actually acquired by the SPECT or PET system. The difference between the actual sinogram and the current sinogram is used to update the current estimate for the image. This cycle continues, as shown in Fig. 15.14, until the changes to the current estimate approach zero.

Different methods exist for updating the current estimate based on the sinogram differences. The most popular methods use the so-called expectation maximization (EM),

Fig. 15.14 Flowchart for an iterative reconstruction algorithm

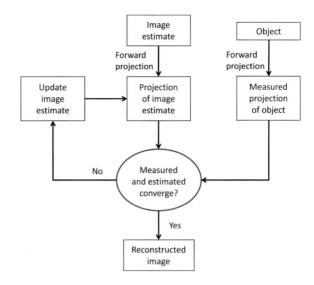

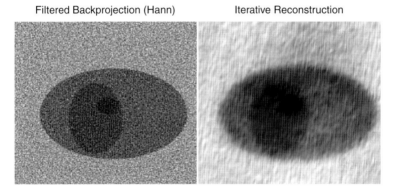

Fig. 15.15 Comparison of filtered backprojection (Hann filter) and iterative reconstruction from a noisy sinogram

whereby each pixel carries a statistical weight factor, as opposed to the uniform weight given to each pixel by backprojection. By initially working with just a subset of all available projections to produce a reasonable estimate before incorporating all projections, the iterative process can be sped up. This popular technique is termed ordered subset EM (OSEM). Figure 15.15 compares images reconstructed by FBP and OSEM.

A good iterative technique remains insensitive to the initial "guess" for the tracer distribution. Either a blank guess or a guess based on FBP can be used as the starting estimate. Figure 15.16 demonstrates iterative reconstruction of the same tracer distribution using a blank image and an image with a solid square centered in the image.

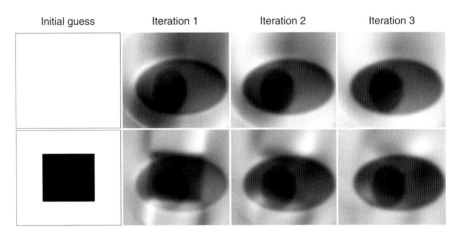

Fig. 15.16 Effect of the initial guess on the iterative reconstruction process via the algorithm in Fig. 15.14

15.4.4
SPECT Attenuation Correction

Photons emitted by SPECT tracers undergo attenuation before reaching the detector. The degree of attenuation depends not only on the amount of material through which the photon must pass, but also on the attenuating characteristics of that material. Additionally, photons can be scattered between their emission and detection. Both of these effects introduce systematic bias into the reconstructed image. Several techniques exist for reducing this bias.

The Chang multiplicative method uses the reconstructed image itself to estimate the length of tissue that attenuates the photon energy before it reaches the detector. It assumes a uniform attenuation coefficient to produce attenuation correction factors based on the Beer-Lambert law. These multiply the reconstructed image to produce the attenuation corrected image. Figure 15.17 demonstrates a uniform cylinder with and without Chang attenuation correction. Note that the assumption of a uniform attenuation coefficient breaks down significantly in the chest, where the mediastinum, lungs, and bones each have quiet different attenuation characteristics. Thus this technique, employed by SPECT imaging in other parts of the body, works poorly for cardiac imaging.

If a true attenuation map could be obtained, then the problems with the uniform attenuation coefficient assumption in the Chang method could be overcome. Two primary methods exist for obtaining an attenuation map: an external radionuclear source (termed a transmission source) or a CT scan. In the transmission source technique, the external radioactive element (typically 153-gadolinium or 123m-tellurium) is placed opposite a camera head either as a line source or a moving point source. Two scans are acquired, one without the patient in the scanner (the reference scan) and one with the patient in the scanner (the transmission scan). Using these two scans, an image of the attenuation coefficients (termed the attenuation map) can be reconstructed. Alternatively, a CT scanner, incorporated into the SPECT camera to simplify coregistration of the images, can image an attenuation map.

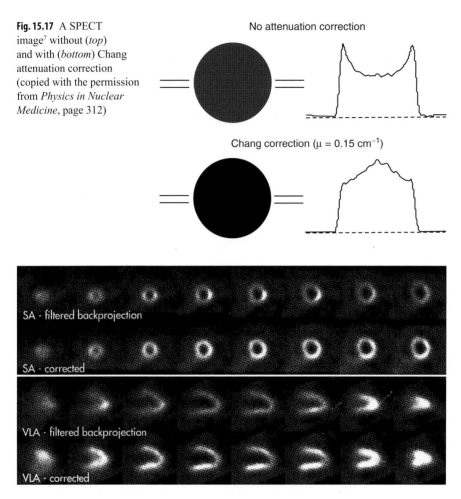

Fig. 15.17 A SPECT image[7] without (*top*) and with (*bottom*) Chang attenuation correction (copied with the permission from *Physics in Nuclear Medicine*, page 312)

Fig. 15.18 Impact of attenuation correction on SPECT images of myocardial blood flow[54] (with and without) (copied with permission from *Nuclear Medicine and PET/CT*, page 296)

In either case, the attenuation map can be used to estimate better the effect of attenuation on a photon emitted from any location within the patient to any detector in the scanner. This overcomes the assumption of a uniform attenuation coefficient of the original Chang method. Figure 15.18 demonstrates an image produced using FBP without an attenuation map and the reconstruction using FBP and the attenuation map.

Scatter reduces both the energy of the photon and alters its direction, making it appear as a photon originating from another location within the patient. Thus, some of the attenuated photons recovered represent events that occurred in a different location within the patient rather than that along the collimated volume. A technique to account for this bias uses one or more "scatter windows" below the highest energy window for the tracer, as diagrammed in Fig. 15.19. Photons within these lower-energy windows are more likely to have undergone scatter interactions than photons detected within the highest-energy window. The lower the energy level,

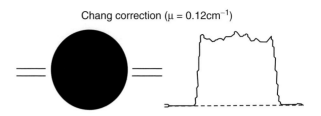

Fig. 15.19 Effect of scatter correction on a SPECT image[7] (copied with the permission from *Physics in Nuclear Medicine*, page 317). Compare to SPECT image without scatter correction in Fig. 15.17

the more likely it is that the photon underwent multiple scatter interactions as opposed to extensive attenuation before being detected. Based on phantom studies, each scatter window can have part of its counts eliminated as being more likely due to scatter than attenuation.

15.4.5
PET Attenuation Correction

Attenuation correction in PET is fundamentally different from that in SPECT as two photons 180° apart are produced by beta decay. The probability of detecting a PET tracer decay event does not depend on the depth at which the decay occurred, as in SPECT, but rather on the total path length through the material between the two cameras. Thus the attenuation correction factor remains constant for all events detected by two cameras, regardless of where the events occur along the path connecting the detectors.

An attenuation map can be created either by a rotating rod source, historically germanium-68, or a CT scan, which is favored on the latest generation scanners. The process is similar to that described for SPECT attenuation maps, as detailed in the proceeding section. The counts for each camera pair are adjusted based on the blank and transmission scan data for that pair.

Scatter correction using the method described for SPECT does not work well for PET imaging, due to the energy accuracy of the detector crystals for these photons. Therefore more complex methods are used, which are beyond the scope of this text but can be found in standard references.[7]

15.4.6
Absolute Activity

The goal of nuclear imaging seeks to recover a reconstructed image of the tracer distribution that is proportional to the actual tracer distribution within the patient. For it is then possible to recover absolute activity by calibrating the proportionality relationship. In general, absolute activity can be routinely obtained from standard PET protocols, as attenuation correction is robust and effective. While attenuation correction for SPECT is maturing, it has not reached the point that standard scanners can recover absolute activity. In fact, due to attenuation artifacts, the tracer distribution in SPECT is often not even proportionally related to the actual tracer uptake in a consistent fashion. This limits the role of SPECT for advanced modeling of the physiologic signals of flow and metabolism.

15.5 Quality Replication of Signal of Interest

15.5.1 Noise in Radiotracer Decay

If a fixed amount of radioactive tracer were placed near a detection counter that could detect all decays perfectly, the number of decays per unit time would still vary. The reason is that radioactive decay is a random process. While the average number of decays over a long period of time obeys the law of exponential decay, characterized by the half-life of the radiotracer, the actual number observed in any given period can differ from this average.

The Poisson distribution describes the probability of observing a certain number of decays as opposed to the expected, average number of decays. For example, assume that 100 atoms of a radiotracer exist, and that the half-life of the tracer is 1 min. Over that 1 min the expected number of decays is 50. However either fewer or more than 50 may be observed during any repetition of the experiment. Figure 15.20 graphs the probability that anywhere from 0 to 100 decays will be observed.

Note three characteristics of Fig. 15.20. First, the Poisson distribution can only be defined for nonnegative integer values. This differs from the Gaussian or normal distribution, which can be computed even for fractional or negative values. Second, the average observed value in the Poisson distribution is equal to the average number of decays. Third, while the Poisson distribution appears roughly "bell-shaped," it differs from a true Gaussian or normal distribution. For comparison, a Gaussian or normal probability distribution has been plotted in Fig. 15.20 with the same mean and variance as the Poisson distribution. When the number of expected counts is large, the Poisson distribution approximates a Gaussian distribution.

Therefore inherent noise exists in nuclear cardiology images due to this variation in decay counts. A useful property of the Poisson distribution is that its standard deviation is

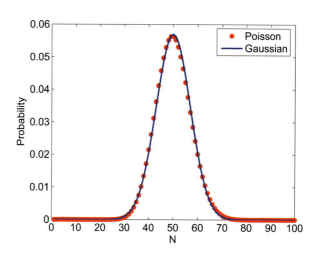

Fig. 15.20 Poisson distribution with mean of 50 with n ranging from 0 to 100. *Solid line* shows a Gaussian distribution of equivalent mean and variance

equal to the square root of the expected, average number of counts. Thus, for Fig. 15.20, the variance is the square root of 50, or approximately 7.1. In general, the acquired image of tracer distribution has an associated standard deviation that varies across the image by the number of observed counts at each point. Thus, dynamic imaging has larger variation compared with static imaging (refer to Figure 15.1) due to Poisson statistics.

15.5.2
Noise and Bias in the Detector System

The response of the camera crystal, photomultiplier tube, analog-to-digital converter, and electrical detector introduce further noise and even systematic bias. Detector design has sought to minimize noise while maximizing signal and several additional corrections are included to avoid systematic bias when detecting radioactive decays. These add a further level of noise to the detector system, although hopefully significant bias has been minimized. This topic is complex and the interested reader is referred to a standard text on nuclear imaging system design.[7]

15.5.3
Cardiac and Respiratory Motion

Cardiac cycle motion of the left ventricle takes place superimposed on diaphragmatic motion during respiration. These phasic movements occur on a much shorter time scale compared to image acquisition. Thus the acquired image looses spatial resolution due to these factors and represents an "average" or "blurring" of the true tracer distribution. While ECG gating[8,9] and respiratory gating[9-12] can be employed, their improved spatial resolution must be balanced against decreased signal-to-noise from worse count statistics.[13] Furthermore, vasodilatory pharmacologic stress agents frequently induce tachypnea.

15.5.4
Physiologic Variation in Flow

Flow through the left ventricular myocardium is the physiologic signal of interest for most of nuclear cardiology. However, flow is a dynamic process, adapting constantly to meet changes in myocardial metabolic demand. Even under apparently stable conditions, heterogeneity of myocardial blood flow exists on a microscopic scale[1] and on a scale observable by PET imaging.[14] The clinical significance of the former, microscopic variability has not yet been determined, while the latter, larger-scale heterogeneity may be due to early manifestations of atherosclerotic disease.

Little work thus far has examined the reproducibility of flow for an individual patient by serial imaging. More information exists on the normal limits for flow at rest and during stress. The following sections of this chapter summarize the current literature on physiologic variation in flow by SPECT and PET. This is followed by a discussion of the estimated flow variations introduced by therapeutic interventions.

15.5.5
Variation in Flow by SPECT

One of the best sources on the reproducibility of relative flow by SPECT for a single patient scanned repeatedly without intervention comes from the control group of a multi-center trial on transmyocardial laser revascularization.[15] These 90 patients underwent serial SPECT imaging at 0, 3, 6, and 12 months while remaining on a stable medication regimen without other intervention. While the average reversible defects for the whole group remained constant, for individual patients these varied by 50% over time. Only 13% of this variability could be ascribed to image reconstruction and analysis, implying a large variation in flow as measured by SPECT. However, smaller, single center studies of SPECT reproducibility suggest better results.[16-18] In summary,[19] the challenge is clear but the solutions are still under development.

Several databases have been published on the variability for relative flow by SPECT for groups of normal patients.[20-22] These have been incorporated into commercially available software packages to assist with the scoring.[23-28]

Data on the variability of relative flow by SPECT after a therapeutic intervention suggests that simple segment matching may be less sensitive than more complex techniques for identifying clinically relevant changes.[29,30] For example, in a study of 49 patients undergoing surgical revascularization after a myocardial infarction, a visual analysis of before-vs.-after SPECT images did not reach statistical significance, unlike a matched voxel analysis.[30] Computer simulation work on serial imaging has suggested a lower limit of 10% relative uptake by t-test when comparing single patients for significant changes.[31]

15.5.6
Variation in Flow by PET

Limited data exist on reproducibility of relative flow by PET for a single patient scanned repeatedly without therapeutic intervention. Table 15.3 shows several relative uptake endpoints for ten patients who were scanned twice.[32] The variability (standard deviation divided by the mean) is on the order of 10%. Table 15.3 also shows absolute flow endpoints for 21 healthy volunteers who were scanned twice 10 min apart.[33] The variability is on the order of 15%. Table 15.3 also shows absolute flow endpoints for 15 patients with chronic stable angina scanned 24 weeks apart.[34] The variability is on the order of 20%.

More data exist on the variability for absolute flow by PET for groups of normal patients. The variability (standard deviation divided by the mean flow) is on the order of 25–30%. Data on the variability of relative and absolute flow by PET after a therapeutic intervention depend on the initial flow as well as the efficacy of the intervention (see Table 5 of deKemp et al).[35]

Table 15.3 Reproducibility of relative and absolute flow by PET

Endpoint	Scan number 1	Scan number 2	Mean Δ as % of scan number 1	Scan number 1 vs. number 2 by paired t-test
From Sdringola et al[32]				
Mean activity of lowest quadrant (%)	62±13	63±11	0.7	NS
% LV>2.5SD	13.9±14.0	12.7±17.2	8.6	NS
% LV<60%	16.7±14.6	15.4±14.8	7.8	NS
Stress/rest relative ratio of mean lowest quadrant	0.89±0.15	0.89±0.10	2.2	NS
From Kaufmann et al[33]				
Resting flow (mL/g/min)	0.89±0.14	0.99±0.15	11.2	NS
Stress flow (mL/g/min)	3.51±0.45	3.83±0.49	9.1	NS
Stress/rest flow reserve	4.05±0.75	3.93±0.72	3.0	NS
Resting flow (mL/g/min)	1.03±0.19	1.10±0.20	7.8	NS
From Jagathesan et al[34]				
Stress flow (mL/g/min)	2.02±0.44	2.09±0.57	3.5	NS
Stress/rest flow reserve	1.98±0.40	1.90±0.46	4.0	NS

LV left ventricle; *NS* not significant; *SD* standard deviation

15.5.7
Physiologic Variation in Metabolism

Metabolism in the left ventricular myocardium reflects the current availability of metabolic substrates as well as recent or ongoing perfusion relative to the metabolic need. Like flow, metabolism is a dynamic process, adapting constantly to meet changes in substrate availability and delivery. Compared to flow, less work has been done on studying the reproducibility of metabolic images. The following sections of this chapter summarize the current literature on physiologic variation in metabolism by SPECT and PET. This is followed by a discussion of the estimated metabolic variations introduced by therapeutic interventions.

15.5.8
Variation in Metabolism by SPECT

No literature exists on the reproducibility of I-123 BMIPP in humans. Metabolic SPECT images only define relative uptake and must be interpreted in relation to flow. Only a handful of studies with a total of less than 30 normal volunteers have studied normal BMIPP kinetics.[36-38] Most of the work on BMIPP has focused on its prognostic significance, as opposed to how therapeutic interventions alter its distribution. A handful of studies exist examining changes in BMIPP uptake after therapy,[39-45] although these are too small to allow for generalization.

15.5.9
Variation in Metabolism by PET

Limited data exist on the reproducibility of serial FDG imaging in individual patients. In 49 cancer patients without manifest cardiac disease, three serial, whole-body oncologic PET scans showed high regional temporal variability on the order of 10% difference in percent uptake.[46]

Approximately 20 studies have both used FDG metabolism by PET to predict which segments would regain contractile function after revascularization and also compared the results after surgical revascularization.[5] A minority of these studies used a fully quantitative tracer model to predict glucose recovery, and based on receiver operating characteristic (ROC) curve cutoff a threshold of 0.25 μmol/min/g yields a 99% sensitivity and 33% specificity. The majority used a semi-quantitative approach with a 50% relative uptake threshold, although specificity increases if higher thresholds are employed. A weighted analysis of these data show a 91% sensitivity and 64% specificity on a per-segment basis, using recovery of function after revascularization as the gold standard.[5]

15.5.10
Image Artifacts

A variety of mechanisms can produce artifacts on the reconstructed image. Some artifacts are intrinsic to the nuclear imaging process, while other artifacts are due to violations of the assumptions behind image reconstruction.

The two most important artifacts that are intrinsic to nuclear imaging are partial volume effects and attenuation. Partial volume effects refer to the inability to recover radioactivity concentration completely from an object that is below the resolution limit of the detector system. Figure 15.21 demonstrates the partial volume effect by showing cylinders of equal activity but decreasing diameter. Once, the diameter falls below twice the spatial resolution of the imaging system, the recovered activity concentration decreases. The proportion of recovery activity concentration, termed the recovery coefficient, thus falls below one when the cylinder diameter falls below twice the spatial resolution. This represents spatial undersampling (Chap. 9).

The thickness of the left ventricular myocardium is approximately 10 mm. Thus SPECT and PET systems need to have a spatial resolution on the order of 5 mm to avoid partial volume artifacts. For the thinner apex, even smaller spatial resolutions are necessary. Current generation PET scanners deliver a spatial resolution of approximately 5–6 mm,[47] which is therefore at the upper limit for producing minimal partial volume effects.

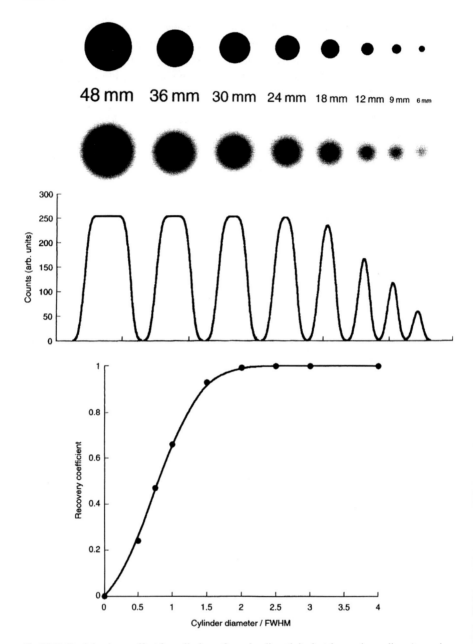

Fig. 15.21 Partial volume effect for cylinders of equal radioactivity but decreasing radius. Assuming a spatial resolution of 12 mm, the count concentrations recovered begin to fall once the diameter falls below twice the spatial resolution (24 mm). The recovery coefficient quantifies how much activity concentration has been lost due to this partial-volume effect[7] (copied with the permission from *Physics in Nuclear Medicine*, pages 318–319, Figs. 17-15 and 17-17)

It is possible for the recovery coefficient to be greater than one. If a small area of low tracer uptake is surrounded by two areas of high tracer uptake, then counts can "spill over" and make the recovered activity greater than the actual activity. This again is due to the partial volume effect and has important implications for hot spot vs. cold spot optimization, as discussed below.

Attenuation can affect all photons produced by radiotracer decay. SPECT is far more prone to attenuation than PET given its single photon production, lower energy levels, and lack of routine attenuation correction. Clinically, attenuation artifact is suspected in SPECT in two common areas: anterior defects in women, due to breast tissue attenuation; and inferior defects due to diaphragmatic attenuation. Methods to overcome attenuation artifacts have been discussed earlier. However, these techniques can produce artifacts of their own.

Proper attenuation correction depends on alignment of the attenuation (transmission) map with the radiotracer (emission) map. Given both the very high signal in the myocardial wall compared with the low signal in the adjacent lungs and the higher attenuation coefficient of the soft tissue mediastinum compared to the mostly air-filled lungs, the transmission/emission alignment in cardiac nuclear imaging is especially crucial. The lateral wall is therefore most prone to misalignment, which creates a false defect.

Transmission/emission misalignment in routine clinical practice occurs in approximately 40% of all PET studies, with moderate-to-severe defects observed in 25% of cases.[48] Figure 15.22 shows the artifact introduced by misalignment, and its resolution following proper registration. A variety of sources for the misalignment exist, including differential breathing between emission and transmission, movement of organs over a period of time when supine, and resolution differences between transmission and emission imaging modalities.

The reconstruction algorithms which use the sinograms (refer to Figure 15.9) assume an infinite number of projection angles and that all points on the detector function properly. While in practice only a finite number of projections are possible, obtaining a smaller number of projection angles will degrade the sinogram and introduce artifact into the reconstructed image. Similarly, if a crystal detector on the camera is not functioning, then the sinogram will have a blank section and this will introduce artifact into the reconstruction. Figure 15.23 demonstrates the impact of too few projections and a malfunctioning detector on the sinogram and its reconstruction. Related artifacts can be caused by incomplete angular sampling and incomplete object sampling.

15.5.11
Hot Spot vs. Cold Spot Optimization

Much of noncardiac nuclear imaging seeks a large signal ("hot spot") within a low signal background. For example, oncologic PET looks for an area of greatly increased metabolic uptake as represented by high FDG signal. In contrast, the majority of cardiac nuclear imaging seeks a small signal ("cold spot") within a high signal background. Normal myocardial blood flow during hyperemia is large, while defects produced by flow-altering lesions appear as areas of relatively lower flow.

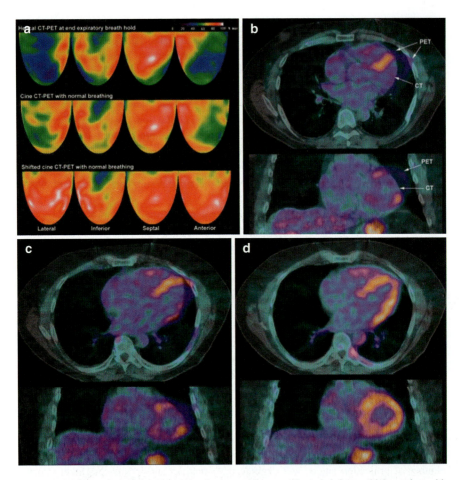

Fig. 15.22 Misalignment of the attenuation image produces artifactual defects which resolve with proper registration (copied with the permission from Gould et al.[48]). (**a**) Polar maps of rubidium uptake using three different registration techniques. The *top two rows* represent suboptimal registration and create artifactual perfusion abnormalities (shown in *blue*). The *bottom row* shows optimal CT-PET registration, identifying only an inferobasal perfusion defect. (**b**) Axial and coronal sections from PET (*purple–orange*) and CT (*blue–green*) during end-expiratory breath hold (*top row*, (**a**)), showing poor registration. PET image of the heart is seen in the CT lung field. (**c**) CT-PET during normal breathing. (**d**) CT-PET during normal breathing but shifted for optimal registration

Therefore, optimizations in camera design, data acquisition, and image reconstruction for hot spot imaging are likely not optimal for cold spot imaging. This area has not been extensively studied as its importance has only recently become appreciated. However, some phantom work demonstrates that OSEM offers not only lower noise but also lower cold spot contrast, while FBP has not only higher noise but also higher cold spot contrast.[49] While the clinical impact of these tradeoffs on myocardial flow and metabolism imaging remain to be determined, it serves as a warning against adopting noncardiac nuclear imaging parameters without testing them in cardiac applications.

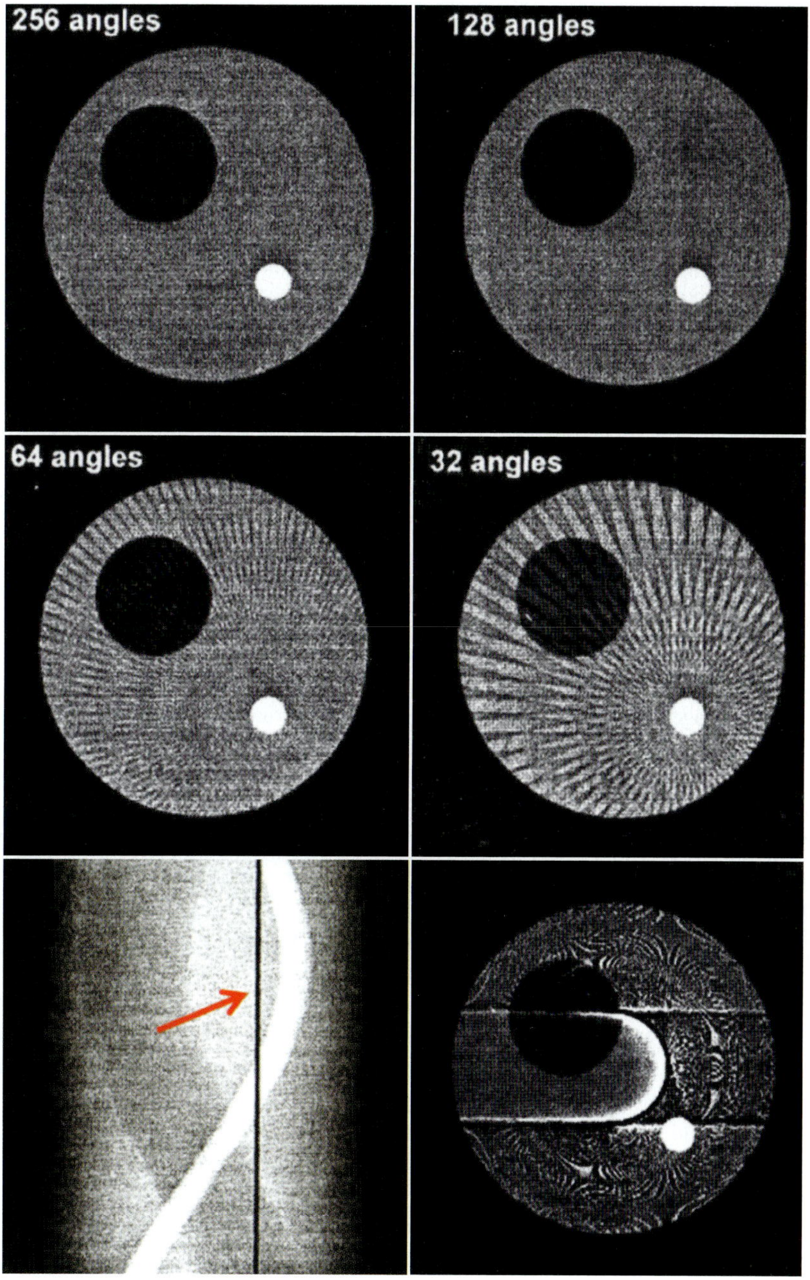

15 Nuclear Cardiology: SPECT and PET	245

Fig. 15.23 Artifacts introduced by sampling too few projections (*top*) and a malfunctioning detector (*bottom*)[7] (copied with the permission from Physics in Nuclear Medicine, pages 286 and 288). In the *top* panel, as the number of projection angles decreases, a star burst artifact appears. In the *bottom*, *left* panel, a single malfunctioning detector creates a vertical artifact (*arrow*) in the sinogram, which creates diffuse artifacts in the backprojected reconstructed image as shown in the *lower*, *right* panel (should appear as in the *top*, *left* of *upper* panel)

15.6
Data Storage

Modern scanners have moved to an industry-wide standard termed DICOM (Digital Imaging and Communications in Medicine).[50] This facilitates exchange of patient scan data among health care providers, interoperability for software vendors, and generally provides the ability to store the data in Picture Archiving and Communication Systems (PACS), making them available to viewing workstations throughout the hospital.

The DICOM standard defines the manner in which the various imaging modalities (nuclear medicine, computed tomography, ultrasound, and so on) encode and define their respective data types (for example, acquired SPECT projections, reconstructed transaxial and orthogonal images slices, static and dynamics acquisition images and regions of interest).

Although interoperability is fairly consistent for the final, postprocessed, reconstructed slice data, the ability to reconstruct the raw data acquired with one vendor system with the software of a second vendor is not as reliable. Although vendors will document conformance to the DICOM standard, variable interpretation of the standard often yields raw data sets that are not directly cross-system compatible. While certain nuclear medicine acquisition data (SPECT and gated-SPECT) are defined in the standard, the raw sinogram data of PET and CT acquisitions are not defined and are therefore encoded and stored in vendor specific, proprietary formats.

Digital images are composed of a matrix of pixels (picture elements). In nuclear image acquisition, each pixel stores a value that defines the number of counts collected in that segment of the imaging field of view. During the reconstruction process, images are created with pixel values to define the relative activity or tracer distribution. These pixel values, when displayed on a computer screen, are assigned an intensity value and displayed as a certain color. The maximum number of values that can be stored in each pixel is defined by the pixel depth (number of bits). An 8-bit byte can store a maximum of $2^8 = 256$ values, whereas a 2-byte word can store $2^{16} = 65,536$.

The stored file sizes of these images (acquisition or reconstructed slice) can easily be calculated as the product of the pixel depth, the number of pixels in each image, and the number of images acquired or slices reconstructed. For example, a typical SPECT acquisition data set would be acquired with a 64×64-matrix projection, 2 bytes per pixel, and 64 projections, producing an approximately 524,288 byte file. Increasing the matrix to 128×128 would produce a file 4 times larger. In general, a few hundred bytes more are used to store information defining the image, when and how it was created, patient demographics, and other header values.

A gated SPECT data set can be considered as eight individual SPECT studies, each imaging the myocardium at a different phase of the cardiac cycle. Therefore its file sizes are on the order of 4MB. The file size of the reconstruction data generated from these data is dependent on the axial extent of the reconstruction (usually only slices containing the myocardium are generated) and the number of time frames per cardiac cycle, but are typically on the order of 200KB for SPECT and 1,600KB for gated SPECT. CT images are generally reconstructed into matrices as large as 512×512, producing single slice files sizes on the order of 549K bytes each.

Several different compression schemas are available for images after reconstruction, including both lossless and lossy techniques (Chap. 8) such as native encoding, run length encoding, JPEG, JPEG-lossy, JPEG 2000, and MPEG2 MP@ML. These compression techniques may also be employed to compact the data before transmission across the computer network to speed transfer. Thus, it is up to the individual workstation preferences after image reconstruction as to which compression technique is employed.

The data acquisition described above for nuclear medicine SPECT can be defined as a frame mode acquisition – computer memory/storage is allocated to collect 64 projections of 8 bytes in 64×64 pixels. Therefore, the file size of the acquired data is known before acquisition begins. At a minimum, PET scanners can acquire data in a similar manner, allocating computer resources into sinograms. The number of sinograms (defining the number of slices through the scanners axial field of view) is dependent on the number of scanner axial rings and detector elements, the in-plane field of view, and scan mode (2D vs. 3D). Eight-frame ECG gating in either mode for a given scanner would produce a raw data set 8 times larger.

Many current PET scanners allow for data acquisition using a method called list mode. In a list mode acquisition, each individual photon event is stored into a file along with its detector element. At periodic intervals and throughout the acquisition, a timing marker is added to the list. If the acquisition is ECG gated, an R-R timing marker is also added to indicate the beginning of the cardiac cycle. The size of the list and file size is also dependent on the amount of tracer used, its decay properties, and the length of the acquisition. Typical file size for a list mode acquisition can range from a few hundred megabytes to 1.5GB.

The benefit of a list mode acquisition is that, at the time of processing, any number of different reconstructions can be performed from the data – ECG gated reconstruction in 8 and/or 16 time bins, single or multiple statics from different time intervals during the acquisition, or multiple dynamic reconstructions each with different temporal resolutions. Reconstructed files sizes will vary depending on the selected reconstruction type. In general, PET produces images of high spatial resolution and larger matrix sizes are employed. For example, a typical FDG cardiac viability study would reconstruct into 111 slices in a 168×168-matrix producing more that 6,400KB of slice data. Again, an eight ECG-frame reconstruction would require 8 times as much storage.

Typically PET data obtained prior to image reconstruction are not part of the DICOM archive. This can often be saved in a vendor-specific format from the scanner itself. Vendors offer different levels of detail which can be stored. Most allow for the sinogram-level data to be saved and retrieved if reconstruction with a different technique or different parameters is desired. Few allow for temporal subsets of the acquisition to be separated and reprocessed or for individual detections to be excluded.

If an attenuation map is created either by a radioactive source or a separate CT image, then this can be stored as part of the vendor-specific archive. However this is not necessarily part of the DICOM file itself, unless the CT scan has itself been reconstructed and stored independently as a DICOM image.

References

1. Bassingthwaighte JB, Beard DA, Li Z. The mechanical and metabolic basis of myocardial blood flow heterogeneity. *Basic Res Cardiol*. 2001;96(6):582–594.
2. Hariharan R, Bray M, Ganim R, Doenst T, Goodwin GW, Taegtmeyer H. Fundamental limitations of [18F]2-deoxy-2-fluoro-D-glucose for assessing myocardial glucose uptake. *Circulation*. 1995;91(9):2435–2444.
3. Sokoloff L, Reivich M, Kennedy C, et al. The [14C] deoxyglucose method for the measurement of local cerebral glucose utilization: theory, procedure, and normal values in the conscious and anesthetized albino rat. *J Neurochem*. 1977;28(5):897–916.
4. Machac J, Bacharach SL, Bateman TM, Bax JJ, Beanlands R, Bengel F, Bergmann SR, Brunken RC, Case J, Delbeke D, DiCarli MF, Garcia EV, Goldstein RA, Gropler RJ, Travin M, Patterson R, Schelbert HR; Quality Assurance Committee of the American Society of Nuclear Cardiology. Positron emission tomography myocardial perfusion and glucose metabolism imaging. *J Nucl Cardiol*. 2006;13(6):e121–e151.
5. Knuuti J, Schelbert HR, Bax JJ. The need for standardisation of cardiac FDG PET imaging in the evaluation of myocardial viability in patients with chronic ischaemic left ventricular dysfunction. *Eur J Nucl Med Mol Imaging*. 2002;29(9):1257–1266.
6. Knuuti MJ, Nuutila P, Ruotsalainen U, et al. The value of quantitative analysis of glucose utilization in detection of myocardial viability by PET. *J Nucl Med*. 1993;34(12):2068–2075.
7. Simon Cherry R, James Sorenson A, Michael Phelps E, eds. *Physics in Nuclear Medicine*. 3rd ed. Amsterdam: Elsevier; 2003.
8. Bateman TM, Berman DS, Heller GV, et al. American Society of Nuclear Cardiology position statement on electrocardiographic gating of myocardial perfusion SPECT scintigrams. *J Nucl Cardiol*. 1999;6(4):470–471.
9. Büther F, Dawood M, Stegger L, et al. List mode-driven cardiac and respiratory gating in PET. *J Nucl Med*. 2009;50(5):674–681.
10. Cho K, Kumiata S, Okada S, Kumazaki T. Development of respiratory gated myocardial SPECT system. *J Nucl Cardiol*. 1999;6(1 Pt 1):20–28.
11. Livieratos L, Rajappan K, Stegger L, Schafers K, Bailey DL, Camici PG. Respiratory gating of cardiac PET data in list-mode acquisition. *Eur J Nucl Med Mol Imaging*. 2006;33(5):584–588.
12. Kovalski G, Israel O, Keidar Z, Frenkel A, Sachs J, Azhari H. Correction of heart motion due to respiration in clinical myocardial perfusion SPECT scans using respiratory gating. *J Nucl Med*. 2007;48(4):630–636.
13. Dawood M, Büther F, Stegger L, et al. Optimal number of respiratory gates in positron emission tomography: a cardiac patient study. *Med Phys*. 2009;36(5):1775–1784.
14. Johnson NP, Gould KL. Clinical evaluation of a new concept: resting myocardial perfusion heterogeneity quantified by markovian analysis of PET identifies coronary microvascular dysfunction and early atherosclerosis in 1, 034 subjects. *J Nucl Med*. 2005;46(9):1427–1437.
15. Burkhoff D, Jones JW, Becker LC. Variability of myocardial perfusion defects assessed by thallium-201 scintigraphy in patients with coronary artery disease not amenable to angioplasty or bypass surgery. *J Am Coll Cardiol*. 2001;38(4):1033–1039.
16. Prigent FM, Berman DS, Elashoff J, et al. Reproducibility of stress redistribution thallium-201 SPECT quantitative indexes of hypoperfused myocardium secondary to coronary artery disease. *Am J Cardiol*. 1992;70(15):1255–1263.
17. Mahmarian JJ, Moyé LA, Verani MS, Bloom MF, Pratt CM. High reproducibility of myocardial perfusion defects in patients undergoing serial exercise thallium-201 tomography. *Am J Cardiol*. 1995;75(16):1116–1119.
18. Alazraki NP, Krawczynska EG, DePuey EG, et al. Reproducibility of thallium-201 exercise SPECT studies. *J Nucl Med*. 1994;35(8):1237–1244.

19. Iskandrian AE, Garcia EV, Faber T. Analysis of serial images: a challenge and an opportunity. *J Nucl Cardiol*. 2008;15(1):23–26.
20. Garcia EV, DePuey EG, Sonnemaker RE, et al. Quantification of the reversibility of stress-induced thallium-201 myocardial perfusion defects: a multicenter trial using bull's-eye polar maps and standard normal limits. *J Nucl Med*. 1990;31(11):1761–1765.
21. Van Train KF, Garcia EV, Maddahi J, et al. Multicenter trial validation for quantitative analysis of same-day rest-stress technetium-99m-sestamibi myocardial tomograms. *J Nucl Med*. 1994;35(4):609–618.
22. Van Train KF, Areeda J, Garcia EV, et al. Quantitative same-day rest-stress technetium-99m-sestamibi SPECT: definition and validation of stress normal limits and criteria for abnormality. *J Nucl Med*. 1993;34(9):1494–1502.
23. Beller GA. Quantitative nuclear cardiology and future directions for SPECT imaging. *J Nucl Cardiol*. 2007;14(4):417–418.
24. Garcia EV, Faber TL, Cooke CD, Folks RD, Chen J, Santana C. The increasing role of quantification in clinical nuclear cardiology: the Emory approach. *J Nucl Cardiol*. 2007;14(4):420–432.
25. Germano G, Kavanagh PB, Slomka PJ, Van Kriekinge SD, Pollard G, Berman DS. Quantitation in gated perfusion SPECT imaging: the Cedars-Sinai approach. *J Nucl Cardiol*. 2007;14(4):433–454.
26. Ficaro EP, Lee BC, Kritzman JN, Corbett JR. Corridor4DM: the Michigan method for quantitative nuclear cardiology. *J Nucl Cardiol*. 2007;14(4):455–465.
27. Watson DD, Smith WH 2nd. The role of quantitation in clinical nuclear cardiology: the University of Virginia approach. *J Nucl Cardiol*. 2007;14(4):466–482.
28. Liu YH. Quantification of nuclear cardiac images: the Yale approach. *J Nucl Cardiol*. 2007;14(4):483–491.
29. Slomka PJ, Berman DS, Germano G. Quantification of serial changes in myocardial perfusion. *J Nucl Med*. 2004;45(12):1978–1980.
30. Itti E, Klein G, Rosso J, et al. Assessment of myocardial reperfusion after myocardial infarction using automatic 3-dimensional quantification and template matching. *J Nucl Med*. 2004;45(12):1981–1988.
31. Faber TL, Modersitzki J, Folks RD, Garcia EV. Detecting changes in serial myocardial perfusion SPECT: a simulation study. *J Nucl Cardiol*. 2005;12(3):302–310.
32. Sdringola S, Loghin C, Boccalandro F, Gould KL. Mechanisms of progression and regression of coronary artery disease by PET related to treatment intensity and clinical events at long-term follow-up. *J Nucl Med*. 2006;47(1):59–67.
33. Kaufmann PA, Gnecchi-Ruscone T, Yap JT, Rimoldi O, Camici PG. Assessment of the reproducibility of baseline and hyperemic myocardial blood flow measurements with 15O-labeled water and PET. *J Nucl Med*. 1999;40(11):1848–1856.
34. Jagathesan R, Kaufmann PA, Rosen SD, et al. Assessment of the long-term reproducibility of baseline and dobutamine-induced myocardial blood flow in patients with stable coronary artery disease. *J Nucl Med*. 2005;46(2):212–219.
35. deKemp RA, Yoshinaga K, Beanlands RS. Will 3-dimensional PET-CT enable the routine quantification of myocardial blood flow? *J Nucl Cardiol*. 2007;14(3):380–397.
36. Takeda K, Saito K, Makino K, et al. Iodine-123-BMIPP myocardial washout and cardiac work during exercise in normal and ischemic hearts. *J Nucl Med*. 1997;38(4):559–563.
37. De Geeter F, Caveliers V, Pansar I, Bossuyt A, Franken PR. Effect of oral glucose loading on the biodistribution of BMIPP in normal volunteers. *J Nucl Med*. 1998;39(11):1850–1856.
38. Caveliers V, De Geeter F, Pansar I, Dendale P, Bossuyt A, Franken PR. Effect of exercise induced hyperlactatemia on the biodistribution and metabolism of iodine-123–15(p-iodophenyl)-3-R, S-methyl pentadecanoic acid in normal volunteers. *Eur J Nucl Med*. 2000;27(1):33–40.
39. Nakajima K, Shimizu K, Taki J, et al. Utility of iodine-123-BMIPP in the diagnosis and follow-up of vasospastic angina. *J Nucl Med*. 1995;36(11):1934–1940.

40. Hashimoto A, Nakata T, Tsuchihashi K, Tanaka S, Fujimori K, Iimura O. Postischemic functional recovery and BMIPP uptake after primary percutaneous transluminal coronary angioplasty in acute myocardial infarction. *Am J Cardiol.* 1996;77(1):25–30.
41. Kim Y, Sawada Y, Fujiwara G, Chiba H, Nishimura T. Therapeutic effect of co-enzyme Q10 on idiopathic dilated cardiomyopathy: assessment by iodine-123 labelled 15-(p-iodophenyl)-3(R, S)-methylpentadecanoic acid myocardial single-photon emission tomography. *Eur J Nucl Med.* 1997;24(6):629–634.
42. Taki J, Nakajima K, Matsunari I, et al. Assessment of improvement of myocardial fatty acid uptake and function after revascularization using iodine-123-BMIPP. *J Nucl Med.* 1997; 38(10): 1503–1510.
43. Sakurabayashi T, Takaesu Y, Haginoshita S, et al. Improvement of myocardial fatty acid metabolism through L-carnitine administration to chronic hemodialysis patients. *Am J Nephrol.* 1999;19(4):480–484.
44. Kuwabara Y, Watanabe S, Nakaya J, et al. Postrevascularization recovery of fatty acid utilization in ischemic myocardium: a randomized clinical trial of potassium channel opener. *J Nucl Cardiol.* 2000;7(4):320–327.
45. Iwado Y, Mizushige K, Manabe K, et al. Suppression of fatty acid metabolism after exercise stress in patients with no electrocardiographic ST segment shift during balloon angioplasty. *Angiology.* 2001;52(12):841–849.
46. Inglese E, Leva L, Matheoud R, et al. Spatial and temporal heterogeneity of regional myocardial uptake in patients without heart disease under fasting conditions on repeated whole-body 18F-FDG PET/CT. *J Nucl Med.* 2007;48(10):1662–1669.
47. Teräs M, Tolvanen T, Johansson JJ, Williams JJ, Knuuti J. Performance of the new generation of whole-body PET/CT scanners: discovery STE and discovery VCT. *Eur J Nucl Med Mol Imaging.* 2007;34(10):1683–1692.
48. Gould KL, Pan T, Loghin C, Johnson NP, Guha A, Sdringola S. Frequent diagnostic errors in cardiac PET/CT due to misregistration of CT attenuation and emission PET images: a definitive analysis of causes, consequences, and corrections. *J Nucl Med.* 2007;48(7):1112–1121.
49. Wollenweber SD, Gould KL. Investigation of cold contrast recovery as a function of acquisition and reconstruction parameters for 2D cardiac PET. *IEEE Nucl Sci Symp Conf Rec.* 5: 2552–2556;23-29 Oct 2005.
50. DICOM. http://medical.nema.org/; 2010 Accessed 06.10.2010.
51. Fred Mettler A Jr, Milton Guiberteau J, eds. *Essentials of Nuclear Medicine Imaging.* 5th ed. Amsterdam: Elsevier; 2006.
52. Ami Iskandrian E, Ernest Garcia V, eds. *Nuclear Cardiac Imaging: Principles and Applications.* 4th ed. New York: Oxford University; 2008.
53. van der Wall EE, eds. *Noninvasive Imaging of Cardiac Metabolism.* Dordrecht, The Netherlands: Martinus Nijhoff; 1987.
54. Paul Christian E, Kristen Waterstram-Rich M, eds. *Nuclear Medicine and PET/CT: Technology and Techniques.* 6th ed. Amsterdam: Elsevier; 2007.

Magnetic Resonance Imaging

16

Daniel C. Lee and Timothy J. Carroll

16.1 Basic Description of the Technique(s)

16.1.1 Magnetic Resonance Image Acquisition

Magnetic Resonance Imaging (MRI) has witnessed a huge amount of growth in its application to cardiac disease in the last ten years due, in part, to developments in signal acquisition and processing. MRI provides clinicians with important information regarding anatomy, function, perfusion, and viability of the myocardium.

16.1.2 Physiologic Parameter/Signal Being Evaluated

The signal being evaluated in clinical MRI of the heart comes from charged *protons* (^{1}H) on water molecules (H_2O) within the body. In this way, MRI differs from other imaging modalities such as X-ray, CT, PET, and echocardiography in that tissues themselves generate the signal rather than an X-ray tube, radioactive tracer, or ultrasound transducer. The nuclei of these protons exhibit *precession*, a rotational motion similar to that of a gyroscope (Fig. 16.1).

The behavior of nuclear spins inside the magnetic field of the MRI scanned can be approximated as a vector which precesses around the direction of the main magnetic field (Fig. 16.2). The frequency at which the spins precess can be calculated from the Larmor equation:

$$F = \text{gamma } B_0,$$

where F is the precessional frequency (in MHz), gamma is the gyromagnetic ratio, a constant specific to each type of nucleus (in MHz T^{-1}), and B_0 is the static magnetic field

---

D.C. Lee (✉)
Division of Cardiology, Feinberg School of Medicine, Northwestern University,
Chicago, IL, USA
e-mail: dlee@northwestern.edu

J.J. Goldberger and J. Ng (eds.),
Practical Signal and Image Processing in Clinical Cardiology,
DOI: 10.1007/978-1-84882-515-4_16, © Springer-Verlag London Limited 2010

Fig. 16.1 The precession of nuclear magnetic spins is similar to the precession of a spinning toy gyroscope

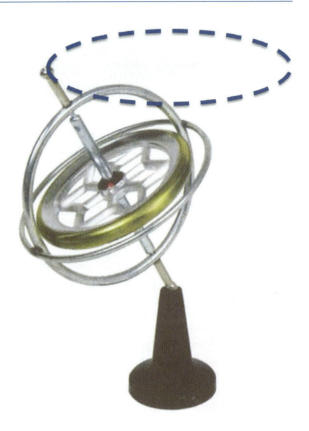

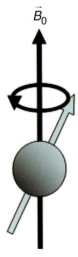
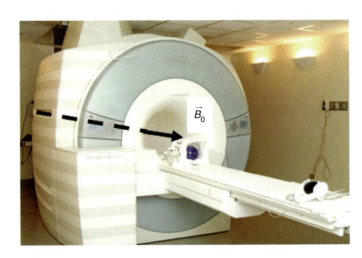

Fig. 16.2 The nuclear spin aligns itself with the MRI scanner's main magnetic field, B_0. In most clinical MRI scanners, the main field is collinear with the bore of the scanner

(in Tesla). For hydrogen protons, the gyromagnetic ratio is 42.58 MHz T^{-1}. Therefore, at the most commonly used field strength of 1.5 Tesla, the precessional frequency is 63.87 MHz. This frequency is also called the *resonant frequency*. This frequency is directly proportional to the strength of the magnetic field, so doubling the field doubles the precessional frequency. For example, the corresponding frequencies for 3.0 T, 4.7 T, and 9.4 T scanners are 127.74 MHz, 200.13 MHz, and 400.25 MHz, respectively. The precessional frequency also corresponds to the frequency of the radiofrequency excitation pulse that stimulates the MRI signal.

16.1.3
Basic Description of the Technique

Under normal circumstances, water protons are oriented randomly so the sum of their magnetic fields (*net magnetization vector*, M) is zero. Clinical MRI scanners employ strong magnetic fields (referred to as the *static field*, B_0, measured in units of Tesla). For most commonly encountered MRI scanners, the direction of the magnetic field is along the axis down the magnet's bore (Fig. 16.2).

When placed within the scanner's magnet bore, these spinning charges align along the axis of the main magnetic field (B_0) in either a parallel (spin up, white arrows) or antiparallel (spin down, yellow arrows) direction (Fig. 16.3). They continue to precess out of phase with one another, so the transverse vectors cancel and M_0 is aligned with B_0.

The degree to which the tissue becomes magnetized determines the strength of the MRI signal. As with the frequency, the signal strength is proportional to the magnetic field so that doubling the strength of the magnetic field will in turn double the MRI signal strength. In 1.5 T scanners, the net bulk magnetization of the tissue is 4.5 parts per million (ppm). In 3.0 T scanners the net magnetization is twice that value, i.e., 9.0 ppm.

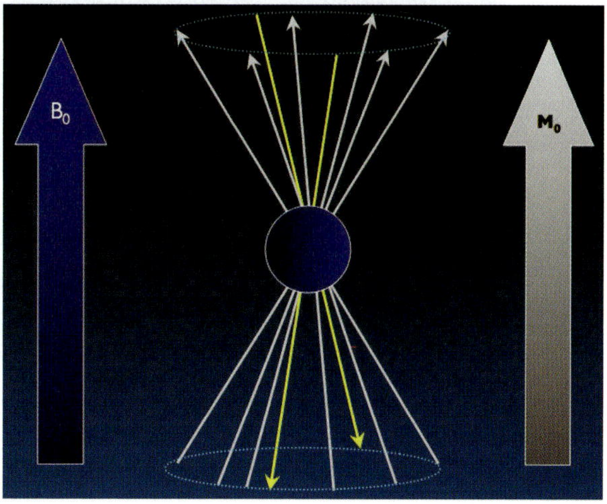

Fig. 16.3 The magnetization of individual water atoms are randomly distributed in the *x–y* plane. However, the presence of a strong external magnetic field, provided by the MRI scanner, imparts a net magnetization, M_0, which aligns itself with the main magnetic field, B_0

In order to create an MRI image, the net, bulk magnetization must be manipulated in some way. A radiofrequency (RF) pulse, tuned to the resonant frequency of the scanner with polarization at right angle to the main magnetic field, is applied to excite the water protons' spins. This RF pulse temporarily perturbs the precessing spins off the axis defined by the direction of the main magnetic field and also brings the spins into phase coherence (resonance). The strength and duration of the RF pulse determine the degree to which M_0 moves away from the z-axis. A 90° pulse tips M_0 into the transverse plane (Fig. 16.4). According to Faraday's laws of induction, the rotation of M_0 in the transverse plane induces voltage in a receiver coil positioned in the transverse plane. The spin will then return to its unperturbed state, precessing around the main magnetic field. As this happens, the resultant decrease in signal measured by the receiver coil is called the *free induction decay (FID)*.

The process by which the perturbed spins return to their unperturbed state is complex, but is well described by a differential equation known as the Bloch equation. The Bloch equation describes the rate at which signal decays and governs the generation of contrast in MRI images. The rate at which spins return to their ground state depends on the interaction of proton spins with neighboring spins and magnetic field inside the local tissue. The local magnetic field will be slightly different from point-to-point inside the body. These slight differences determine how rapidly the spins "relax" back to normal longitudinal position along the main magnetic field. Longitudinal magnetization recovers according to an exponential function and the rate at which this occurs can be expressed as a time constant, T1, in milliseconds (Fig. 16.5). Differences in local T1 values are the basis for T1 image contrast in MRI.

A voxel of tissue will have a large number of protons included in it. These protons will tend to precess at slightly different rates, depending on the uniformity of the field in the tissue. The rate at which transverse magnetization decays due to protons dephasing follows a different exponential function and is known as the transverse relaxation rate or T2 (Fig. 16.5).

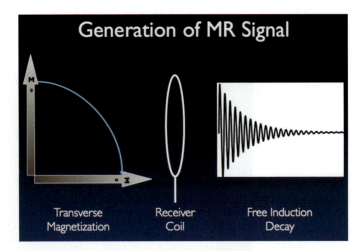

Fig. 16.4 The magnetization that is created by the main magnetic field must be tipped into the transverse plane to create the MRI signal. A receiver coil detects the MRI signal as the magnetization "relaxes" to its original orientation. The detected signal is referred to as the "free induction decay"

16 Magnetic Resonance Imaging

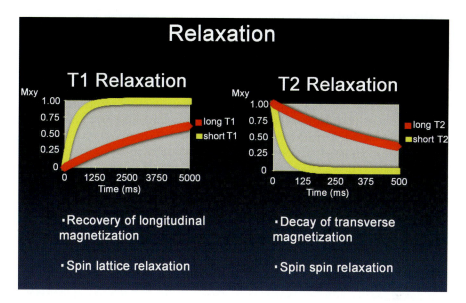

Fig. 16.5 As the net magnetization, M_0, returns to its original orientation, the rate of return is described by two parameters: T1 (longitudinal relaxation rate) and T2 (transverse relaxation rate). These two values are tissue-dependent and provide the basis for MRI contrast

MRI image contrast is based upon creating images when the contrast between two tissue types is greatest. If the MRI pulse sequence is designed to sample when T1 differences are greatest, it is said to be a T1-weighted image. If a sequence is designed to acquire the MR image when T2 differences are greatest, the image is said to be T2-weighted. The adjustable image contrast (i.e., T1 vs. T2 weighting) is what sets MRI apart from other imaging modalities.

16.2
Key Signal Processing Techniques Used

16.2.1
Fourier Transform

The MRI signal is an electromagnetic wave which emanates from the patient's body. This wave is made up of a number of different frequencies. The raw MRI signal is sometimes referred to as the FID. Multiple FIDs must be sampled in order to collect enough information to create an MRI image. To transform the raw MRI signals into an image, a Fourier transformation must be performed. A detailed description of the Fourier transform is presented in Chapter 3. The raw MRI data are stored in 2D or 3D arrays referred to as "k-space" data in reference to the wave nature of the electromagnetic waves that produced the signal. In k-space, low frequencies occupy the center where high frequencies appear at the edges of k-space. The low frequency, center of k-space is the most important component of the image data for determining image contrast. The periphery of k-space is responsible for improving the sharpness of an image.

In MRI images, in addition to the static magnetic field imparted by the magnet bore, another magnetic field known as a *spatial gradient* can be applied to create different magnetic fields at different positions within the object being scanned. Gradients alter the magnetic field in a linear fashion, and the strength of a gradient is expressed in mT/m. Protons at different positions along the spatial gradient are exposed to different magnetic fields and will, therefore, precess at different frequencies as predicted by the Larmor equation (Fig. 16.6).

The *phase* of the magnetic moment of a proton refers to its position along the precessional path around B_0 at any given time, measured in degrees or radians. This can be visualized either as a sine wave or a hand moving around a clock face. The temporary application of a spatial gradient changes the precessional frequency resulting in a change in the phase of the magnetic moment with respect to the magnetic moment of protons not exposed to the change in precessional frequency (Fig. 16.7). When the gradient is switched off, the precessional frequencies of the protons will return to their original frequencies, but the accumulated phase shift will remain.

Alterations in the frequency and phase of protons imparted by gradients oriented in the x, y, and z-axes can, therefore, be used to localize the position of these signals within the image (Fig. 16.8).

Following the application of an RF pulse, the MRI signal is acquired as a series of echoes. Each echo is slightly different due to the application of phase encoding gradients (Gy) and frequency encoding (read) gradients (Gx). The loud banging noise associated with an MRI scanner is due to the turning on and turning off of the phase encode and read gradients. Figure 16.9 shows an example of one signal echo acquired from a 1.5 T MRI scanner. The echo is acquired from a range of frequencies ($-K_{max}$ to K_{max}) with the zeroth frequency located in the center of the echo. It is important to note that most of the signal that goes toward making an MRI image is contained in the center of k-space. This is demonstrated by the large peak located at the center of the echo shown in Fig. 16.9.

During the performance of a scan, spatial gradients are applied in a specific manner that is defined by the *pulse sequence*. A series of echoes, each with different phase encoding history, are sampled and digitized using an analog-to-digital converter (ADC) and used to

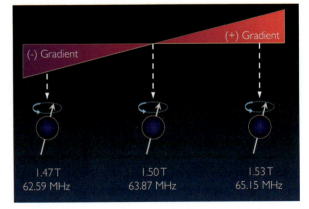

Fig. 16.6 Application of a spatial gradient causes an increase (*right*) or decrease (*left*) in the local magnetic field and a concomitant change in the precessional frequencies of protons. Protons positioned along the spatial gradient can, therefore, be selectively excited or localized based on their characteristic precessional frequency

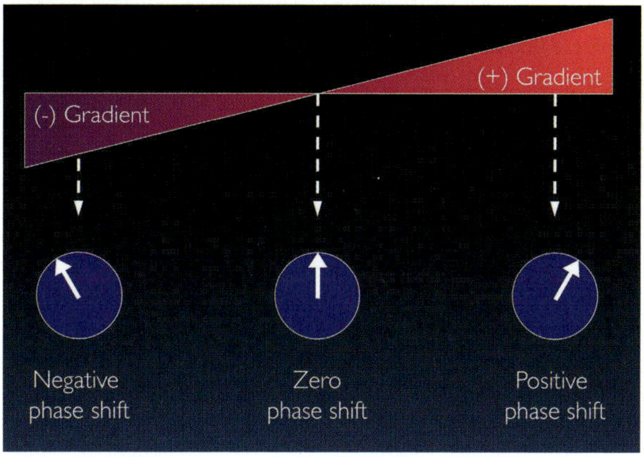

Fig. 16.7 As protons precess, the position along the rotational path can be expressed as phase. Temporary application of a spatial gradient causes proton spins to speed up or slow down, resulting in a proportional change in phase. Because the strength of the applied magnetic field varies along a spatial gradient, the magnitude of the phase shift is dependent on the location of the protons along the spatial gradient

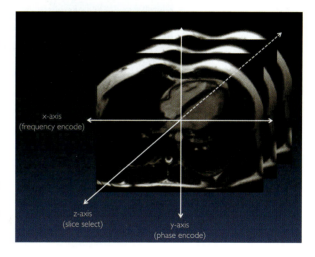

Fig. 16.8 A spatial gradient oriented in the *z*-axis is used to prescribe the imaging slice by selectively exciting protons at a specific precessional frequency. Application of a second spatial gradient imparts different phase shifts to protons depending on their position along the *y*-axis. A third spatial gradient causes protons to precess at different frequencies depending on their position along the *x*-axis

form a 2D *k-space* matrix. *K*-space is rectangular in shape with the frequency axis running horizontally, the phase axis running vertically, and both axes centered (zero value) in the middle of the rectangle (see Fig. 16.10). For each echo, the phase encoding gradient is activated to a differing degree to fill a specific horizontal line of *k*-space. When all the horizontal lines of *k*-space are filled, the scan of that slice is complete.

It is important to note that *k*-space is not the image, in that data from the top line do not correspond to the top of the image. Each echo contains phase and frequency information measured from the entire slice by the receiver coil during read out. The *k*-space representation of the image is uninterpretable to the human eye prior to postprocessing with Fourier

Fig. 16.9 One MRI echo corresponding to a single line in k-space

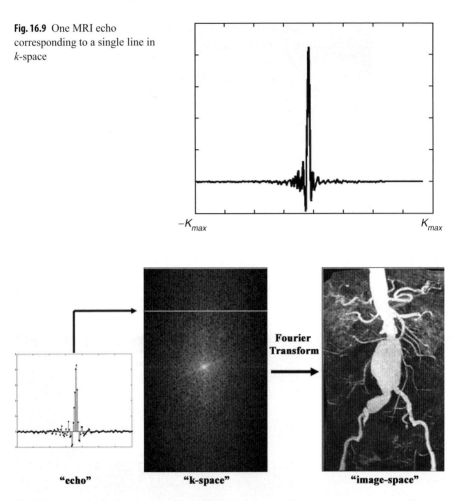

Fig. 16.10 A series of echoes acquired in an MRI scan are stored in computer memory as a 2D array known as k-space. The application of a mathematical Fast Fourier Transform (FFT) results in the familiar MRI image

transformation. The Fourier transform is a mathematical operation which transforms the acquired MRI signals into a weighted sum of position-dependent grey-scale values. The mathematical algorithm is known as the Fast Fourier Transform (FFT) and is the basis of all modern imaging systems. Figure 16.10 shows an example of a frequency space representation of an MRI image and the corresponding image after a 2D Fourier transform. Fourier transform and signals in the frequency domain are discussed in Chapter 3.

There are a number of important properties of the k-space representation of the image, which are commonly exploited in image acquisition. First is the fact that most of the signal intensity that is acquired in an MRI scan exists at low frequency. In other words, since frequencies are acquired from $-K_{max}$ to $+K_{max}$, the low-spatial frequencies appear at the center of the *k*-space image. This means that the center of *k*-space accounts for most of the information contained in the image and the acquisition of the center of *k*-space is of prime importance when signal acquisitions schemes are derived. Second, the periphery of *k*-space, i.e., the signal acquired near kmax, are the high-spatial frequencies. The high-spatial frequencies provide detail to the image. In other words, the spatial resolution of an image will depend on the high-spatial frequencies. Figure 16.11 shows how the low- and high-spatial frequencies contribute to the formation of an MRI image. Forming an image using only the lowest spatial frequencies (i.e., setting the outer portion of the *k*-space matrix to zero) gives a rough, low-resolution version of the image. Forming an image using only the high-spatial frequencies, which are located on the periphery of the *k*-space matrix, is shown in the middle column. The high-spatial frequencies provide edge detail to the image and are needed for high-resolution images.

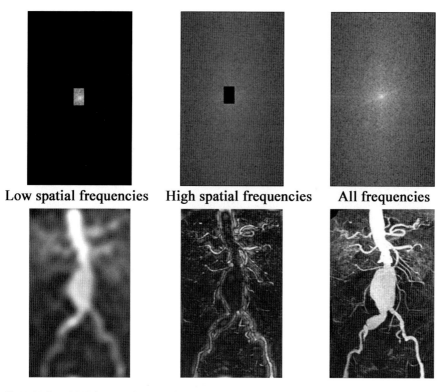

Fig. 16.11 Raw MRI data, or "*k*-space" data (*top row*), and the corresponding MR image that results after the application of a FFT (*bottom row*). In the left panels, only the central, low frequencies are used to generate the image. The central part of *k*-space (indicated by the *central rectangle*) provides the overall image contrast. In the middle panels, only the peripheral, higher frequencies are used to generate the image (central rectangle set to zero). In the right panels, when both the outer edges of *k*-space and the central region of *k*-space are used to generate the image, a high-resolution MR image results

16.2.2
Filtering

Corruption of the acquisition of either the low- or high-spatial frequencies will degrade image quality. This is particularly problematic in cardiac image acquisition since the heart will contract, changing its position and shape between the acquisition of low- and high-spatial frequencies. Finally, low- and high-spatial frequencies provide complementary information. The fact that low- and high-spatial frequencies can be adjusted independently in *k*-space allows the possibility to filter images or enhance edge details based upon altering the high and/or low-spatial frequencies prior to the Fourier transformation required by the image reconstruction software.

The imaging signal acquired by the MRI scanner is recorded in *k*-space and converted into an image through the process of Fourier transformation. There are well-defined mathematical relations between the spatial domain signal, i.e., the image, and the frequency domain signal (Chapter 3). Understanding these relations can aid in understanding the physical limitation imposed on image acquisition. For example, the spatial resolution of an image is determined by high-spatial frequencies. There is an inverse relationship between *k*-space and image space. The following relation holds

$$K_{max} \propto \frac{1}{\Delta x},$$

where K_{max} is the highest spatial frequency acquired and Δx is the spatial resolution. A qualitative explanation of this relation is that as higher spatial frequencies are added to an image, the spatial resolution increases. In a similar fashion, the field of view of an image, i.e., the largest object that can be included in the image, is inversely proportional to the separation between two *k*-space samples:

$$FOV \propto \frac{1}{\Delta k}.$$

Combining these two relations yields an expression that describes how spatial resolution is related to imaging time for 2D cardiac imaging. The time to acquire an image (TA) is determined by the number of *k*-space lines acquired and the time to acquire them. For example, if one line of space is acquired for each repetition time of the image acquisition (TR), we can simply calculate the scan time. If we assume a 320 mm Field of View and require 1.0 mm spatial resolution, we require 320 mm spaced by 1 mm or 320 samples.

$$TA = Nsamples * TR$$

For our 320 samples and assuming a 3.0 ms TR, TA=960 ms, roughly 1 s.

The time to acquire even a low-resolution MRI image is, therefore, longer than the beat-to-beat interval for typical heart rates. Cardiac motion must be compensated for in some way. The simplest approach to freezing cardiac motion is to acquire images very rapidly. This is known as "real time" imaging. With echo-planar imaging, a 2D image slice can be acquired in as little as 40 ms. Real-time cardiac MRI images are played in succession to depict the contraction of the heart. Multiple slices can be acquired to cover the whole heart within a single breath-hold. These are typically acquired with either echo- planar images

(EPI) or balanced steady state free precession (SSFP) images. These two approaches differ in how the MRI signal is manipulated and acquired.

In EPI acquisitions, the signal from the echo is read out and refocused multiple times through the use of reverse polarity phase encoding gradients. This has unwanted consequences on image quality. The signal can be refocused, but on each successive echo, the signal diminishes in proportion to the T2* of the tissue. The T2*-decay of the EPI signal has the effect of multiplying the acquired signal by an exponential modulation function resulting in image blurring. The resulting real-time images are of lower spatial resolution than the prescribed image matrix.

Recently, balanced gradient SSFP pulse sequences have been developed to improve the image quality of real-time MRI. The SSFP image acquisition refocuses the magnetization by alternating RF pulses and balanced gradients. Unlike EPI readouts, balanced SSFP does not suffer from T2* signal modulation and images are generally of higher image quality than EPI images.

16.2.3
Gating

In cardiac MRI, the motion of the heart can be frozen by synchronizing acquisition of the image data to the cardiac cycle. These acquisitions are known as being "cardiac gated." Cardiac gated MRI scans are generally used to make cine images, which depict the contraction of the heart, or to make high-resolution images of one point in the cardiac cycle. For example, MRI-based coronary artery images are acquired using gated acquisitions.

The basic premise behind cardiac gating is that MRI image data are made up of a set of distinct lines of k-space. If the heart returns to roughly the same position each cardiac cycle, it does not matter which cycle the k-space data are acquired in. Therefore, only some small fraction, or segment, of the MRI image needs to be acquired in each cardiac cycle. For example, if a particular 2D MRI image is acquired on a 128×128 matrix, it requires 128 lines of k-space to be acquired. A cardiac gated scan, acquiring 10 lines of k-space per cardiac cycle, would require 13 heart beats to acquire the image. For a heart rate of 72 bpm, this is a 15.6 s scan time, which is easily performed within a single breath-hold. Assuming a TR=3.0 ms, the ungated scan would take $128 \times 3.0 \text{ e}^{-10} \text{ s} = 0.384 \text{ s}$.

From the example given above, it is clear that the number of k-space lines acquired per segment will determine the number of heartbeats needed to acquire the MRI image. The number of lines per segment is determined by the size of the acquisition window. For high-spatial resolution images, the goal is to minimize the amount of blurring caused by cardiac motion. Minimizing cardiac motion during the acquisition of the segment of k-space in a segmented acquisition, the acquisition window is initiated in the most quiescent part of the cardiac cycle – mid diastole. The width and position of the data acquisition (DAQ) window within the cardiac cycle are adjustable parameters and adjusted during the scan to optimize image quality and minimize scan time. For patients with compromised pulmonary function, the size of the window may be increased to reduce the length of the breath-hold. For a typical patient, an acquisition window of 50–100 ms is used and acquired 800 ms after the detection of the R-wave. Figure 16.12 shows a schematic diagram of cardiac gating.

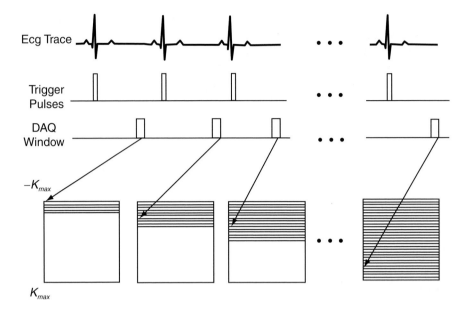

Fig. 16.12 In cardiac gated MRI scans, the acquisition of the images is synchronized to the cardiac cycle. The MRI k-space is divided into a number of segments. Within each cycle, a single segment consisting of 10 to 20 lines of the image is acquired. In this approach, the image is acquired over several heartbeats

Cardiac gating requires leads to be placed on the patient's chest. The ECG signal is detected by the scanner hardware and real-time feedback allows the scanner to synchronize image acquisition to the detection of the R-wave. Once the R-wave is detected, a trigger pulse is sent to the scanner to signal the acquisition of image data.

16.3
Factors Interfering with Quality Replication of the Signal of Interest

16.3.1
Signal-to-Noise Ratio

The Signal-to-noise ratio (SNR) of an MRI signal is a widely used parameter to quantify image quality. For an MRI image, the signal itself depends on the type of desired image contrast (i.e., T1, T2, SSFP), the details of the equipment used (type of receiver coils, coil placement), and scanner adjustment (local field shim, center frequency). We will focus only on those which are controllable at the time of the scan.

The SNR of an MRI image depends on: (1) the number of elements emitting the MRI signal; in other words, the number of signal producing water molecules in the image voxel, (2) the size of the signal each molecule produces, (3) the quality of the signal detection, and (4) the amount of spurious noise and the statistics of noise averaging.

As a general rule of thumb, the SNR of an MRI image depends on the square root of the scan time and the size of the voxel that is producing the signal. By increasing the spatial resolution of an MRI signal, we are decreasing the voxel's size, the number of protons contributing to the signal, and consequently the SNR. For example, if we prescribe a 1.2 × 1.2 × 1.2 mm MRI scan and compare that to a 1.0 × 1.0 × 1.0 mm scan, all other things being equal, we would see a SNR decrease of

$$\Delta \text{SNR} = \frac{(1.0\,\text{mm} \times 1.0\,\text{mm} \times 1.0\,\text{mm})}{(1.2\,\text{mm} \times 1.2\,\text{mm} \times 1.2\,\text{mm})} = 0.58.$$

In other words, a modest increase in the spatial resolution of an MRI image results in a nearly 60% drop in SNR. Signal averaging is one method to improve SNR with increased spatial resolution. In this way, we increase imaging time in order to boost SNR. By effectively doubling the imaging time, we gain $\sqrt{2}$ or roughly 40% in SNR.

The size of the MRI signal emitted by each water molecule is controllable through altering the main magnetic field. Currently, most clinically used MRI scanners employ a 1.5 Tesla magnetic field to produce the MRI signal. We can simply double the size of the signal that each voxel produces by doubling the size of the magnetic field. For example, an MRI scanner that uses a 3.0 Tesla magnet will have twice the SNR of the same MRI image acquired at 1.5 T. This is a very rough approximation because as the field strength increases, the resonant frequency, the signal receiver electronics, and the magnetic properties of the tissue (T1, T2 etc.) are also affected. Consequently, almost all the MRI pulse sequence parameters must be retuned for higher field scanners. However, the starting point of a twofold increase in SNR is desirable for many applications and the adaptation of cardiac MRI to 3.0 T is well under way.

16.3.2
Artifacts

An understanding of MRI signal processing techniques is necessary for the recognition and elimination of imaging artifacts.

16.3.2.1
Phase Wrap

Phase wrap refers to the folding of anatomy from outside the field of view (FOV) onto anatomy within the FOV (Fig. 16.13). This occurs when signal from protons positioned outside the FOV are detected by the receiver coil. Because every phase value from 12:00 through 11:59 (or all 360°) is allocated to protons within the FOV, protons from outside the FOV are assigned overlapping values resulting in mismapping of those pixel values onto pixels within the field of view. Scanning a larger FOV will correct the phase wrap, but this requires increasing the number of phase encoding steps, which increases the scan time. Alternatively, the number of phase encoding steps can be held constant by dropping the resolution.

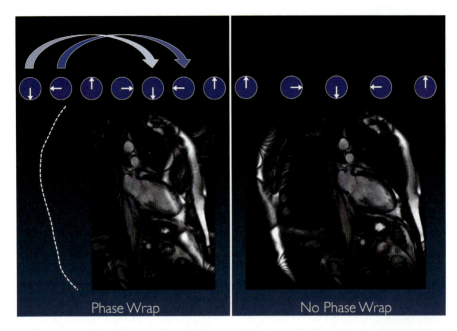

Fig. 16.13 The left panel demonstrates phase wrap which causes anatomy from the posterior thorax to be folded onto the anterior thorax. All phase values from 0 to 360° are assigned to protons within the narrow field of view. However, protons outside of the field of view are still affected by the gradient and still detected by the receiver coil, and their phase values overlap with those within the field of view. Sampling a wider field of view in the phase direction (anterior–posterior in this case) corrects the phase wrap, as seen in the right panel

16.3.2.2 Phase Mismapping

Phase mismapping is caused by anatomy moving in the phase encoding direction during the scan. Because each phase encoding step happens sequentially, moving anatomy may erroneously be assigned multiple phase values. This results in duplication of the anatomy in the image, also referred to as a ghosting artifact (Figs. 16.14 and 16.15).

16.3.3 Magnetic Resonance Image Analysis

Although visual interpretation of CMR studies may sometimes suffice, image processing techniques for the quantification of wall motion, perfusion, and infarction can improve the accuracy and reproducibility of results. Quantification also allows for clearer communication of findings and easier comparison between studies for follow-up or research. Most importantly, clinical decisions are often made based on quantitative indices such as ejection fraction, left ventricular volume, and infarct size. Therefore, the clinician should have

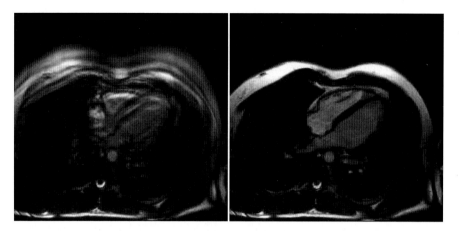

Fig. 16.14 During free-breathing (*left panel*), the heart and chest wall move in the phase encoding direction (anterior–posterior) resulting in phase mismapping artifact. By scanning during a breath-hold (*right panel*), the artifact is eliminated

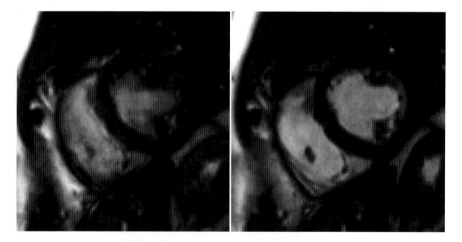

Fig. 16.15 Contraction and relaxation of the heart can also lead to phase mismapping (*left panel*). Gating the image acquisition to the ECG extends the scan time, but results in a crisp image

an understanding of image processing techniques used in the analysis of CMR studies in order to recognize the strengths and limitations of quantitative CMR indices.

The first step in image processing of CMR images is the input of image data into a software analysis program. These programs may be designed specifically for CMR image analysis by MR scanner manufacturers and third party vendors, or they may be general digital image analysis programs which can be modified to analyze CMR images. The most basic functions of these programs are to allow the user to define a region of interest (ROI) on an image, count the pixels within that region of interest, register the grayscale intensity of each pixel, and report statistics regarding the pixels in the ROI such as mean signal intensity. More sophisticated programs automatically trace the contours of the left ventricle and calculate cardiac specific indices such as ejection fraction, left ventricular volume, and infarct size.

A typical mid short-axis cine CMR image is shown in Fig. 16.16. Using ImageJ (a digital image analysis program available from the NIH), two regions of interest (ROI's) have been defined. ROI 1 has been drawn in the left ventricular blood pool and ROI 2 in the anterior myocardium. The number of pixels, maximum signal intensity, minimum signal intensity, mean signal intensity, and standard deviation of signal intensity are displayed by the program. Note the intrinsically higher signal of blood relative to the myocardium.

16.3.4
Quantification of Volumes and Mass from Cine CMR Images

Cine CMR images are ideal for the quantification of left ventricular volumes and mass because of the excellent delineation between blood, myocardium, and surrounding structures. This results in a higher interstudy reproducibility for CMR than echocardiography in the measurement of left ventricular mass and volume,[1] which can translate into reduced sample size requirements for clinical trials designed to demonstrate changes in mass, volume, or ejection fraction.

According to Simpson's rule, the volume of an object can be approximated by dividing the object into multiple slices and summing the volumes of the individual slices. CMR data sets used for volumetric analysis are typically composed of multiple short-axis slices acquired every 10 mm spanning the entire ventricle from base to apex. Figure 16.17 depicts a stack of short-axis cine images and their relationship to the four-chamber cine slice. This type of volumetric approach is preferable to a biplane approach such as the modified Simpson's rule of an ellipsoid model because the assumptions built into geometric models may not be met in abnormal hearts. This concept was illustrated in a study of 25 patients with dilated cardiomyopathies by Chuang et al. Volumetric measures of ejection fraction and left ventricular volume by 3D echocardiography and MRI agreed well. However, for both echocardiography

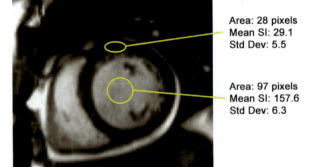

Fig. 16.16 Postprocessing of CMR images based on Region of Interest (ROI) analysis. Postprocessing programs report local image statistics to enhance the interpretation of images

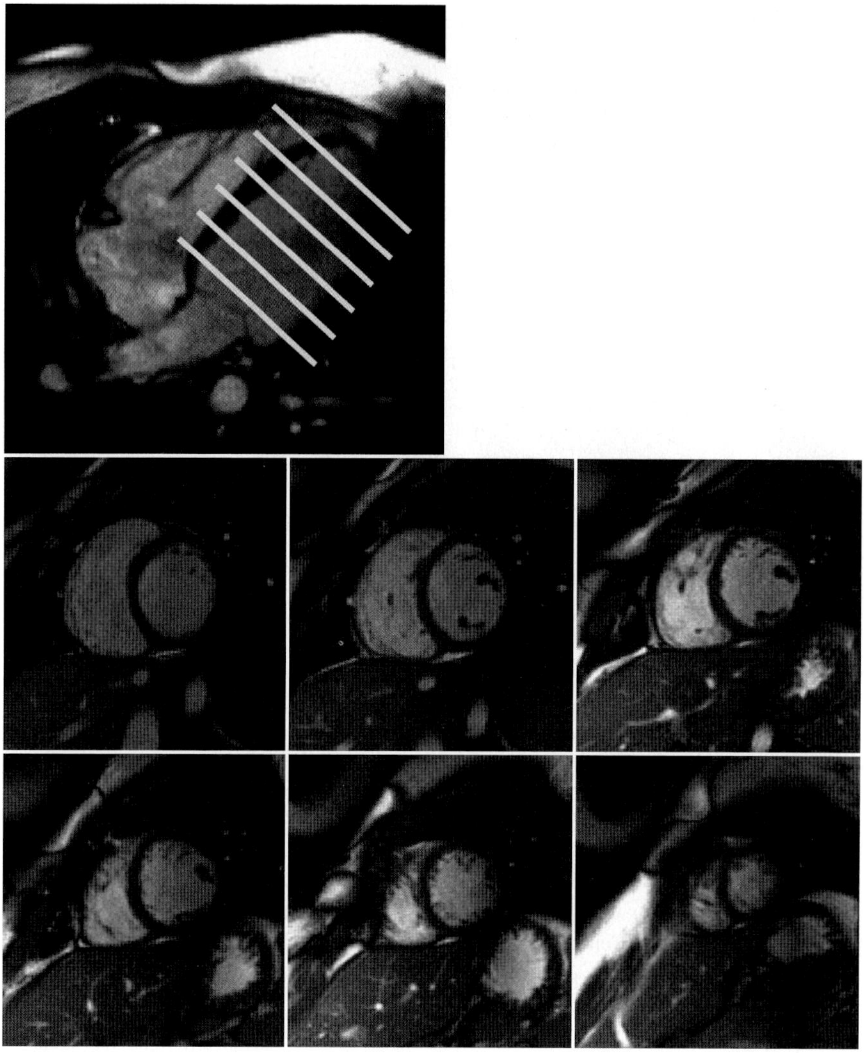

Fig. 16.17 Several consecutive short-axis image slices are combined to provide accurate determination of left ventricular volume. Note the excellent image contrast between the blood pool and myocardium

and MRI, the agreement was poor between biplane and volumetric methods, and the agreement was even worse between echocardiographic and MRI biplane methods.[2]

The first step in quantification involves defining the endocardial and epicardial contours for each short-axis image (Fig. 16.18). The volume of a slice is calculated by multiplying the number of pixels in the slice by the known area of each pixel and the slice thickness. The sum of volumes for the individual slices represents the total volume for the left ventricle. The volume within the endocardial contours represents the blood pool volume and

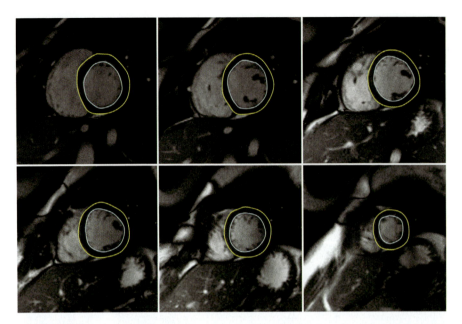

Fig. 16.18 Endocardial and epicardial contours are drawn to define the area of the myocardium. Volume and mass are calculated from the area and slice thickness

the volume between the endocardial and epicardial contours represents the myocardial volume. Myocardial mass can then be calculated by multiplying the myocardial volume (in ml) by the density of myocardium (1.05 gm/ml).

A typical short-axis cine is composed of 20–25 images acquired at equally spaced time intervals over the cardiac cycle. Calculation of ejection fraction requires contouring the endocardial border for each short-axis slice at end systole and end diastole. Some more sophisticated programs can incorporate contours from long-axis images to account for the effect of longitudinal contraction (i.e., from base to apex).

16.3.5
Automated Contouring of Cine Images

At a minimum, quantification of ejection fraction on cine CMR images requires contouring of the endocardial borders on each of 8–10 short-axis images at systole and diastole. Mass measurements require additional contouring of the epicardial borders, and analysis of changes over time requires additional contours propagated over some or all of the cardiac cycle. This can be a laborious task which can take up to 1 h. Obviously, this is impractical for routine clinical care. Therefore, automated contour detection algorithms have been developed to speed up the analysis of studies.

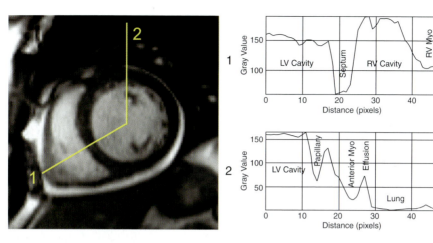

Fig. 16.19 Automated image contouring algorithms use line plots to determine the myocardial border. Sharp changes in signal intensity along the profile demark the borders between the bright blood pool and myocardium

A common algorithm begins by generating line profiles from the center of the left ventricle in order to detect tissue transitions based on changes in grey value. Figure 16.19 illustrates a short-axis cine with two radial line profiles. Each line profile plots the signal intensity along the length of a line. Note how the variability in the grey value of intracavitary and surrounding structures may pose difficulties for the detection algorithm. Profile 1, which travels through the midinferoseptum, demonstrates very clear transitions because of the sharp delineation between blood and myocardium. Profile 2 is more challenging. The sharpest transition from bright to dark occurs at the interface of blood and a papillary muscle. Small trabeculations along the surface of the anterior myocardium cause some blurring of the endocardial blood myocardial border. The epicardial border is marked by an effusion, but often the transition from myocardium to lung can be difficult to discern. The variable appearance of different line profiles may cause this step of the algorithm to select inappropriate endocardial and epicardial borders. Therefore, additional constraints can be used to improve contour selection. For example, the contours of the heart should be relatively smooth, so the algorithm will attempt to minimize dramatic changes in contour position between neighboring line profiles. Similarly, tissue transitions for a line profile taken at the same position over multiple phases throughout the cardiac cycle should not vary too much from one cardiac phase to the next. The algorithm can, therefore, utilize a cost function to define the tissue borders by balancing changes in grey value on the line profile with smoothness of the contours within a single frame and smoothness in border changes from frame-to-frame.

Good image quality is probably the most important factor influencing the success of automated algorithms. However, success of the algorithm can also be improved by increasing the amount of information entered into the algorithm. Increasing the number of radial line profiles in each frame will improve the propagation of borders around the LV in each frame. Reducing the time interval between frames (i.e., more frames per cardiac cycle) will improve the propagation of borders from frame-to-frame. The algorithm may also utilize user-defined seed points to refine border selection. However, the improvement in contour selection resulting from this increased data must be balanced against the cost of increased computing time and increased user interaction. The development of accurate automated contour detection algorithms remains a challenging issue, and some user interaction is still required to ensure consistently accurate results.

16.3.6
Analysis of Delayed Enhancement CMR Images

One of the unique strengths of CMR is the ability to visualize viable and irreversibly injured myocardium, enabling assessment of myocardial viability.[3] Several minutes following the administration of gadolinium contrast, areas of myocardial infarction become bright (hyperenhanced) when imaged using a T1-weighted segmented inversion recovery gradient echo pulse sequence (Fig. 16.20). Animal studies have demonstrated a close correlation between the area of contrast enhancement by CMR and the area of infarct by histological studies in both the acute [4] and chronic settings.[5]

The development of the segmented inversion recovery gradient echo sequence improved the visualization of myocardial infarction by creating a signal difference between infarcted and normal myocardium of 1,080% in animals and 485% in humans.[6] The transmural extent of hyperenhancement can be visually graded based on the percentage of a region of the myocardial wall that is hyperenhanced (Fig. 16.21). Clinical studies have demonstrated that segments with a lower transmural extent of hyperenhancement have a higher likelihood of wall motion recovery following revascularization, and segments with a greater transmural extent of hyperenhancement have a lower likelihood of wall motion recovery following revascularization.[7]

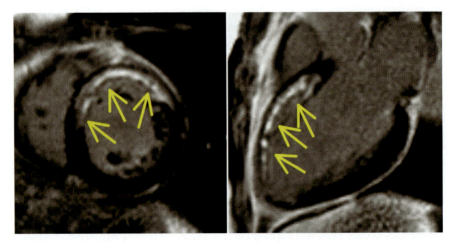

Fig. 16.20 In this T1-weighted image, contrast agent uptake appears bright. The uptake of MRI contrast agent has been shown to demark areas of infarct

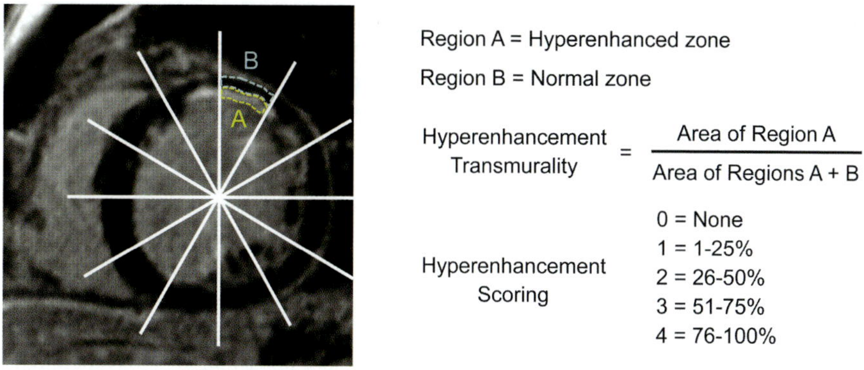

16 Magnetic Resonance Imaging

Region A = Hyperenhanced zone

Region B = Normal zone

$$\frac{\text{Hyperenhancement}}{\text{Transmurality}} = \frac{\text{Area of Region A}}{\text{Area of Regions A + B}}$$

Hyperenhancement Scoring
- 0 = None
- 1 = 1-25%
- 2 = 26-50%
- 3 = 51-75%
- 4 = 76-100%

Fig. 16.21 Segmented gradient echo MRI scans have been developed that produce excellent image contrast between normal and infarcted myocardium. Hyperenhancement scoring has been shown to be predictive of recovery following revascularization

16.3.7
Automated Infarct Quantification

The pixels bounded by endocardial and epicardial contours can be dichotomized into normal and infarcted pixels by thresholding. This method defines a signal intensity threshold above which pixels are counted as infarct and below which pixels are counted as normal myocardium. Some investigators have defined this threshold as greater than two standard deviations above the mean signal value for a user-defined area of normal myocardium. Others define the threshold as 50% of the maximum signal value within the infarct, referred to as "full width half max." This technique was found to be highly accurate when compared to pathologic measures of infarct size.[8]

Although thresholding is an objective and reproducible method for classifying pixels as infarct or noninfarct, suboptimal image quality or improper contouring of endocardial and epicardial borders may lead to erroneous measurements. For example, if an area of epicardial fat is not completely excluded, these high signal pixels will be included as infarct pixels. Some newer algorithms attempt to exclude false positive pixels by requiring pixels to be either adjacent to the endocardial border or to a larger area of infarct.[9]

16.4
How are Data Stored

MRI scanners typically store images in a similar manner to all medical images following the Digital Imaging and Communications in Medicine (*DICOM*) standard.[10] The DICOM standard allows for easy transfer of image data between vendors and storage devices. Once the images have been acquired and reconstructed in the MRI scanner's host computer, they must be transferred and stored. Each 2D image has an image "header" associated with the pixel data. The header for an image can be thought of a small file that contains all the relevant patient information, the details of the examination (time, date, location, image size, etc.), as well as the coordinates that describe the orientation at which the image was required. The coordinates stored within the image header are in the RAS coordinate system (RAS=Right/Left, Anterior/ Posterior, Superior/Inferior). These coordinates are calculated based upon the information provided by the technologist at the time when the patient enters the MRI magnet in a process called "Land marking." The DICOM header for each image is attached and stored to the image pixel data so that an MRI image file contains both the header and the pixel data. At this point, the image file can be transmitted, stored, and retrieved without loss of critical information.

The size of the images that must be stored depends on the number of pixels in the image, i.e., the spatial resolution of the image, and the complexity of the MRI exam. As the number of images acquired in an MRI exam grows, so does the complexity of image storage and retrieval. In cardiac exams where several thousand images are acquired, hardcopy filming and review become impossible. Most modern departments have access to *picture archiving and communication systems* (PACS) computer networks. These networks are computers, storage disks, and viewing stations that are designed specifically for medical images.

16.5
Appendix: MRI Image Formation

The basis of the signal in MRI is the excitation of nuclear spins which emit a RF signal. When returning to their unperturbed state, water molecules emit an electromagnetic signal that is slightly different, depending on the local environment. This process is known as relaxation. The process by which the perturbed spins return to their unperturbed state is complex, but is well described by a differential equation known as the Bloch equation,

$$\frac{d\vec{M}}{dt} = \vec{M} \times \gamma\vec{B} - \frac{M_x \hat{i} + M_y \hat{j}}{T_2} - \frac{(M_z - M_0)\hat{k}}{T_1}.$$

In the Bloch equation, M is the magnetization vector of a small macroscopic volume of tissue (or "Voxel"). Magnetization is a vector quantity, and changes in this vector are accompanied by the emission of electromagnetic waves that are detected in the MRI receiver coils. The Bloch equation consists of three terms. The first term:

$$\vec{M} \times \gamma\vec{B}$$

is a mathematical representation of the RF excitation pulse which tips the magnetization from its unperturbed state. The second and third terms describe the transverse and longitudinal relaxation of the magnetization. The rate of the transverse relaxation or "dephasing" depends on the T2 rate constant. In other words, the second term describes the rate at which spins lose phase coherence. T2 will vary from tissue to tissue and this term describes T2 image contrast. The last term describes the rate at which the magnetization realigns itself with the main magnetic field. It is referred to as the longitudinal relaxation rate (T1).

The MRI signal that is acquired, $S(t)$, by the scanner is the frequency space representation of the image, $I(x,y)$. Spatial localization of the MRI signal is achieved by shifting the frequency and phase of the local magnetic field. These slight differences in frequency are sufficient to localize the signal to better than 1 mm. The amount of phase and frequency shift is controlled by the MRI pulse sequence through the application of local field gradients, Gx and Gy. The MRI signal is recorded as segments of an electromagnetic signal S(t, ty). This signal is related to the true MRI image by:

$$S(t;t_y) = \int_x \int_y I(x,y)e^{-i\gamma G_y y t_y} e^{-i\gamma G_x x t} dy dx.$$

The expression shown above is well known in the engineering literature as the Fourier Transformation of the Image. Fast Fourier transform algorithms for the calculation of the image, I(x, y), have existed since the early 1960s. After a signal is acquired, a Fast Fourier Transform must be performed by the scanners image reconstruction computer prior to review.

References

1. Grothues F, Smith GC, Moon JC, et al. Comparison of interstudy reproducibility of cardiovascular magnetic resonance with two-dimensional echocardiography in normal subjects and in patients with heart failure or left ventricular hypertrophy. *Am J Cardiol*. 2002;90(1):29–34.
2. Chuang ML, Hibberd MG, Salton CJ, et al. Importance of imaging method over imaging modality in noninvasive determination of left ventricular volumes and ejection fraction: assessment by two- and three-dimensional echocardiography and magnetic resonance imaging. *J Am Coll Cardiol*. 2000;35(2):477–484.
3. Bucciarelli-Ducci C, Wu E, Lee DC, Holly TA, Klocke FJ, Bonow RO. Contrast-enhanced cardiac magnetic resonance in the evaluation of myocardial infarction and myocardial viability in patients with ischemic heart disease. *Curr Probl Cardiol*. 2006;31(2):128–168.
4. Kim RJ, Fieno DS, Parrish TB, et al. Relationship of MRI delayed contrast enhancement to irreversible injury, infarct age, and contractile function. *Circulation*. 1999;100(19): 1992–2002.
5. Fieno DS, Kim RJ, Chen EL, Lomasney JW, Klocke FJ, Judd RM. Contrast-enhanced magnetic resonance imaging of myocardium at risk: distinction between reversible and irreversible injury throughout infarct healing. *J Am Coll Cardiol*. 2000;36(6):1985–1991.
6. Simonetti OP, Kim RJ, Fieno DS, et al. An improved MR imaging technique for the visualization of myocardial infarction. *Radiology*. 2001;218(1):215–223.
7. Kim RJ, Wu E, Rafael A, et al. The use of contrast-enhanced magnetic resonance imaging to identify reversible myocardial dysfunction. *N Engl J Med*. 2000;343(20):1445–1453.
8. Amado LC, Gerber BL, Gupta SN, et al. Accurate and objective infarct sizing by contrast-enhanced magnetic resonance imaging in a canine myocardial infarction model. *J Am Coll Cardiol*. 2004;44(12):2383–2389.
9. Hsu LY, Natanzon A, Kellman P, Hirsch GA, Aletras AH, Arai AE. Quantitative myocardial infarction on delayed enhancement MRI. Part I: Animal validation of an automated feature analysis and combined thresholding infarct sizing algorithm. *J Magn Reson Imaging*. 2006; 23(3):298–308.
10. The DICOM Standard available at http://medical.nema.org/medical/dicom/2009/

Computed Tomography

17

John Joseph Sheehan, Jennifer Ilene Berliner, Karin Dill, and James Christian Carr

17.1 Introduction

Cardiac imaging was previously confined to plain film, invasive coronary angiography (ICA), nuclear medicine and echocardiography. Non invasive imaging of the heart with computed tomography (CT) and magnetic resonance imaging (MRI) has changed our approach to imaging cardiac disease. The advent of multidetector computed tomography (MDCT) with electrocardiographic (ECG) synchronization has established several clinical roles in the evaluation of coronary artery disease (CAD), coronary artery anomalies, coronary stent, coronary by-pass analysis and coronary plaque characterization. In addition, MDCT can assess myocardial perfusion, myocardial viability, valves, coronary veins and pulmonary veins.

This chapter will focus on three sections: the technical aspects of cardiac CT, the relative merits of computed tomography angiography (CTA) in imaging the coronary vessels and the role of MDCT in imaging the remaining cardiac structures.

17.2 Section 1: Technical

17.2.1 X-Ray Hardware

17.2.1.1 X-Ray Generator

An X-ray generator and an X-ray tube are required to produce X-rays. X-ray generators are made up of high-voltage transformers, filament transformers, rectifier circuits along with voltage and current meters. Generators use 440 V compared to the 120 V alternating

---

J.J. Sheehan (✉)
Department of Cardiovascular Imaging, Feinberg School of Medicine, Northwestern University, Chicago, IL, USA
e-mail: johnsheehan999@gmail.com

current (AC) used at the home. The generator increases the voltage and rectifies the waveform from AC to direct current (DC). The generator controls three parameters: tube voltage (kilovolts, or kV), which affect the X-ray energy; tube current (milliamperes, or mA), which affects the radiation quantity; and exposure time (seconds). The voltage is applied across the X-ray tube, and current flows through the X-ray tube. The power dissipated is the product of the X-ray energy (kV) and of the tube current (mA) and is measured in kilowatts (kW).

Transformers (step-up and step-down) change the magnitude of the input voltage by electromagnetic induction. A step-up transformer has more turns in the secondary coil (e.g., 1:400) resulting in a higher voltage across the tube. Rectification changes AC voltage (sinusoidal) to DC voltage across the X-ray tube using diodes. Three phase generators have replaced single-phase generators, which receive three lines of current, each 120° out of phase with one another, resulting in a more constant waveform. This results in less voltage variation or waveform "ripple."[1]

17.2.1.2
X-Ray Tube

An X-ray tube converts electric power produced by the generator into X-ray photons. The tube consists of an evacuated tube housing containing a negatively charged cathode containing the filament that serves as an electron source and a positively charged copper anode which is partly composed of a tungsten target where the X-rays are produced and exit via a window in the housing. The cathode's filament is composed of a coiled tungsten wire. When the current passes through the high resistance filament, the temperature rises, resulting in thermionic emission of electrons. At saturation voltage, all electrons are pulled away from the filament and strike the tungsten imbedded in the circular, rotating positively charged anode. The anode is angled, ranging from 7 to 20° to permit larger heat loading. Only about 1% of the electric energy supplied by the generator to the X-ray tube is converted into X-rays, the remainder is converted to heat.[1]

17.2.2
X-Ray Production

When electrons strike the tungsten in the anode, electromagnetic radiation in the form of X-rays is produced. X-rays are generated by two different processes known as bremsstrahlung (radiation) and characteristic K-shell emission (ionization). The majority of radiation is produced via the bremsstrahlung process. This involves a free electron traveling past a tungsten atom nuclear field, which slows down and changes the direction of the electron. The resultant loss of energy of the electron is released as an X-ray photon. Characteristic radiation is the result of ionization and results when free traveling electrons with energies >69.5 keV, strikes a tungsten atom and ejects an inner shell electron. A lower energy outer shell electron fills the vacancy and the energy difference is emitted as characteristic radiation.

Intensity refers to the quantity or number of X-ray photons produced. X-ray output is directly proportional to the current (mA) and the exposure time (s). It is proportional to the square root of the tube potential (kV). The effective photon energy reflects the quality of the X-ray beam and is proportional to the penetrating power. Increasing the kV by 15% has the same effect as that of doubling milliamperes. The focal spot is the apparent source of X-rays in the tube and it determines the spatial resolution. Filters made of aluminum and copper are placed between the patient and the X-ray source to remove low energy photons, which do not contribute to the final image. Filtration results in beam hardening which changes the shape of the polychromatic X-ray spectra, but does not reduce the maximum photon energy.[1]

17.2.2.1
X-Ray Interactions and Detectors

Information captured by X-ray detectors are the sum of the interactions or lack of interactions of the X-ray photons as they pass through the patient. When X-rays travel through the body they can be transmitted, absorbed or scattered. When photons are absorbed there is transfer of energy to the tissue, which contributes to image contrast and the radiation dose. If a photon changes direction and loses energy, it is called scatter, resulting in loss of image contrast and increased patient dose. When photons interact, the energy transferred to electrons is measured in kiloelectron volts (keV). The two most important interactions in diagnostic radiology are the photoelectric effect and Compton scatter.

The photoelectric effect occurs when an X-ray photon is totally absorbed by a tightly bound inner K-shell electron, resulting in the ejection of a photoelectron. When an outer shell electron fills the inner-shell electron vacancy, the excess energy is emitted as characteristic radiation. In order for the photoelectric effect to occur, the X-ray photon must have energy greater or equal to the binding energy of the inner shell electron. The K-edge of an element is the energy level just above the binding energy of the K-shell electrons. If an X-ray photon has energy just above, there will be a sudden increase in the attenuation coefficient of the X-ray photons interacting with the electron of an atom. The X-ray contrast media iodine has a K-shell binding energy for absorption of X-rays of 33 keV, which is close to the mean energy of most diagnostic X-ray beams. In other word the photoelectric effect predominates at energies just above the K-edge of an element. Examples of K-shell binding energies include: calcium 4 keV, iodine 33 keV, barium 37 keV, and lead 88 keV. Compton scatter occurs when X-ray photons interact with loosely bound outer shell electrons, resulting in a scattered photon, which has less energy and travels in a new direction. The likelihood of these interactions are inversely proportional to the X-ray photon energy.[1]

CT uses rows of scintillators to detect the transmitted X-ray photons and the photoelectrons ejected during the photoelectric effect. Scintillators are materials that emit light when exposed to radiation and are coupled to a light detector (photodiode). The standard CT detectors are gadolinium oxysulfide (GOS) scintillators. Newer generation, garnet based gemstone scintillator material can transfer light more efficiently to the detector diode and speed processing times by shortening the afterglow period significantly compared to GOS.

17.2.2.2
Attenuation of Radiation

The linear attenuation coefficient is the extent to which the intensity of X-ray photons are reduced as it passes through a specific material, over a given distance. It takes account of all interactions including the photoelectric effect and Compton scatter. It is proportional to the atomic number of the absorbing medium and inversely proportional to the photon energy, with the exception of the K-edges.

CT images are maps of relative linear attenuation values of tissues. The relative attenuation coefficient (μ) is expressed in Hounsfield units (HU). The HU of material x is $HU_x = 1,000 \times (\mu_x - \mu_{water})/\mu_{water}$. The HU of water is always zero. The following are approximate HU values: air $=-1,000$, lung $=-300$, fat $=-90$, water $= 0$, white matter $= 30$, gray matter $= 40$, muscle $= 50$, and cortical bone $= 1,000+$.[1]

17.2.2.3
Image Acquisition and Reconstruction

X-ray tubes in a CT scanner produce a fan beam of X-ray photons, which after passing through the patient are measured by an array (row) of detectors. The sum of all the attenuation by all tissues is referred to as the ray sum. The collection of the ray sums for all of the detectors at a given tube position are called projections which will have up to 1,000 individual data points. Projection data sets (ca. 1000) are acquired throughout the 360° rotation angles of the X-ray tube around the patient. Filtered back projection (FBP) mathematical algorithms converts the 1000^2 projection data points (raw data) and converts them into a CT image (image data), using array processors. New reconstruction algorithms such as adaptive statistical iterative reconstruction (ASIR) are able to extract additional spatial resolution and suppress noise at lower patient doses.

Different mathematical filters can be used to suit the clinical task, offering tradeoffs between spatial resolution and noise. Soft tissue filters reduce image noise and improve the contrast to noise ratio, resulting in better visualization of low contrast lesions (e.g., soft plaque). The tradeoff is decreased spatial resolution. Bone and stent filters result in increased noise but improved fine detail visualization.

17.2.2.4
Image Display and Storage

The image data is displayed as individual picture elements called pixels, as a two-dimensional (2D) image. Each of the pixel intensity is coded using either 1 or 2 bytes. The total number of pixels in an image is the product of the number of pixels in the horizontal and vertical, x and y-axes. The total number of pixels in each axis is referred to as matrix size. The field of view (FOV) is the diameter of the body region. The CT pixel size is the FOV divided by the matrix size (typically 512). For example the CT pixel sizes are 0.8 mm for a 40 cm FOV thorax (40 cm divided 512). A voxel is the volume element in the patient, which is calculated by product of the pixel and slice thickness. The brightness of each pixel is related to the relative attenuation coefficient of the tissue in the voxel.

Each pixel is normally represented by 12 bits, or 4,096 gray levels. A bit (binary digit) is the fundamental information element used by computers and can be assigned one of two discrete values. One bit can code for two values corresponding to black and white. n bits can code for 2^n gray levels. As a result 12 bits codes for 2^{12} or 4,096 shades of gray. If there are 512 pixels in the x-axis and 512 in the y-axis, the matrix size is $512 \times 512 = 512^2$. If each pixel uses 2 byte coding in a 512×512 matrix the image data would be 1 MB.

Window width and level optimize the appearance of CT images by determining the contrast and brightness levels assigned to the CT image data. Window width refers to the range of grayscale values displayed. All pixels with values below the range register as black and all of those above as white. Window level defines the center value of the window width and, therefore the overall image brightness. A CT image with a window width of 100 HU and a window level (center) of 50 HU displays an image in which HU values of zero or less appear black, HU values of 50 appear midgray and HU values greater that 100 appear white. Interpolation is the mapping of an image of one matrix size to the display of another size.[1]

17.2.2.5
Image Quality

Factors affecting image quality and characteristics of cardiac images include temporal and spatial resolution. Temporal resolution is defined as the required time for data acquisition per slice. It represents the length of the reconstruction window during each heart cycle, which is determined by the gantry speed. The primary challenge required to image a rapidly beating heart is that the imaging modality should provide high temporal resolution.

Spatial resolution refers to the degree of blurring in the image and the ability to discriminate objects and structures of small size. Axial resolution within the scan plane can be improved by using a small FOV, larger matrix size, smaller focal spot and smaller detectors. The demand for high spatial resolution that enables the visualization of various coronary segments that run with decreasing diameter to the apex is high. One of the major goals of MDCT technology development has been to obtain similar spatial resolution in all directions, also expressed as isotropic spatial resolution.[2]

Noise is the random fluctuations of pixel values in a region that receives the same radiation exposure of another. Noise is an important determinant of CT image quality and limits the visibility of low contrast structures. It is determined primarily by the number of photons used to make an image (quantum mottle). It can be reduced by increasing tube current and voltage. It can also be reduced by increasing voxel size (decreasing matrix size, increasing FOV, or increasing slice thickness).

Contrast is the difference of the intensity of the one area relative to another. Image contrast is the difference in the intensity of a lesion and that of the surrounding background. CT is superior to conventional radiography for detecting low contrast differences. CT contrast is the difference in the HU values between tissues. CT contrast increases as tube voltage (kV) decreases and is not affected by tube current (mA). Contrast can be increased by adding a contrast medium such as iodine. The displayed image contrast is determined by the CT window (width and level).

17.2.2.6
Scanner Design

Since the first pencil beam EMI scanner in 1972, there have been numerous generations of CT scanners. The first four generations of scanners all had a single row of detectors (single slice) with evolving X-ray tube and detector configurations. Initially, for these generations, the image data were acquired one slice at a time. This involved scanning a slice and then moving the patient table to the next slice position and scanning again, otherwise known as "step and shoot." The next advancement was the introduction of helical (spiral) CT, which involved the patient's table moving continuously through the CT gantry, as the tube rotated around the patient. The relationship between the patient and tube motion is called pitch, which is defined as table movement (mm) during each full rotation of the X-ray tube divided by the collimation width (mm). A faster pitch means thicker slices, reduced resolution but lower scan time and lower patient dose. A pitch of greater than 1 will leave gaps between slabs and a pitch of less than 1 will allow necessary overlap among slabs.

Electron beam computed tomography (EBCT) technology, also known as fifth generation CT, provides excellent temporal resolution that allows freezing cardiac motion through very short acquisition times. In EBCT, the detectors are stationary. The X-ray source is fixed. It consists of 210° ring of tungsten. This is bombarded by an electromagnetically focused beam of electrons fired from an X-ray gun. The patient is placed between the X-ray source and detector, obviating the need for moving any part of the scanner during the exam. While EBCT has better temporal resolution at the present time (50 ms), the spatial resolution is not nearly as good as MDCT because the collimators are too thick.

17.2.2.7
Detectors

The next major advancement was the development of MDCT. This incorporated the use of multiple rows of detectors to detect wider fan beams. This configuration makes more efficient use of X-ray tube output and covers a larger area in the patients' z-axis (long axis) for every tube rotation. Unlike, conventional CT, MDCTs slice thickness is determined by detector width and not collimator thickness. The number of rows has increased at a rapid pace over the recent years, covering 2, 4, 8, 16, 32, 64, 128, 256 and now 320 slices. The current driving force behind this rapid evolution is CAD.

Flying focal spot technology allows improvement in spatial resolution without decreasing detector elements' size by utilizing two overlapping X-ray beams without a corresponding increase in dose. Detector elements of 0.6 mm can be utilized to acquire 0.33 mm spatial resolution images.

Diagnostic performance in coronary CTA is primarily determined by temporal resolution, which is the required time for data acquisition per slice. The determinant of this is the gantry rotational speed. For the typical setup of a single tube and detector, half a gantry rotation is necessary to acquire the date for volume reconstruction, i.e., temporal resolution is equal to half gantry rotation. The temporal resolution of a 64-slice CT with a gantry rotation of 330 ms is 166 ms. In order to obtain motion free images at any phase in the cardiac cycle, a temporal resolution of 10 ms is required. To achieve such high TR is impossible with CT. As a result cardiac CT phase reconstruction is centered on the quiescent or low motion window in end diastole. The postulated required temporal resolution for reliable cardiac imaging is in the range of 65 ms.[3] Philips has developed a 256-slice CT (128×0.625) with a rotation time of 270 ms and temporal resolution of 135 ms. However, with automatic multisegmental reconstructions with voxel-based optimization, temporal resolutions up to 68 ms are achieved.

Siemens has developed dual source computed tomography (DSCT) technology, which comprises of two X-ray tubes and two corresponding detectors. The two acquisition systems are mounted on the rotating gantry, with an angular offset of 90°. For cardiac imaging a detector configuration of 64×0.6 mm is used, whereby two subsequent 64-slice readings with a flying focal spot are combined into two 128-slice projections, with isotropic spatial resolution of 0.33 mm. With the tube rotation time of 280 ms, data can be sampled over only 90° of a gantry rotation (as opposed to 180° with single source systems), resulting in the industry's fastest temporal resolutions of 75 ms. The ultrafast tube rotation and table feed enables acquisition of the entire heart in 250 ms within a single diastolic phase without a breathhold, resulting in reduced dose down to an unprecedented 1 mSv or less.

Toshiba has developed a 320-slice CT scanner with 0.5 mm detectors (16 cm coverage along the patients z-axis), which images the body in a cylindrical fashion and can scan the entire heart prospectively, in one heart beat without any table movement. This is expected to reduce the likelihood of both cardiac and respiratory motion artifacts.

17.2.2.8
Dual Energy

One of the more recent advances in CT has been the introduction of dual energy. When operated in dual energy mode, the two tubes emit X-ray spectra of different energy levels that are simultaneously registered in their corresponding detector array. At any given time point, this provides synchronous dual-energy image formation for the entire anatomy encompassed by the scan range. This enables differentiation of scanned tissues with different spectral properties. There is early evidence that this technique can be successfully applied for analyzing the iodine signature within the myocardial blood pool.[4]

17.2.3
Image Acquisition and Protocols

Two types of triggering or ECG gating exist: retrospective and prospective.

17.2.3.1
Retrospective Gating

Cardiovascular MDCT imaging is currently predominantly performed in the spiral (helical) mode, with data being acquired by constant rotation of the X-ray tube/detector system throughout the entire cardiac cycle (continuous scanning). The data acquired are linked to the ECG tracing, allowing retrospective reconstruction of multiple cardiac phases, when the study is complete. A specific phase within the RR interval can be chosen to create a stack of images.

There are two techniques to retrospectively gate the scan to the ECG for image reconstruction. In one technique, the images are collected from one particular point in time in the cardiac cycle which is defined as a percentage of the R-R interval. Alternatively, this point in time is defined at an absolute fixed time in milliseconds (ms) before or after the R-R interval. This latter method is better for irregular heart rhythms.

Retrospective gating allows for faster coverage of the heart than does prospective triggering because images are reconstructed at every heart beat. Continuous spiral acquisition allows overlapping of image sections and therefore permits 20% greater in plane spatial resolution than that allowed by the collimator itself, resulting in a resolution of 0.6 mm for a 0.75 mm section and 0.4 mm for a 0.6 mm section.

Continuous acquisition throughout the cardiac cycle also allows retrospective reconstruction at different phases of the cardiac cycle. This permits selection of the best phase(s) for each of the coronary arteries and their segments where there is the least motion and the best image quality. Retrospectively, individual heart beats may be deleted or the reconstruction interval for an individual beat can be shifted manually if there are arrhythmias or variable heart rates. Retrospective triggering is the preferred method of triggering for assessing cardiac function and valve pathology.

17.2.3.2
Prospective Gating

Prospective ECG triggering is a sequential scan in which data acquisition is prospectively triggered by the ECG signal in diastole. Data is only collected at a predefined cardiac phase, established by the operator before the acquisition.

With this technique, tube current is turned on only at a predefined point after the R wave (a constant cardiac phase). At all other times between each RR interval no radiation is emitted. This triggering method requires a regular heart rhythm; otherwise the image created during each heart beat will occur at a different part of the cardiac phases, resulting in artifacts. Prospective gating is most often used for calcium scoring. Prospective gating reduces the radiation dose by up to 10 times. However, this occurs at the expense of unavailability of systolic phases for additional image reconstruction (which may be needed if diastolic images are suboptimal). In addition, assessment of cardiac function is not possible.

Hsieh et al developed a new approach for CTA referred to as prospectively gated axial (PGA). This technique uses a combined "step-and-shoot" axial data acquisition and an incrementally moving table with prospective adaptive ECG triggering. This method takes advantage of the large volume coverage available with the 64-slice MDCT scanner that enables complete coverage of the heart in 2–3 steps. With this technique, the table is stationary during the image acquisition. It then moves to the next position for another scan initiated by the subsequent cardiac cycle. The result is very little overlap between the scans, significant 50–80% reduction in radiation dose, and more robust and adaptive ECG gating.[5] Earls et al reported an effective dose for the PGA group (mean 2.8 mSv) which was significantly lower than for the retrospectively gated helical (RGH) group (mean 18.4 mSv). This represents a reduction in mean effective dose to the patient by up to 80% from the RGH to the PGA.[6]

17.2.3.3
ECG Dose Modulation

Dose modulation is utilized to help reduce the radiation exposure. During retrospective scanning, the tube current (milliampere-mA) is turned on continuously during the exam. The tube current or mA is dialed down by 80% during systole (Fig. 17.1). Although the lower mA may result in a suboptimal quality image, this may not be of clinical consequence. Overall, this dose modulation technique reduces the radiation dose by up to 40% of the

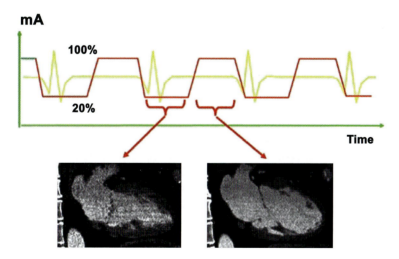

Fig. 17.1 Tube current may be lowered to 20% of the nominal current value in the systolic phase, yielding a noisy systolic image (*left*). Full dose is applied in diastolic phase, allowing high quality images when the heart is still (*right*)

usual dose. With most machines, dose modulation is the default mode and needs to be turned off if not desired. With increased heart rates, dose modulation cannot be used.

17.2.3.4
Image Acquisition and Reconstruction

X-ray tubes in a CT scanner produce a fan beam of X-ray photons, which after passing through the patient are measured by an array (row) of detectors. The sum of all the attenuation by all tissues is referred to as the ray sum. The collection of the ray sums for all of the detectors at a given tube position are called projections which will have up to 1,000 individual data points. Projection data sets (ca. 1000) are acquired throughout the 360° rotation angles of the X-ray tube around the patient. FBP mathematical algorithms converts the 1000^2 projection data points (raw data) and converts them into a CT image (image data) using array processors.

There are four different CT reconstruction algorithms using different approaches to calculate the slice image given the set of its views. The first approach solves numerous simultaneous linear equations; however it is impractical due to the extensive computational time required. The second approach uses several different iterative techniques including: algebraic reconstruction technique (ART), simultaneous iterative reconstruction technique (SIRT), and iterative least squares technique (ILST). These iterative techniques are generally slow. A third technique uses Fourier reconstruction entailing Fourier transformation in the spatial and frequency domain. FBP, however is the method most widely used. This is a modification of an older technique, called back projection or simple back projection. An individual sample is backprojected by setting all the image pixels along the ray pointing to the sample to the same image in the direction it was originally acquired. The final back projection image is then taken as the sum of all the backprojected views. Back projected images however, result in blurry images. FBP is a technique to correct the blurring encountered in simple back projection, resulting in a reconstructed imaged that closely resembles the actual image. See Chap. 15 for a more detailed discussion on FBP. New reconstruction algorithms such as ASIR are able to extract additional spatial resolution and suppress noise at lower patient doses.

Different mathematical filters can be used to suit the clinical task, offering tradeoffs between spatial resolution and noise. Soft tissue filters reduce image noise and improve the contrast to noise ratio, resulting in better visualization of low contrast lesions (e.g., soft plaque). The tradeoff is decreased spatial resolution. Bone and stent filters result in increased noise but improved fine detail visualization.

17.2.4
Radiation and Dose

Medical imaging has undergone tremendous technologic advances in recent decades, particularly affecting cardiac imaging. There has been rapid evolution in MDCT technology with increasing temporal and spatial resolution, allowing rapid imaging of a greater patient population than in previous years. With this evolution, the scientific and public awareness of the radiation risks associated with this technology has been increasing. Therefore, it is essential for operators to understand the effects of the radiation exposure delivered and to implement techniques that reduce this exposure.

Radiation effects can be divided into two categories, stochastic and deterministic. Stochastic refers to the probability of the effect, rather than its severity and increases with dose. This is assumed to occur without threshold, so even minor exposures may carry some increased risk. For example, the probability of radiation induced leukemia is substantially greater after 100 rad than after 1 rad, but the severity of disease is the same if it occurs. Deterministic defines that the severity of injury increases with dose. This is assumed to occur only above a dose threshold; requiring higher doses to produce effect. For example, development of cataractogenesis is known to occur after a dose exposure of 200 rad.

Potential biological effects from ionizing radiation depend on the radiation dose and the biological sensitivity of the tissue or organ system irradiated. Effective dose (E) is the descriptor that reflects this difference in biologic sensitivity. The units of E are Sieverts (Sv), often expressed as millisieverts (mSv). Not all tissues are equally sensitive to the effects of ionizing radiation. Therefore, tissue weighting factors (Wt) assign a particular organ or tissue the proportion of the risk of stochastic effects (e.g., cancer and genetic effects) resulting from irradiation of that tissue compared to uniform whole body irradiation. The X-ray radiation that everyone is exposed to each year from natural sources amounts to 2–5 mSv.

CT contributes a significant portion of the total collective dose from ionizing radiation to the public (Table 17.1). The goal is to keep doses "as low as reasonably achievable"

Table 17.1 Relative radiation doses for different imaging modalities

Examination	Effective dose (mSv)
Average annual background U.S.	3.6
General	
PA and lateral CXR	0.04–0.06
Head CT	1–2
Chest CT	5–7
Abdomen/pelvis CT	8–11
Calcium score	1–3
Invasive coronary angiography	3–5
Cardiac nuclear SPECT (dual isotope: sestamibi/thal)	10–15
Cardiac CT (retrospectively gated)	11–22
Cardiac CT (prospectively gated)	1–5

(ALARA). This represents a practice mandate adhering to the principle of keeping radiation doses to patients and personnel as low as possible. Among the most widely known protocols such as calcium scoring studies, the effective dose is relatively small, 1–3 mSv.[7] The effective radiation dose with retrospectively gated coronary angiography by 64-slice MDCT is estimated to be approximately 11–22 mSv.[8]

Operating within the ALARA guideline, obtaining diagnostic images with the minimum exposure to the patient is critical in cardiac CT. Several techniques of automated exposure control exist to achieve this goal. It is feasible for CT systems to adjust the current based on variations in X-ray intensity at the detector. Depending on the system, this can be performed in either the z axis or as the X-ray tube travels around the patient. Combining both approaches in an algorithm that "chooses" the correct tube current to achieve a predetermined level of noise is ideal.[9]

Strategies for reduction of radiation dose in cardiac MDCT include the following[10]:

Optimize scan parameters
- Weight adjusted tube current (mA)
- Reduce kV to 100 in low-body mass indices (BMI) patients
- Limit z-axis coverage to heart
- Reduce FOV (25 cm)

ECG dose modulation
- Up to 40% dose reduction

Prospective gated axial (PGA)
- Up to 80% dose reduction

Adaptive scanning
- Up to 40% dose reduction to the breast
- Up to 25% reduction by eliminating pre and post spiral radiation

Garnet-based gemstone scintillator detectors
- Up to 50% dose reduction

Dual source detectors
- With temporal resolution of 75 ms, table feed of 43 cm/s, entire heart scan in 250 ms with <1 mSv

New Reconstruction Algorithms (ASIR)

Bismuth Breast Shields

Clinically, studies performed using higher mA have less noise and higher signal-to-noise ratio and contrast-to-noise ratio which is visually more appealing and useful in heavily calcified vessels or intracoronary stents. However, doubling the tube current doubles the radiation dose. Lowering the tube voltage allows for significant reduction in effective dose as increasing the kV by 15% has the same effect as that of doubling mA. The trade-off for lower tube voltage is increased noise, however using 100 kV for low-BMI patients results in increased intensity of iodinated contrast as 100 kV is closer to the K-edge of iodine.

Adaptive scanning reduces the radiation exposure of dose-sensitive anatomical regions, such as the female breast. This is done by switching the X-ray tube assemblies off during the rotation phase in which the anatomical regions, concerned, are most directly exposed to radiation. In this way, it is possible to reduce the radiation exposure of individual anatomical regions such as the breasts by up to 40%. Furthermore, an adaptive dose shield can block irrelevant prespiral and postspiral radiation with dynamic diaphragms, thus ensuring that only a minimum and clinically essential radiation exposure occurs. This enables an additional 25% reduction of the dose required for routine examinations.

The implementation of these techniques and other dose reduction strategies evolving industry-wide will greatly minimize the radiation risks associated with these cardiac scans.

17.2.5
Patient Selection and Preparation

Patients who are not good candidates for CTA include those with unstable acute coronary syndrome who may need percutaneous coronary intervention (PCI), patients in atrial fibrillation, those with renal failure or iodinated contrast allergy. Obesity limits the ability to obtain diagnostic examinations due to the increased soft tissue attenuation and image noise. With BMI over 30 kg/m^2, it has been shown that the accuracy of the test falls below that for patients of normal weight.[11] Coronary artery calcification also reduces the diagnostic accuracy of CTA.

To conduct a coronary CTA examination, intravenous access is obtained, ideally with an 18 G antecubital catheter in the right arm. Next, breath holding is practiced with the patient and they are instructed to avoid swallowing and movement, to avoid step artifact in the resultant image. Beta blockade is used to achieve slower heart rates, either intravenously or orally, depending on the clinical setting. A sample protocol includes Metoprolol intravenous injection 5 mg IV repeated up to 3 times depending on the heart rate. Alternatively, oral dosing can be administered the night before and morning of the exam. Slowing the heart rate is essential for image quality in 16 and 64 slice CT. A recent study of DSCT demonstrated slightly lower per-segment evaluability for high heart rates without beta-blockade but no decrease in diagnostic accuracy for the detection of coronary artery stenosis.[12] Nitroglycerin 0.4 mg sublingual is given to vasodilate the coronary arteries and to improve visualization.

Iodinated contrast is then administered. Bolus timing is critical to ensure that imaging is performed with maximum contrast intensity in the coronaries. This can be achieved by one of two methods, bolus tracking or the timing bolus method. The bolus tracking method tracks density of contrast in a region of interest (ascending aorta for coronary evaluation). When the contrast density reaches a pre-specified Hounsfield value, imaging is begun. The timing bolus method involves two injections, one of small volume (20 mL) to allow measurement of the time to peak intensity of contrast in the ascending aorta. The full injection is then administered with the time of imaging being determined by the test bolus.

A similar protocol used to image the coronary arteries can be applied to assess the pulmonary and cardiac veins. To assess the pulmonary vein ostia, a contrast bolus of greater than 100 mls is recommended with gating optional. The time to scan will be slightly earlier than for the coronaries, with a scan duration of only 2 s necessary. The bolus tracking technique can be used with the region of interest placed within the left atrium to optimize opacification of the pulmonary vein ostia.

The volume of contrast to be used is determined by the scan time according to the following formula:

$$\text{Scan time} \times 5 + 10 \text{ mls} = \text{volume of contrast}$$
$$\text{E.g., } 14 \text{ s scan} \times 5 \text{ mls} + 10 \text{ mls} = 80 \text{ mls total}$$

A popular contrast administration protocol utilizes a triphasic injection; the first phase is contrast, the second phase is an admixture (70% saline/30% contrast) with the third phase being a bolus chaser of saline alone. The advantage of this triphasic technique is that it will produce enough contrast in the right ventricle to allow visualization of the septum for left ventricular functional assessment. The rate of infusion of contrast is a critical determinant of the quality of image. A minimal flow rate of 5 mls/s is optimal for the general population. For obese patients, higher rates should be attempted.[13]

Personalized, computerized, patient-based dosing of contrast media delivery protocols are showing promise, helping to produce diagnostic quality images more consistently. They personalize the scan delay, flow rate and volume for each of the three phases of injection based on patient weight, scan time, time to aorta peak, HU peak number and the concentration of iodine used (300 or 350).

17.2.6
Artifacts, Pitfalls and Solutions

Many unique artifacts can result from imaging the rapidly moving heart, the most common of which is the result of cardiac pulsation.[2] This results in an image with horizontal slabs of the image in displaced alignment (Fig. 17.2). The second type is banding artifacts which result from an increased heart rate during the scan. These are similar in appearance to pulsation artifacts. These artifacts especially occur in patients with high heart rates, heart rate variability, and in the presence of irregular or ectopic heart beats (e.g., premature ventricular complexes (PVCs) and atrial fibrillation). These can be minimized by scanning with higher temporal resolution on the order of 50 ms or by multi-second reconstruction with MDCT. A beta-blocker should be used to reduce the heart rate to less than 65 beats/min.[14] Recent data support high diagnostic accuracy for the detection of coronary artery stenosis with the use of DSCT without beta blockade, attributed to the improved temporal resolution (75–83 ms) compared to single source MDCT (166 ms).[15] However, in clinical practice, the exact role of beta blockade in dual source imaging is yet to be determined, especially at high heart rates.

Other types of artifacts commonly observed are due to incomplete breath holding, observed on sagittal or coronal views. These are seen as "stair-step" artifacts through the entire data set, including nonmoving structures, such as the bones. Adequate patient instruction prior to imaging is essential to avoid such artifacts.[8]

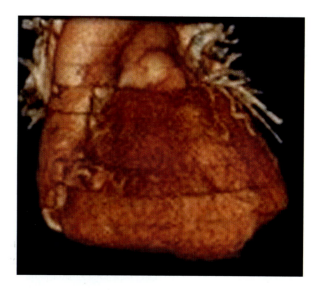

Fig. 17.2 Misregistration or stairstep artifact. Multiple horizontal slabs appear as displaced segments in this 3D volume rendered image

Streak artifacts can be noted around high attenuation structures, such as coronary stents, pacing wires and coils and can obscure adjacent structures. These are difficult to avoid and can be reduced with special artifact reduction software developed by the manufacturers.

High attenuation structures such as stents and calcified plaques can appear enlarged ("bloomed") because of partial-volume averaging effects. This results in overestimation of the size of the calcified plaque. This can obscure the coronary lumen, limiting the estimation of stenosis in the affected segments (Fig. 17.3). Although sharper filters or kernels and thinner slices (0.5–0.6 mm) may reduce the artifact with stents, this has little effect on calcification. Therefore, eliminating calcium blooming artifacts is of utmost importance for the success of coronary CTA.

Beam hardening is important to recognize. This artifact is a low density focus in a reconstructed image, appearing similar to noncalcified coronary atherosclerotic plaque. It is a result of low-energy photon absorption as the X-ray beam crosses a high-density structure, such as a surgical clip or calcification. In areas neighboring the dense structure, the high energy beam passes through with little absorption, resulting in a low density focus. It occurs in one direction of the scan plane.

17.2.7
Reconstruction and Post Processing

Multiplanar reconstruction (MPR) is the simplest method of reconstruction. A volume is built by stacking the axial slices. The software then cuts slices through the volume in a different plane (usually orthogonal). Curved planar reformations (CPR) of the vessel along its entire length are generated by creating a center line through the long axis of the vessel. Center line calculation is based on values of Hounsefield units within the lumen of the

Fig. 17.3 Invasive coronary angiography (ICA) (*left*) demonstrates mild luminal irregularities of the proximal left anterior descending artery. The computed tomography (CT) coronary angiogram demonstrates significant calcified plaque disease that appears larger than the vessel lumen due to blooming artifact

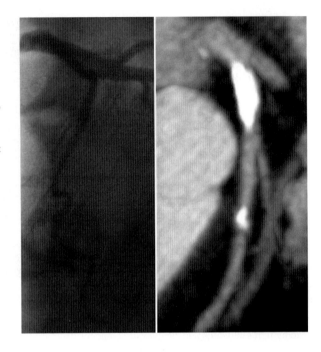

vessel. Modern post-processing algorithms for depicting the coronary vasculature automatically reconstruct the vessels producing three dimensional (3D) models of the coronary tree along with CPR for each vessel (Fig. 17.4). Optionally, a special projection method, such as maximum-intensity projection (MIP) can be used to build-up the reconstructed slices. A 3D data set is a group of contiguous 2D slices. Volume rendering techniques (VRT) allows 3D visualization for clearer depiction of complex anatomy and their relationship (Fig. 17.5). Volume rendered vessel views can be combined with axial and CPRs to allow more intuitive vessel analysis (Fig. 17.6).

17.3
Section 2: Coronary Vessels

17.3.1
Coronary Calcium Scoring

CAD is the leading cause of death in the United States. The Framingham Heart Study risk score is used for CAD risk prediction in the US based on the patient's age and sex along with the presence of established coronary risk factors such as hypertension, hyperlipidemia, diabetes mellitus and cigarette smoking. Noninvasive cardiac risk stratification, measuring coronary artery calcification deposition, can be used independent of the standard risk factors to predict atherosclerotic cardiovascular disease events in healthy middle-aged persons.

Fig. 17.4 A curved planar reformatted (CPR) image of a normal left anterior descending artery

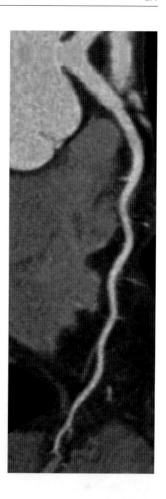

A large prospective cohort study evaluated the relationship of coronary artery calcification to standard coronary disease risk factors and C-reactive protein. CT coronary calcium scores predicted CAD events independent of standard risk factors, and more accurately than standard risk factors and C-reactive protein. This may refine the Framingham risk stratification in patients with intermediate risk.[16]

A coronary calcium score can act as a surrogate marker when assessing the burden of coronary artery atherosclerosis. EBCT has been established for over 15 years in the detection and quantification of coronary calcium deposits. Agatston et al in 1990 first described the original semi quantitative scoring system (Agatston score) based on the number of calcium deposits and the deposit density.[17] This is identified on a prospectively gated, non contrast cardiac CT by high X-ray attenuation values (Hounsfield units >130) (Fig. 17.7). Calcified lesions are quantified by section-by-section, semi quantitative analysis of the CT images. The accepted cut-off values for calcium score are: 0, no identifiable calcium; 1–100, mild atherosclerosis; 101–400, moderate atherosclerosis; >400, extensive coronary calcium depositions. MDCT has replaced EBCT and has been shown to correlate well.[18]

Fig. 17.5 Volume rendered technique to view the coronary arteries and their relationships

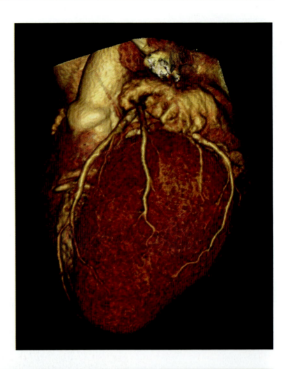

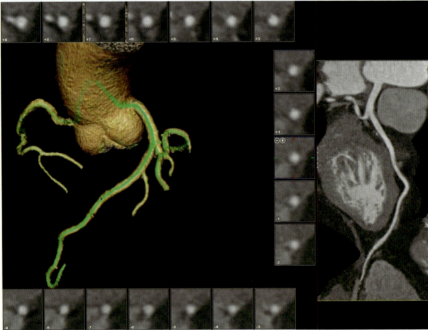

Fig. 17.6 Volume rendered technique vessel only view of the left anterior descending artery along side the curved planar reformat. The *blue dot* on the distal LAD corresponds to the central axial image

Fig. 17.7 A non contrast calcium scoring CT demonstrates extensive calcification along the proximal and mid left anterior descending artery

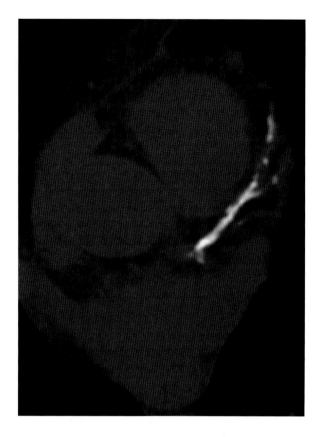

The Multi Ethnic Study of Atherosclerosis (MESA) has reported that all MDCT systems are at least reliable as EBCT for performing and reproducing coronary calcium measurements. Prospective ECG-gating is the technique commonly employed to minimize the radiation dose. Retrospective ECG-gating is associated with higher effective radiation dose (2.6–4.1 mSv).[19] Utilization of ECG-based tube current modulation can however reduce radiation levels that are more comparable with prospective gating.[20–25]

MDCT calcium scoring has a high sensitivity and high negative predictive value for CAD (>80%). Calcified plaque usually corresponds to the late stage in the evolution of atherosclerosis. It does not identify soft plaque and does not attribute vulnerability. The earlier and more active stages are more associated with noncalcified (lipid and fibrous tissue) or mixed plaque.[22–25] Acute coronary syndromes are most often related to non calcified or mixed plaque, while extensive coronary artery calcification is more typical of stable CAD.[26,27] A zero coronary calcium score has a high negative predictive value for ruling out atherosclerosis in selected patient populations, particularly patients with symptomatic atypical chest pain.[28,29] This combined with a low risk stress test can provide reassurance, particularly in anxious patients. Detection of calcified CAD, unlike other risk factors, is direct evidence that CAD exists and may have a more significant impact on the patients' appreciation of the disease, resulting in improved compliance with dietary, exercise and medical therapies recommended.

Table 17.2 The role of CT coronary calcium scoring according to the American College of Cardiology/American Heart Association Expert Consensus

A negative CT test makes the presence of atherosclerotic plaque, including unstable plaque, very unlikely.
A negative test is highly unlikely in the presence of significant luminal obstructive disease.
Negative tests occur in the majority of patients who have angiographically normal coronary arteries.
A negative test may be consistent with a low risk of a cardiovascular event in the next 2–5 years.
A positive CT confirms the presence of a coronary atherosclerotic plaque.
The greater the amount of calcium, the greater the likelihood of occlusive CAD, but there is not a 1-to-1 relationship and findings may not be site specific.
The total amount of calcium correlates best with the total amount of atherosclerotic plaque, although the true "plaque burden" is underestimated.
A high calcium score may be consistent with moderate to high risk of a cardiovascular event with in the next 2–5 years.

The use of coronary calcium score as a risk assessment tool should improve the physician's ability to stratify individuals at high risk of events, to whom aggressive treatment of risk factors for CAD can be more appropriately directed, and help direct the admission or discharge of emergency department patients.[28]

The American College of Cardiology/American Heart Association has outlined the role of CT coronary artery calcium (Table 17.2).

17.3.2
Coronary Artery Disease

ICA remains the gold standard for determining the precise location and degree of stenosis due to its high spatial and temporal resolution (0.13–0.30 mm and 20 ms). It also allows for therapeutic angioplasty and stenting. However it is an expensive procedure with significant radiation exposure and carries a small risk of serious complications.[30] Furthermore, only one third of these examinations are performed in conjunction with an interventional therapeutic procedure.[31] Twenty percent of patients have normal or minimal CAD. Thus, a non-invasive assessment of coronary arteries is highly desirable for the diagnosis of CAD.

CAD is a more systemic, diffuse condition, and the treatment is likewise often systemic. While discrete significant obstructive lesions are important to identify, quantify and treat, it may also be just as important to determine whether or not atherosclerotic plaque is present in the coronary arteries, so that systemic therapies and life style modifications can be initiated. Until the development of MDCT, CT in the assessment of CAD was restricted to the detection and quantification of coronary artery calcification. CT has a number of advantages over ICA. It is a non-invasive, 3D technique that can obtain a calcium score, has a high negative predictive value for CAD, has the potential to characterize plaque components, provides additional anatomical information and entails no recovery time after the study.

However, coronary CTA has several limitations and should not be expected to widely replace ICA in the foreseeable future. Firstly, the radiation exposure is higher than conventional ICA (15.2 mSv for males and 21.4 mSv for females vs. 6.0 mSv[20] and limits its application for serial measurements (for example during stress, at rest and delayed scans) and follow-up examinations (such as for plaque assessment) as well as use in young patients.[32] However, recent advances in scanner design now allow for sub mSv CTA, making this very much less of an issue. Second, the spatial resolution limits the ability of coronary CTA to provide exact, quantitative measures of stenosis severity. Thirdly, patients with atrial fibrillation or other arrhythmias as well as patients with contraindications to iodinated contrast media cannot be studied. Finally, the blooming artifacts from high density materials such as coronary calcifications or stents may hamper accurate assessments of the integrity of the coronary lumen.

17.3.3
Indications and Appropriateness Criteria

The American College of Cardiology, in collaboration with other professional societies, released new appropriateness criteria to help guide usage of CTA for diagnosis and management of cardiovascular disease.[33] A panel comprising radiologists and cardiologists were asked to assess whether the use of CTA for various indications was appropriate (A), uncertain (U), or inappropriate (I). In rating each indication, the panel was provided the following definition of appropriateness: An appropriate imaging study is one in which the expected incremental information, combined with clinical judgment, exceeds the expected negative consequences (radiation or contrast exposure, false negatives or false positives) by a sufficiently wide margin for a specific indication that the procedure is generally considered acceptable care and a reasonable approach for the indication.

The technical panel scored each indication as follows: score 7–9 (appropriate test for specific indication: test is generally acceptable and is a reasonable approach for the indication). Score 4–6 (uncertain for specific indication: test may be generally acceptable and may be a reasonable approach for the indication). Uncertainty also implies that more research and/or patient information is needed to classify the indication definitively. Score 1–3 (inappropriate test for that indication: test is not generally acceptable and is not a reasonable approach for the indication).

17.3.4
Effects of Calcification, Obesity and Heart Rate

Factors that reduce the diagnostic accuracy include coronary artery calcification, obesity, and high heart rates. Severe coronary artery calcification seems to be the factor affecting the visualization and diagnostic accuracy of MDCT. In one study, the sensitivity, specificity, positive predictive value and negative predictive value with an Agatston score <400 were 100%, 99.5%, 83%, and 100% compared to 96%, 95%, 86%, and 99% with an Agatston score ≥400.[34] Severe, coronary artery calcification, obscures the coronary lumen and can lead to overestimation of the severity of the lesions due to blooming artifacts, making quantification of the degree of coronary artery stenosis difficult. Thus, caution should be taken into account in imaging patients with severe calcification.[35]

Relationship between body mass index (BMI) and the diagnostic accuracy of 64-slice CTA in coronary artery calcification was investigated in one study.[11] When body mass index was normal (<25 kg/m^2), sensitivity, specificity, and positive and negative predictive values were all 100% compared to overweight (25–29.9 kg/m^2) which were 100%, 91%, 93%, and 100%, and for obese (body mass index ≥30 kg/m^2) were reduced to 90%, 86%, 91%, and 86%.

The ability to detect a significant stenosis can vary according to heart rate. When heart rates were compared in one study evaluating 64-slice CT, those that were <70 beats/min had sensitivity, specificity, positive predictive value and negative predictive values of 97%, 95%, 97%, and 95%, compared to 88%, 71%, 78%, and 83% when they were 70 beats/min or higher.[11] In order to reduce motion artifact, β-blocking agents are used to keep patients' heart rates below 60 bpm producing better results. The latest development of DSCT has been reported to improve temporal resolution when compared to early 64-slice scanners, and coronary arteries were visualized without motion artifacts at any heart rate and beta-blocker utilization could be discarded.[15] In both heart-rate subgroups, diagnostic accuracy for the assessment of coronary artery stenosis is similar and the rate of false ratings was comparable.[34]

17.4
Section 3: Non-Coronary Cardiac

In addition to the established use of cardiac CT to evaluate the coronary artery anatomy and the degree of CAD MDCT can be useful in assessing the entire heart, including valvular structures, the myocardium, intracardiac masses and the pulmonary veins emptying into the heart.

17.4.1
Valvular Structures

Although echocardiography is the most established imaging modality to evaluate the cardiac valves, MDCT may provide additional information, especially in patients with limited acoustic windows. While the temporal resolution of MDCT is inferior to that of cardiac MRI, the spatial resolution is superior, estimated at approximately 0.4–0.6 mm as compared to an estimated 1–2 mm spatial resolution with cardiac MRI.[35] Further technological advances, including the use of a dual-source CT scanner may prove to decrease the current gap in the temporal resolution. In the current era, CT allows for a more detailed depiction

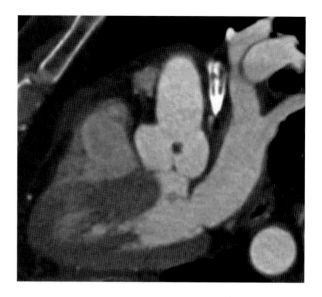

Fig. 17.8 A 3-chamber view from a contrast enhanced electrocardiographic (ECG) gated cardiac CT demonstrates a 5 mm well defined spherical papillary fibroelastoma arising from the left coronary cusp

of the valvular anatomy, whereas MRI can better visualize valvular motion. Therefore, MDCTs utility is in its ability to detect the detailed structure of cardiac valves including the valve leaflets, chordae tendinae and papillary structures.[35] MDCT is useful in identifying more complex valvular pathology, including proper function or dysfunction of prosthetic valves,[36] aortic valve fibroelastomas (Fig. 17.8), valvular endocarditis and abscesses. It is also helpful in determining the feasibility of percutaneous coronary sinus valvuloplasty in patients being evaluated for mitral valve repair.

17.4.2
Myocardial Scar and Viability

Initial attempts to evaluate the myocardium with single detector CT were limited due to poor spatial and temporal resolution, artifact secondary to cardiac motion and unreliable intravascular contrast volume due to a significant first-pass effect.[37] With improved spatial and temporal resolution and decreased artifact due to ECG gating, the use of ECG gated MDCT allows for a more realistic opportunity to assess myocardial scar, viability and perfusion.

Two techniques are available to assess the myocardium: (1) First pass contrast enhanced multidetector computed tomography (CE-MDCT) and (2) delayed contrast enhanced multidetector computed tomography (DE-MDCT). In first pass imaging, MDCT is performed during the administration of contrast. A region of hypoenhancement, or a lower than normal signal intensity, indicates a region of microvascular obstruction or obstructive epicardial coronary disease.[38] Delayed enhanced MDCT is typically performed 10–15 min after the administration of contrast. A region of hyperenhancement, or higher than normal

Fig. 17.9 A delayed enhanced ECG gated CT demonstrates hyperenhancement of the lateral wall of left ventricle consistent with a transmural non-viable infarct in the left circumflex territory

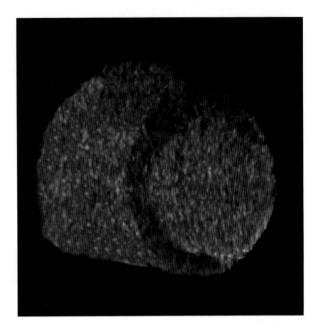

signal density, represents the presence of abnormal myocardium (Fig. 17.9). In the acute setting, it is thought to represent cellular and microvascular damage with leakage of contrast into the intracellular space coupled with reduced outflow rates of contrast into the infarcted myocardium. In the chronic setting, hyperenhancement is thought to be due to an accumulation of contrast in the interstitial space. In the limited human studies available to date, approximately 120–140 mL of contrast is necessary. The radiation doses range from 7 to 8 mSv for men and 7 to 11 mSv for women for the first-pass scan and 2–3 mSv for men and 2–4 mSv for women for the DE-MDCT.

17.4.3
Myocardial Masses

Similar to the assessment of valvular structures, echocardiography is the initial imaging modality of choice in evaluating cardiac masses. Although the temporal resolution of MDCT is inferior to echocardiography, the soft tissue contrast is superior on MDCT. Additionally, MDCT may allow for a more accurate assessment of the size and location of intracardiac masses as well as the evaluation of the surrounding mediastinum. Cardiac MDCT also identifies calcification within the mass, which aids with mass characterization.[39] Although MRI is better able to characterize tissue, the use of HU, which is a number assigned to a region of interest describing the relative difference in signal density differences, may help in the determination of mass composition. The HU of neoplasms and thrombi may overlap with that of normal myocardium, which may result in false-negative results.

17.4.4
Pulmonary Veins

The use of MDCT is helpful in defining pulmonary vein anatomy before percutaneous atrial fibrillation after ablation. The number of pulmonary veins and, the configuration of pulmonary vein anatomy, including the presence of accessory pulmonary veins (Fig. 17.10), or conjoined pulmonary veins, can be identified on MDCT.[40] Additionally, systemic venous variants including partial azygous continuation of the inferior vena cava, partial anomalous pulmonary venous return, persistent left sided superior vena cava or any anatomic abnormality that will cause a mass effect on the left atrium, including a dilated descending aorta or esophagus are important to identify pre-procedure.[41] Pre-procedural MDCT to define the pulmonary vein anatomy may also improve the success of wide area circumferential ablation.[42] Furthermore, MDCT may identify non-pulmonary vein pathology, including unknown malignancies, pulmonary fibrosis, cardiac thrombus or pericardial disease, which may alter the treatment course.[43]

Post procedural MDCT can be useful to document the presence of complications following the procedure, especially in the setting of a symptomatic patient. MDCT can be helpful in the diagnosis of pulmonary vein stenosis, which may occur in up to 3% of patients undergoing catheter ablation for atrial fibrillation. The rate of pulmonary stenosis can be decreased by real-time imaging during the ablation procedure.[44,45] MDCT is also useful in diagnosing rarer, but devastating complications of atrio-esophageal fistulas, veno-occlusive disease, thromboembolic disease resulting in strokes, systemic emboli or pulmonary emboli, pulmonary vein dissection, cardiac perforation, pulmonary vein infarction or phrenic nerve damage.

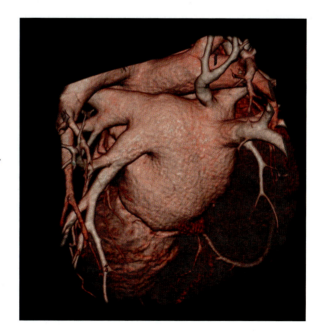

Fig. 17.10 An ECG gated CT pulmonary vein mapping study demonstrates an anomalous left middle lobe pulmonary vein arising adjacent to the ostia of the left superior pulmonary vein (Image provided courtesy of Stephan Achenbach, Deter Ropers, Tobias Pflederer, and Mohammed Marwan.)

17.5 Conclusion

MDCT is increasingly being used for non-invasive assessment of the coronary arteries. Even though its exact clinical role has not yet been firmly established, it promises to become a useful test for excluding significant disease particularly in low to intermediate risk patients with atypical symptoms. CT is also useful for evaluating non-coronary diseases of the heart. While investigation of cardiac masses, valvular disease and congenital heart disease are currently accepted indications for cardiac CT, other areas such as CT perfusion and viability will remain the focus of intense research work over the next few years. Radiation exposure remains a limitation to the development of cardiac CT, however several recently developed techniques allow significant reductions to radiation dose thereby facilitating the acceptance of this modality as a safe and accurate alternative to currently used conventional diagnostic tests.

Summary of Key Terms

- Cardiac.
- Computed Tomography (CT).
- Computed Tomography Angiography (CTA).
- Multi Detector CT (MDCT).
- Coronary Artery Disease (CAD).

References

1. Huda W, Slone RM. *Review of Radiologic Physics*. 2nd ed. Baltimore, MD: Lippincott Williams and Wilkins; 2003:16–130.
2. Mahesh M, Cody DD. Physics of cardiac imaging with multiple-row detector CT. *Radiographics*. 2007;27(5):1495–1509.
3. Jahnke C, Paetsch I, Achenbach S, et al. Coronary MR imaging: breath-hold capability and patterns, coronary artery rest periods, and beta-blocker use. *Radiology*. 2006;239(1):71-78.
4. Ruzsics B, Lee H, Zwerner PL, et al. Dual-energy CT of the heart for diagnosing coronary artery stenosis and myocardial ischemia-initial experience. *Eur Radiol*. 2008; 18(11):2414–2424.
5. Hsieh J, Londt J, Vass M, et al. Step-and-shoot data acquisition and reconstruction for cardiac x-ray computed tomography. *Med Phys*. 2006;33(11):4236–4248.
6. Earls JP, Berman EL, Urban BA, et al. Prospectively gated transverse coronary CT angiography versus retrospectively gated helical technique: improved image quality and reduced radiation dose. *Radiology*. 2008;246(3):742–753.
7. Hunold P, Vogt FM, Schmermund A, et al. Radiation exposure during cardiac CT: effective doses at multi-detector row CT and electron-beam CT. *Radiology*. 2003;226(1):145–152.
8. Hoffmann U, Ferencik M, Cury RC, et al. Coronary CT angiography. *J Nucl Med*. 2006; 47(5):797–806.

9. Schoepf UJ. *CT of the Heart – Principles and Applications*. Totowa, NJ: Humana Press; 2005 [chapter 3].
10. Paul JF, Abada HT. Strategies for reduction of radiation dose in cardiac multislice CT. *Eur Radiol*. 2007;17(8):2028–2037.
11. Raff GL, Gallagher MJ, O'Neill WW, et al. Diagnostic accuracy of noninvasive coronary angiography using 64-slice spiral computed tomography. *J Am Coll Cardiol*. 2005; 46(3):552–557.
12. Johnson TR, Nikolaou K, Wintersperger BJ, et al. Dual-source CT cardiac imaging: initial experience. *Eur Radiol*. 2006;16(7):1409–1415.
13. Rodriguez-Granillo GA, Rosales MA, Degrossi E, et al. Modified scan protocol using multislice CT coronary angiography allows high quality acquisitions in obese patients: a case report. *Int J Cardiovasc imaging*. 2007;23(2):265–267.
14. Leschka S, Wildermuth S, Boehm T, et al. Noninvasive coronary angiography with 64-section CT: effect of average heart rate and heart rate variability on image quality. *Radiology*. 2006;241(2):378–385.
15. Achenbach S, Ropers D, Kuettner A, et al. Contrast-enhanced coronary artery visualization by dual-source computed tomography – initial experience. *Eur J Radiol*. 2006;57(3):331–335.
16. Arad Y, Goodman KJ, Roth M, et al. Coronary calcification, coronary disease risk factors, C-reactive protein, and atherosclerotic cardiovascular disease events: the St. Francis Heart Study. *J Am Coll Cardiol*. 2005;46(1):158–165.
17. Agatston AS, Janowitz WR, Hildner FJ, et al. Quantification of coronary artery calcium using ultrafast computed tomography. *J Am Coll Cardiol*. 1990;15(4):827–832.
18. Schoepf UJ, Becker CR, Ohnesorge BM, et al. CT of coronary artery disease. *Radiology*. 2004;232(1):18–37.
19. Morin RL, Gerber TC, McCollough CH. Radiation dose in computed tomography of the heart. *Circulation*. 2003;107(6):917–922.
20. Jakobs TF, Becker CR, Ohnesorge B, et al. Multislice helical CT of the heart with retrospective ECG gating: reduction of radiation exposure by ECG-controlled tube current modulation. *Eur Radiol*. 2002;12(5):1081–1086.
21. Poll LW, Cohnen M, Brachten S, et al. Dose reduction in multi-slice CT of the heart by use of ECG-controlled tube current modulation ("ECG pulsing"): phantom measurements. *Rofo*. 2002;174(12):1500–1505.
22. Burke AP, Kolodgie FD, Farb A, et al. Healed plaque ruptures and sudden coronary death: evidence that subclinical rupture has a role in plaque progression. *Circulation*. 2001; 103(7):934–940.
23. Kolodgie FD, Burke AP, Farb A, et al. The thin-cap fibroatheroma: a type of vulnerable plaque: the major precursor lesion to acute coronary syndromes. *Curr Opin Cardiol*. 2001; 16(5):285–292.
24. Virmani R, Burke AP, Kolodgie FD, et al. Vulnerable plaque: the pathology of unstable coronary lesions. *J Interv Cardiol*. 2002;15(6):439–446.
25. Virmani R, Kolodgie FD, Burke AP, et al. Lessons from sudden coronary death: a comprehensive morphological classification scheme for atherosclerotic lesions. *Arterioscler Thromb Vasc Biol*. 2000;20(5):1262–1275.
26. Shemesh J, Apter S, Itzchak Y, et al. Coronary calcification compared in patients with acute versus in those with chronic coronary events by using dual-sector spiral CT. *Radiology*. 2003;226(2):483–488.
27. Beckman JA, Ganz J, Creager MA, et al. Relationship of clinical presentation and calcification of culprit coronary artery stenoses. *Arterioscler Thromb Vasc Biol*. 2001;21(10): 1618–1622.
28. Georgiou D, Budoff MJ, Kaufer E, et al. Screening patients with chest pain in the emergency department using electron beam tomography: a follow-up study. *J Am Coll Cardiol*. 2001;38(1):105–110.

29. Shemesh J, Tenenbaum A, Fisman EZ, et al. Absence of coronary calcification on double-helical CT scans: predictor of angiographically normal coronary arteries in elderly women? *Radiology*. 1996;199(3):665–668.
30. Scanlon PJ, Faxon DP, Audet AM, et al. ACC/AHA guidelines for coronary angiography. A report of the American College of Cardiology/American Heart Association Task Force on practice guidelines (Committee on Coronary Angiography). Developed in collaboration with the Society for Cardiac Angiography and Interventions. *J Am Coll Cardiol*. 1999;33(6):1756–1824.
31. American Heart Association (ASA). *Heart and Stroke Statistical Update*. Dallas, DX: The American Heart Association; 2002.
32. Brenner DJ, Hall EJ. Computed tomography – an increasing source of radiation exposure. *N Engl J Med*. 2007;357(22):2277–2284.
33. Hendel RC, Patel MR, Kramer CM, et al. ACCF/ACR/SCCT/SCMR/ASNC/NASCI/SCAI/SIR 2006 appropriateness criteria for cardiac computed tomography and cardiac magnetic resonance imaging: a report of the American College of Cardiology Foundation Quality Strategic Directions Committee Appropriateness Criteria Working Group, American College of Radiology, Society of Cardiovascular Computed Tomography, Society for Cardiovascular Magnetic Resonance, American Society of Nuclear Cardiology, North American Society for Cardiac Imaging, Society for Cardiovascular Angiography and Interventions, and Society of Interventional Radiology. *J Am Coll Cardiol*. 2006;48(7):1475–1497.
34. Scheffel H, Alkadhi H, Plass A, et al. Accuracy of dual-source CT coronary angiography: first experience in a high pre-test probability population without heart rate control. *Eur Radiol*. 2006;16(12):2739–2747.
35. Vogel-Claussen J, Pannu H, Spevak PJ, et al. Cardiac valve assessment with MR imaging and 64-section multi-detector row CT. *RadioGraphics*. 2006;26(6):1769–1784.
36. Faletra FF, Alain M, Moccetti T. Blockage of bileaflet mitral valve prosthesis imaged by computed tomography virtual endoscopy. *Heart*. 2007;93:324.
37. Canty JM Jr, Judd RM, Brody AS, et al. First-pass entry of nonionic contrast agent into the myocardial extravascular space. Effects on radiographic estimates of transit time and blood volume. *Circulation*. 1991;84:2071–2078.
38. Lardo AC, Cordeiro M, Silva C, et al. Contrast enhanced multidetector computed tomography viability imaging after myocardial infarction: characterization of myocyte death, microvascular obstruction, and chronic scar. *Circulation*. 2006;113:394–404.
39. Araoz PA, Mulvagh S, Tazelaar HD, et al. CT and MR imaging of benign primary cardiac neoplasms with echocardiographic correlation. *RadioGraphic*. 2000;20(5):1303–1317.
40. Jongbloed MR, Dirksen M, Bax JJ, et al. Atrial fibrillation: multi-detector row CT of pulmonary vein anatomy prior to radiofrequency catheter ablation – initial experience. *Radiology*. 2005;234:702–709.
41. Lacomis JM, Goitein O, Deible C, et al. CT of the pulmonary veins. *J Thorac Imaging*. 2007;22:63–76.
42. Martinek M, Nesser H, Aichinger J, et al. Impact of integration of multislice computed tomography imaging into three-dimensional electroanatomic mapping on clinical outcomes, safety, and efficacy using radiofrequency ablation for atrial fibrillation. *Pacing Clin Electrophysiol*. 2007;30(10):1215–1223.
43. Lobel R, Lustgarten DL, Spector PS. Multidetector computed tomography guidance in complex cardiac ablations. *Coron Artery Dis*. 2006;17:125–130.
44. Scharf C, Sneider M, Morady F, et al. Anatomy of the pulmonary veins in patients with atrial fibrillation and effects of segmental ostial ablation analyzed by computed tomography. *J Cardiovasc Electrophysiol*. 2003;14:150–155.
45. Saad EB, Rossillo A, Saad CP, et al. Pulmonary vein stenosis after radiofrequency ablation of atrial fibrillation, functional characterization, evolution, and influence of the ablation strategy. *Circulation*. 2003;108:3102–3107.

ECG Telemetry and Long Term Electrocardiography

18

Eugene Greenstein and James E. Rosenthal

18.1 Types of Recorders

Long term electrocardiographic (LTECG) recording is a method of recording the ECG over a designated period of time. This technology allows detection of intermittent arrhythmias, ST segment changes, and repolarization abnormalities. It provides a method for determining whether periodic symptoms are associated with cardiac arrhythmias. Technological advances in the past few years have provided a diversity of recording, transmitting, and analysis systems. Four general types of devices are currently available: continuous recorders, intermittent or event recorders, instruments for real-time recording and transmission of ECGs, and implantable recorders. Types of electrocardiographic recorders are shown in Table 18.1.

18.1.1 Continuous Recorders

Continuous recorders are referred to as Holter recorders, after their inventor, Norman "Jeff" Holter. Historically, the ECG was recorded continuously on reel-to-reel or cassette tape via a battery-powered tape recorder with a very slow tape speed. The recorder was small enough to be suspended by a strap over the shoulder or around the waist. Improvements in solid-state memory have allowed for greater miniaturization and lower power consumption of digital systems. As a result solid-state memory systems have largely replaced cassette tape recording. These systems are capable of storing full ECG data (so-called *full disclosure*) from periods that are usually no longer than 48 h.

All digital recording systems filter, amplify, digitize, and store the ECG in solid-state memory. Two types of digital systems exist. In the first, every QRS complex is recorded.

E. Greenstein (✉)
Division of Cardiology, Northwestern University,
Feinberg School of Medicine, Chicago, IL, USA
e-mail: egreenst@md.northwestern.edu

Table 18.1 Types of electrocardiographic recorders (modified from[8] Hurst's the Heart, 12th ed)

Type	Recording	Scanning	Transmitting
Continuous			
Analog	All ECG complexes "full disclosure"	Technician with computer assistance, area determination, and superimposition	None
Digital-continuous recording	All ECG complexes "full disclosure"	Technician with computer assistance, area determination, and superimposition	Transtelephonic
Digital – real time analysis	Computer analysis of ECG and selected ECG printouts	Real time by microprocessor with retrospective technician editing	None
Event recorder			
"Postevent" nonlooping, without memory, handheld or worn	ECG, selected by patient activation	Direct visualization	Transtelephonic
"Preevent," looping, with memory, monitor worn with attached electrodes	ECG, selected by patient activation, with memory of event	Direct visualization	Transtelephonic
Continuous mobile outpatient telemetry system	ECG, selected by patient or automatic	Direct visualization, technician with computer assistance	Transtelephonic
Implantable devices			
Subcutaneous, implanted digital recorder	ECG, selected by patient activation with memory of event or automatic	Direct visualization	Direct telemetry
Automatic electronic sensor in ICD or pacemaker	ECG, when activated by ICD or recognized by sensor in pacemaker, with memory	Direct visualization of analysis or ECG	Direct telemetry
Real time			
Real-time transtelephonic monitoring	ECG at central monitoring station – no recording at device	Direct visualization	Transtelephonic

"Full disclosure" of the ECG is possible and ECG strips corresponding to any specific moment can be viewed. The second type of recording system allows for onboard electronics to analyze the data and record only the items of interest (usually maximal and minimal rate, changes in RR intervals, arrhythmias, etc). Brief segments of the patients' ECG can also be stored – usually in areas of interest or during major changes. In this system, the full ECG is not recorded and "full disclosure" is not possible.

Holter monitors are predominantly useful in the evaluation of suspected arrhythmias that occur frequently and are expected to occur in the typical 24–72 h window that the patient wears the monitor. They are not dependent on the patient for activation.

18.1.2
Event Recorders

Event recorders differ from continuous recorders in that they collect ECG data only when the patient or, with some models, when a perturbation in the rhythm activates the device. There are two types of event recorders – those that store data for a predetermined time after the patient activates the device (postevent) and those that record data continually. The latter type, referred to as looping event monitors, continually record and discard data until they are activated by the patient. When that occurs, they store the ECG data for a selected period of time (from seconds to minutes) before and after the patient's activation. Some of these devices capture information only when the patient activates them while others are automatically triggered by predetermined cutoffs for high or low heart rate. The ECG recording is stored on the device until it is transferred, usually trans-telephonically, to a recorder. Patients are instructed to activate the device by pressing a button when they experience symptoms. Devices are limited by error in activation of the device by patients. Those devices that are not automatically triggered by arrhythmias are incapable of capturing asymptomatic arrhythmias.

18.1.3
Telemetry/Mobile Cardiac Outpatient Telemetry

Mobile cardiac outpatient telemetry (MCOT) systems consist of a three-electrode, two-channel sensor transmitting wirelessly to a portable monitor which analyzes and stores ECG data. Significant arrhythmias, whether symptomatic or asymptomatic, are transmitted automatically by the wireless network to a central monitoring station and analyzed by trained personnel. In a study of 100 patients using this system, a clinically defined significant arrhythmia was found in 51 patients, in 25 of whom (49%) the arrhythmia was asymptomatic. MCOT should be used when continuous ECG information is required for longer periods than Holter monitoring, patient activation is not required (though a symptom diary should be kept for correlation with findings) and when the processing delay of Holter information is unacceptable (i.e., in suspected serious ventricular arrhythmias).

18.1.4
Implantable Recorders

A miniaturized event recorder, referred to as an implantable loop recorder (ILR) can be implanted subcutaneously on the precordium. The patient can activate this device manually when symptoms occur. Additionally, high and low heart rate cutoffs can be programmed to capture the ECG. These devices are particularly useful to capture events that occur relatively infrequently – for example, a few times per year. A recent study by Gaida et al compared ILR monitoring vs. conventional monitoring (24 h Holter, 4 week mobile cardiac telemetry, and Electrophysiology study). ILR was significantly more effective at making a diagnosis (73 vs. 21%) and more cost efficient. Event recording is also provided by newer-generation pacemakers and implantable cardioverter defibrillators that automatically recognize and record abnormal rhythms.

18.1.5
Real Time Monitoring

These devices acquire data and transmit the ECG information directly and transtelephonically, in real time, without recording the data in the unit carried by the patient. The patient's ECG can be transmitted daily, or even multiple times each day, to a recording station. Patients use a "wand" to communicate with their implanted device, which then transmits the electrocardiographic information over a standard telephone line (similar to a computer modem) to a central monitoring station. Standard transtelephonic pacemaker and ICD interrogation uses this technology. Newer technology (Medtronic Carelink™) allows clinicians to preprogram the device to wirelessly send electrocardiographic data and data regarding pacing system parameters and function without the need of a "wand." This can be done in lieu of or to supplement office visits, or the device can be programmed to transmit data should a preprogrammed event occur (e.g., tachycardia or bradycardia).

18.2
Principles of Telemetry

Biotelemetry is defined as the transmission of biological or physiological data from a remote location to a facility that has the capability to interpret and record the data. In 1903 Einthoven transmitted electrocardiograms from a hospital to his laboratory using immersion electrodes that were connected to a remote galvanometer by telephone lines. Current telemetry systems continue to use the telephone grid but many use radio waves. Infrared (IR) and ultrasonic systems have been pioneered as well.

IR biotelemetry systems are used in hospitals in a similar fashion to radiofrequency systems (for transmission of ECG signals and patient's clinical information). IR systems have the advantages of being more miniaturizable (without the need for antennas), being subject to less interference and not being limited to a specific radiofrequency spectrum.

18 ECG Telemetry and Long Term Electrocardiography

However, IR systems have much shorter ranges (often limited to one room), require more power, and have difficulty with multisystem transmission (e.g., multiple patients in one room). Ultrasonic systems have largely been limited to zoological telemetry – specifically for tracking animals in the oceans.

18.2.1
Components of a Telemetry System

The ECG signal is obtained from the patient via electrodes. It then undergoes a process called modulation that converts the signal and "attaches" it to the carrier of interest (Fig. 18.1). For hospital telemetry the carrier is a radiofrequency signal and for event monitoring it is often a sound wave.

If multiple data signals (e.g., multiple leads) are required, then subcarriers of different frequencies can be generated as well, in a process called frequency multiplexing. Frequency multiplexing is more efficient than employing a separate transmitter for each signal. A transmitter (usually a box carried by the patient) then sends the modulated signal to a receiver at the nursing station or a centralized telemetry center. The receiver de-modulates the carrier to separate the signal of interest and display it in real time on the telemetry computer. Similar to broadcast radio stations, signals can be on the frequency modulated (FM) or amplitude modulated (AM) band. In-hospital telemetry systems commonly employ frequency modulation techniques.

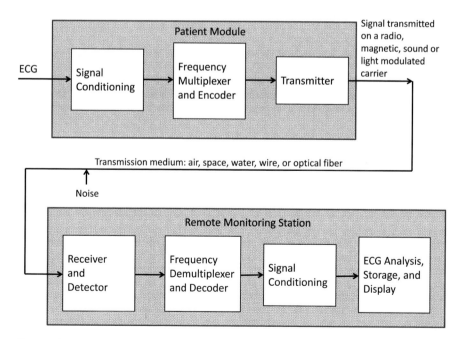

Fig. 18.1 Components of a telemetry System (adapted from[11])

18.2.2
Physiologic Signal

The physiologic signal is the same as described in the ECG section of this book.

18.2.3
Basic Description of the Technique

The goal of these techniques is to capture as much of the electrical information from the heart (with as little noise) as possible. To achieve this, meticulous preparation of the patient to allow for ideal interface between the electrodes and the patient's skin is crucial. In some cases, this requires shaving the chest wall to remove excess body hair that may interfere with electrode contact. If necessary, the skin can also be abraded with emery tape, cleaned with an alcohol swab or similarly treated with commercial devices that are made for this purpose. To identify better the low frequency ST segment, an impedance meter can be used to register skin resistance. Ideal values are <2 kΩ and should be at least <5 kΩ.

Depending on the technique being deployed, varying numbers of electrodes are connected in two to three different possible configurations depending on how many leads are required. Should reproduction of a specific finding be requested (e.g., stress ECG with inferior ST depression) leads that best show the vector of interest may be applied. After the leads have been applied and prior to the patient leaving the laboratory, the patient should be placed in various positions (lateral decubitus, supine, etc) to observe for artifactual ST segment deviation. This is particularly important when telemetry is used to monitor for asymptomatic or "silent" ischemia, where artifactual ST segment shifts can lead to false positive results (Fig. 18.2).

With real time monitoring and ambulatory telemetry, electrocardiographic information is continuously or intermittently transmitted to a central processing service. With event monitoring, data are transmitted periodically by the patient via telephone using a small transmitter that encodes the data as sound waves. With older techniques, such as Holter

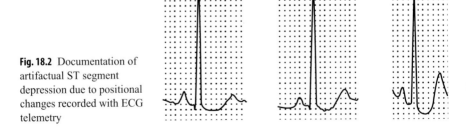

Fig. 18.2 Documentation of artifactual ST segment depression due to positional changes recorded with ECG telemetry

monitoring, the monitor, which has stored the ECG data on its microchip (formerly on magnetic tape) is returned to the central processing service at the end of the observation period. For all techniques, data are automatically analyzed via proprietary algorithms, often with significant participation by technicians that are proficient in the interpretation of arrhythmias. The preliminary findings are then "over-read" by a physician and a final report is generated.

18.2.4
Key Signal Processing Techniques

As the physiologic signal is the same in long term as in surface ECG systems, the recording systems use the same processes to filter the physiologic signal (see section on filtering of the ECG in Chap. 10). Each company designates slightly different low pass and high pass filter cut-offs to optimize the ECG. Filtering cut-offs in general are similar to surface ECG with low pass filters set between 60 and 100 Hz and high pass filters set at 0.05 Hz. Sampling rates also vary and have increased in parallel with the progressive miniaturization of digital storage devices. They are typically at least 128 samples per second. As sampling rates increase the amount of data generated and the amount of storage required increase. Current systems can be programmed to sample at up to 1,000 samples per second.

18.2.5
Motion Correction/Noise Reduction

A major difference between the ECG and long term ambulatory systems is the greater need for motion correction in ambulatory systems as the signal is obtained while patients are engaged in their daily activities, including exercise. Companies use proprietary motion correction algorithms that tend to improve with each successive generation of their devices. Figure 18.3 shows an example of motion correction using the finite residual filter (FRF) algorithm developed by GE Marquette.

18.3
Playback Systems and Analysis

18.3.1
Holter Recording

The ECG recording can be analyzed by playing back the tape or digital data at high speed after the recording has been made ("offline") or by software in the recorder while it is

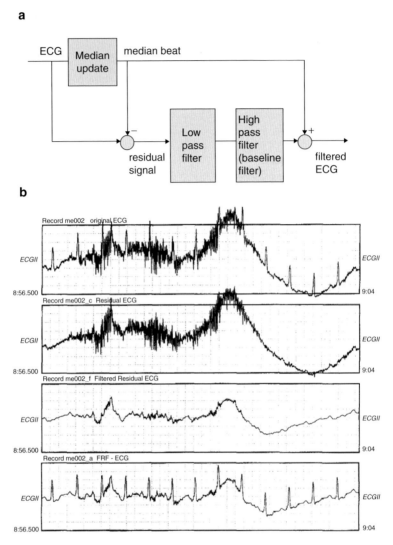

Fig. 18.3 Finite residual filter (copied with Permission from[14]). (**a**) Block Diagram. This system analyzes the surface ECG and determines a median beat (refer to Median beat discussion in Chap. 10) for the lead in question. It then subtracts that median beat from the signal, performs low and high pass filtering, and then returns the median beat to the signal. (**b**) FRF filter applied to electrocardiographic recording. The top panel shows the recorded signal. The second panel shows the signal with the median beat subtracted (residual ECG). The third panel is the filtered residual ECG. The fourth panel restores the median beats to the filtered, residual ECG, providing an improved tracing relative to the original signal

being recorded ("online"). Systems use dedicated or generic personal computers and proprietary software for data analysis and report generation. With techniques that record continuous data, modern systems have sufficient memory to allow "full disclosure" of every beat during the recording memory. Systems analyze the data using various techniques that include:

- Audio-visual superimposition ECG presentation (AVESP), in which, rapidly played beats are superimposed on a screen, allowing beats that are different – either in timing or morphology to "pop" out to the observer.
- R-R histogram generation, in which, a visual tabular representation of heart rates is generated.
- Template matching, in which, a template for the patient's native QRS morphology is created and beats that differ from the template are classified as abnormal (with percentage confidence). This automatic classification can later be over-read and corrected by the operator, who can also analyze specific times of interest (for example when the patient has reported symptoms) on the long term ECG via full disclosure. Template matching is commonly used in more recent systems.

The computer usually provides summaries of heart rates, pauses, frequency of premature supraventricular and ventricular beats, runs of tachycardia and other arrhythmias, and variations in QRS, ST, QT, or T-wave.

18.3.2
Reliability of the Arrhythmia Analysis

AVSEP analysis of long-term ECG (LTECG) recordings by a trained physician usually allows recognition of serious rhythm disturbances. However, even skilled operators sometimes miss arrhythmias using this method. Electronic analysis systems improve the sensitivity and specificity of the LTECG recordings. The techniques employed are different for different manufacturers and are not disclosed in detail for competitive reasons. As a result, there are little data comparing different analysis systems. However a commercially available dataset is maintained by the National Institute of Biomedical Imaging and Engineering and all modern electronic analysis systems must achieve sensitivity and specificity levels for arrhythmia analysis against this data set. In addition, the positive predictive value of these systems depends largely on the rhythm disturbance being identified. In a 1981 study by von Leitner et al the positive predictive value for identification of asystole was only 46%, while in the same system it was 97% for identification of ventricular premature beats. Table 18.2 includes more recent studies with similar results.

Modern systems are able to identify ventricular premature beats based on their measured QRS width. Atrial premature beats are often identified based on prematurity and the sensitivity to identify these beats can be improved by technician dependent alterations to the prespecified prematurity intervals cut-off. Current computer analysis systems cannot accurately identify supraventricular ectopy with aberrancy or intermittent preexcitation, which makes "over-reading" critical for accurate reporting. Even in well-run laboratories, intra-and inter-observer variability's may lead to 10–25% differences in quantification of ventricular beat estimations for the same recording.

Table 18.2 Sensitivity and positive predictive accuracy for different arrhythmias and different analysis systems (modified from 5)

Arrhythmia	Author	Patients (n)	Sensitivity (%)	Positive predictive accuracy (%)	False positive
PVC	Leitner	37	95.3	97.2	
	Lanza	152	92.9	94.9	
	Kennedy	164	92	92	8
	Cooper	50	96	99	0.9
PVC couplets	Leitner	37	93.4[a]	91.8[a]	
	Lanza	152	90.1	87.8	
	Kennedy	164	80	97	3
	Cooper	50	92	92	7
VT	Leitner	37	91[b]	91.8[b]	
	Lanza	152	80	82.3	
	Kennedy	164	81	92	8
	Cooper	50	86	90	10
More than three PVC	Leitner	37	97.4	82.1	
	Lanza	152	88.6	56.6	
	Kennedy	164	81	82	18
SVT	Lanza	152	43.7	60.2	
	Kennedy	164	75	89	11

VT ventricular tachycardia; *SVT* supraventricular tachycardia
[a]Including VT
[b]Including PVC couplets

18.3.3 Ischemia Analysis

LTECG's ability to detect shifts in the level of the ST segment changes was first introduced in 1974 to great skepticism, as the ST segment is a low frequency component of the ECG and clinicians were concerned that signal filtering would make detection of this low frequency component unreliable. Its purpose was to identify symptomatic and asymptomatic (so-called silent) periods of ischemia. Subsequent research in patients with known coronary artery disease has compared silent ST segment changes in LTECG with ischemia on positron emission tomography (PET) and found a high degree of correlation. To optimize the quality of recordings of the ST segment, skin resistance should be measured with an impedance meter and register less than 5 kΩ. Lanza et al found that the lead Chest Modified (CM)5 had the highest sensitivity for detecting ischemia at 89%, and addition of various leads in multiple combinations could increase the sensitivity for detecting ischemia to 96%.

One of the major technical limitations in ischemia detection is the frequent presence of an unstable baseline isoelectric line due to factors such as patient's motion. As a result the baseline QRS-T morphology must be carefully analyzed to ensure that it is suitable for interpretation. As described above (see section basic description of the technique) meticulous skin preparation and testing of the recording quality with the patient's movement is critical to the success of this technique).

18.3.4
Data Storage

Modern LTECG systems digitize the analog ECG signal in the recorder and store the data in a digital format via solid-state memory devices. The direct digital recording avoids all of the biases introduced by the mechanical features of tape recording devices, increases memory capacity and eliminates distortion of an analog system during transfer from the recorder to the central computer. Modern LTECG systems can record at up to 1,000 samples per second, which allows for excellent fidelity in reproduction of the signal required for advanced ECG analysis. Solid-state memory acquisition also expedites electronic data transfer to a central facility. A major limitation to this technology is the cost of the memory itself – which decreases with each subsequent generation.

Historical limitations of storage capacity were overcome by developing compression techniques of two types: "Lossy" and "loss-less." With "lossy" compression microchips in the patient recorder identify arrhythmias and determined which signals to retain. Such systems provided greater compression ratios, but physicians were hesitant to use them because they were relatively inaccurate in distinguishing true arrhythmias from baseline wander and artifact, and didn't allow for retrospective "full disclosure" analysis due to lack of recording of the original signal in its entirety. This led to uncertainty as to whether the absence of a significant arrhythmia meant that it didn't occur or that it failed to be identified and stored by the system. Much of the original resistance to the use of solid-state memory systems was related to lack of faith in these original "lossy" systems. With improvements in solid state memory, modern enhanced storage systems retain the benefits of solid-state recording and now allow for "full disclosure" by using "loss-less" compression methods in which all beats are retained in the memory. Improved data compression algorithms reduce the amount of storage required by 3–5 times but still permit reconstruction of the waveform with no loss of information. Storage methodologies include flash memory cards or portable hard drives which are then "read" by playback system. Figure 18.4 illustrates the data generated by different sampling rates, duration, and number of leads.

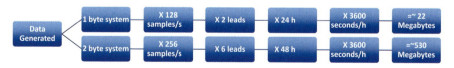

Fig. 18.4 Data generated by different sampling rates, duration, number of leads. Calculation of the data generated in an 8 bit (1 byte), two lead system, with 128 samples per second, over 24 h. Compare this to the amount of data generated in a 16 bit (2 byte), six lead system, with 256 samples per second over 48 h

18.4 Artifacts

Electrocardiographic artifacts have mimicked every type of cardiac arrhythmias and have led to misdiagnosis and inappropriate treatment. Artifacts can occur at each level in the recording process. Patient-related artifacts may results from involuntary muscle contractions (tremors, hiccups) and body movements (changing position, brushing teeth). Figure 18.5 shows an example where motion artifact in the ECG could be mistaken for ventricular tachycardia. Data recording and processing artifacts occur as a result of loose skin-electrode contact, lead fractures, processing errors (human or computer based), and, during the era of tape based recording systems, altered tape speed and incomplete tape erasure.

Occasionally, software processing of the signal may introduce artifacts. For example, current telemetry systems were designed when pacemaker impulse stimuli were unipolar and easily seen on hospital telemetry. However, newer generation pacemakers have been developed with low amplitude, narrow pulse width; bipolar impulses that have higher frequencies (>150 Hz) and are occasionally filtered out by the low pass filters of telemetry systems. To improve pacemaker impulse detection sensitivity, software solutions were developed that look at the analog telemetry signal (prior to filtering) and artificially insert

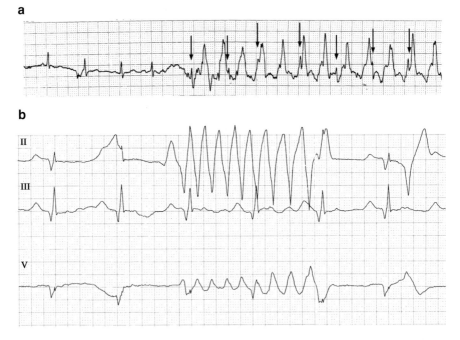

Fig. 18.5 Hospital telemetry strips showing electrocardiographic artifact that mimicked ventricular tachycardia. In (**a**), the artifact is due to the patient shaking his albuterol inhaler. QRS complexes can be marched out within the artifact as indicated by the *arrows*. In (**b**), the QRS complexes in lead III prove that the apparent rapid run in leads II and aVF represents artifact

a pacemaker stimulus in front of the QRS. Very rarely this software can oversense a high frequency portion of the QRS and insert a pacing stimulus. As a result, if this pacemaker detection mode is activated, artifactual pacing stimuli can be seen on telemetry in patients without an implanted pacemaker (Fig. 18.6).

External interference is also a common cause of ECG artifacts. "Noise" can occur in the recordings because of external sources. Examples include signals from, 50 to 60 Hz alternating current (Fig. 18.7.), artifact from arc-welding electromagnetic signals, and artifact from a variety of medical equipment (transcutaneous nerve stimulators, infusion pumps).

Most of these artifacts are readily identifiable from their characteristic nonphysiologic appearances (such as nonphysiologic coupling intervals, "spike like" nature, inconsistencies between recording leads). The reader should "look through" the artifacts for normal ECG appearance. Often QRS complexes within the section containing the artifact can be detected by using ECG calipers to identify the location on the recording of their expected occurrence. Lack of a clinical correlation may be a useful distinguishing feature between artifact and arrhythmia, but can lead to errors since some serious arrhythmias may be asymptomatic. Ultimately, the key to distinguishing artifact from arrhythmia is the clinician's familiarity with the various types of artifacts and a careful analysis of the ECG. Current research

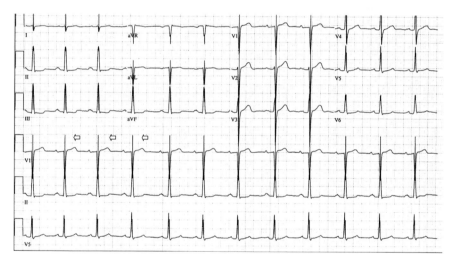

Fig. 18.6 Erroneous pacemaker stimuli (*arrows*) simulating actual cardiac pacing (Copied with permission from[24]). Note that when the apparent pacing stimuli are inscribed, they are temporally associated with a high-frequency potential at the onset of the QRS complex seen in several leads including II, aVF, and V1

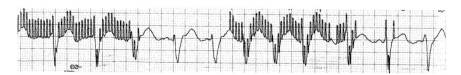

Fig. 18.7 Rhythm strip of 60 Hz alternating current noise

directions in the field of interference artifact reduction includes using accelerometers to detect body position and motion, adaptive filtering that incorporates an "artifact filter" that correlates linearly with the amount of artifact (motion, stretch etc) generated and implantable sub-epidermal electrodes which avoid the artifact from skin-stretch.

References

1. Bragg-Remschel DA, Winkle RA. Ambulatory monitoring of electrocardiograms – current technology of recording and analysis. *Physiologist*. 1983;26(1):39–42.
2. Castells F et al. Principal component analysis in ECG signal processing. *EURASIP J Adv Signal Process*. 2007;2007:1–22.
3. Crawford MH et al. ACC/AHA Guidelines for Ambulatory Electrocardiography. A report of the American College of Cardiology/American Heart Association Task Force on Practice Guidelines (Committee to Revise the Guidelines for Ambulatory Electrocardiography). Developed in collaboration with the North American Society for Pacing and Electrophysiology. *J Am Coll Cardiol*. 1999;34(3):912–948.
4. DiMarco JP, Philbrick JT. Use of ambulatory electrocardiographic (Holter) monitoring. *Ann Intern Med*. 1990;113(1):53–68.
5. Enseleit F, Duru F. Long-term continuous external electrocardiographic recording: a review. Europace: European pacing, arrhythmias, and cardiac electrophysiology: journal of the working groups on cardiac pacing, arrhythmias, and cardiac cellular electrophysiology of the European Society of Cardiology. *Europace*. 2006;8(4):255–266.
6. Eveloy V et al. Developments in ambulatory electrocardiography. Biomedical instrumentation and technology/association for the advancement of medical instrumentation. *Biomedical Instrumentation and Technology*. 2006;40(3):238–245.
7. Fetter RJG et al. Electromagnetic interference from welding and motors on implantable cardioverter-defibrillators as tested in the electrically hostile work site. *J Am Coll Cardiol*. 1996;28(2):423–427.
8. Fuster V, O'Rourke RA, Walsh RA, Poole-Wilson P. *Hurst's the Heart*. 12th ed. New York: McGraw-Hill; 2009.
9. Giada F, Gulizia M, Francese M, et al. Recurrent unexplained palpitations (RUP) study comparison of implantable loop recorder versus conventional diagnostic strategy. *J Am Coll Cardiol*. 2007;49(19):1951–1956.
10. Gibson CM et al. Diagnostic and prognostic value of ambulatory ECG (Holter) monitoring in patients with coronary heart disease: a review. *J Thromb Thrombolysis*. 2007; 23(2):135–145.
11. Güler NF, Ubeyli ED. Theory and applications of biotelemetry. *J Med Syst*. 2002;26(2):159–178.
12. Heilbron EL. Advances in modern electrocardiographic equipment for long-term ambulatory monitoring. *Card Electrophysiol Rev*. 2002;6(3):185–189.
13. Kadish AH et al. ACC/AHA clinical competence statement on electrocardiography and ambulatory electrocardiography: a report of the ACC/AHA/ACP-ASIM task force on clinical competence (ACC/AHA Committee to develop a clinical competence statement on electrocardiography and ambulatory electrocardiography) endorsed by the International Society for Holter and noninvasive electrocardiology. *Circulation*. 2001;104(25):3169–3178.
14. Kaiser W, Findeis M. Artifact processing during exercise testing. *J Electrocardiol*. 1999; 32(suppl):212–219.
15. Kennedy H. The history, science, and innovation of Holter technology. *Ann Noninvasive Electrocardiol*. 2006;11(1):85–94.

16. Kligfield P et al. Recommendations for the standardization and interpretation of the electrocardiogram: part I: the electrocardiogram and its technology: a scientific statement from the American Heart Association Electrocardiography and Arrhythmias Committee, Council on Clinical Cardiology; the American College of Cardiology Foundation; and the Heart Rhythm Society: endorsed by the International Society for Computerized Electrocardiology. *Circulation.* 2007;115(10):1306–1324.
17. Knight BP et al. Clinical consequences of electrocardiographic artifact mimicking ventricular tachycardia. *N Engl J Med.* 1999;341(17):1270–1274.
18. Lee S, Lee M. A real-time ECG data compression algorithm for a digital holter system. Conference proceedings: Annual International Conference of the IEEE Engineering in Medicine and Biology Society. *IEEE Eng Med Biol Soc Conf.* 2008;2008:4736–4739.
19. Lloyd MS et al. Pacing features that mimic malfunction: a review of current programmable and automated device functions that cause confusion in the clinical setting. *J Cardiovasc Electrophysiol.* 2009;20(4):453–460.
20. Mason JW et al. Recommendations for the standardization and interpretation of the electrocardiogram: part II: electrocardiography diagnostic statement list a scientific statement from the American Heart Association Electrocardiography and Arrhythmias Committee, Council on Clinical Cardiology; the American College of Cardiology Foundation; and the Heart Rhythm Society Endorsed by the International Society for Computerized Electrocardiology. *J Am Coll Cardiol.* 2007;49(10):1128–1135.
21. Morganroth J. Ambulatory Holter electrocardiography: choice of technologies and clinical uses. *Ann Intern Med.* 1985;102(1):73–81.
22. Pawar T et al. Impact of ambulation in wearable-ECG. *Ann Biomed Eng.* 2008;36(9):1547–1557.
23. Rothman SA et al. The diagnosis of cardiac arrhythmias: a prospective multi-center randomized study comparing mobile cardiac outpatient telemetry versus standard loop event monitoring. *J Cardiovasc Electrophysiol.* 2007;18(3):241–247.
24. Smelley MP, Childers R, Knight BP. Pseudo Pacemaker Stimuli. *PACE.* 2008;31:513–516.
25. Stone PH, Chaitman BR, McMahon RP, et al. Asymptomatic Cardiac Ischemia Pilot (ACIP) Study. Relationship between exercise-induced and ambulatory ischemia in patients with stable coronary disease. *Circulation.* 1996;94:1537–1544.
26. Stone PH. ST-segment analysis in ambulatory ECG (AECG or Holter) monitoring in patients with coronary artery disease: clinical significance and analytic techniques. *Ann Noninvasive Electrocardiol.* 2005;10(2):263–278.
27. Szilagyi L et al. Quick QRS Complex Detection for On-Line ECG and Holter Systems. Conference proceedings: Annual International Conference of the IEEE Engineering in Medicine and Biology Society. *IEEE Eng Med Biol Soc Conf.* 2005;4:3906–3908.
28. Szilágyi L et al. Quick ECG analysis for on-line holter monitoring systems. Conference proceedings: Annual International Conference of the IEEE Engineering in Medicine and Biology Society. *IEEE Eng Med Biol Soc Conf.* 2006;1:1678–1681.
29. Tai SC et al. Designing better adaptive sampling algorithms for ECG Holter systems. *IEEE Trans Biomed Eng.* 1997;44(9):901–903.
30. Trigano A et al. Arc welding interference recorded by an implanted cardiac pacemaker. *Int J Cardiol.* 2006;109(1):132–134.

Intracardiac Electrograms

19

Alexandru B. Chicos and Alan H. Kadish

In this chapter, we are summarizing the basic principles underlying intracardiac electrogram recording and interpretation, some of their technical and clinical applications in cardiac electrophysiology, and the signal processing steps required in various applications.

Electrograms[1] are recordings of cardiac potentials from electrodes directly in contact with the heart. An electrode is an electrical conductor used to make contact with a nonmetallic part of a circuit – in this case the cardiac extracellular fluid. The word was coined by Michael Faraday from the Greek words *elektron* (meaning amber, from which the word electricity is derived) and *hodos*, a way.[2] Electrodes transduce ionic currents generated by the heart (ions moving through transmembrane channels) into electric currents (electrons moving in metal) that can be detected by electronic devices. In order to accurately transduce, an ideal electrode would respond instantaneously to changes in potential, and without altering them. The silver–silver chloride electrode closely approximates an ideal electrode and is used for research purposes; common materials for recording electrodes used in the electrophysiology laboratory are stainless steel, titanium, or platinum. Recordings are most commonly made from contact endocardial or epicardial electrodes, in bipolar or unipolar configurations. Other types of recordings include the monophasic action potential (MAP) and non-contact recordings.

All devices that measure electrical potentials are actually measuring differences in potential between two points or surfaces; therefore, two inputs, from two electrodes, are necessary. *Unipolar electrograms* represent the potential difference between an "exploring electrode" in contact with the extracellular space of the active tissue, and a reference "indifferent electrode," which is at a distance from the heart. Ideally, this is placed at infinite distance, resulting in all field lines radially directed towards it. In practice, a chest patch, or, more commonly, the "Wilson central terminal" have been used as approximations of indifferent electrodes. For the "Wilson central terminal,"[3] the right arm, left arm,

---

A.B. Chicos (✉)
Division of Cardiology, Department of Medicine,
Feinberg School of Medicine, Northwestern University,
Chicago, IL, USA
e-mail: a-chicos@northwestern.edu

J.J. Goldberger and J. Ng (eds.),
Practical Signal and Image Processing in Clinical Cardiology,
DOI: 10.1007/978-1-84882-515-4_19, © Springer-Verlag London Limited 2010

and left leg are connected to a common point through equal resistances of at least 5,000 Ω. It has been reported that an electrode catheter placed in the IVC provides a better reference, being less affected by noise.[4-6] However, as this involves an additional or custom-made catheter, the Wilson central terminal is more commonly utilized.

The potential being recorded is extracellular (except in the case of the MAP-electrodes), but is a direct result of the transmembrane currents generated during the action potential of excited myocardial cells in a volume conductor (represented by the myocardial extracellular space, intracardiac blood, and surrounding tissues).[7,8] The separation of electrical charges generated at the border between activated and resting myocardium ("in front" of the leading edge of activation) creates moving *electric dipoles*. A dipole is defined as equal and opposite charges q, separated by a small distance d, and is described by the dipole moment, a vector oriented from negative charge towards positive charge, and with amplitude equal to $q \times d$. The wavefront is modeled as the vectorial sum of multiple dipoles perpendicular to the wave front (Fig. 19.1). Figure 19.2 illustrates that when the activation front moves towards the exploring electrode it will result in a positive deflection, and will generate a negative deflection when it moves away from the electrode. The amplitude of the unipolar electrogram decreases as the distance between the dipole and the sensing

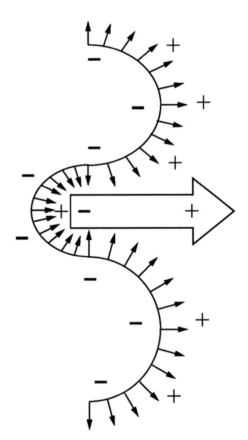

Fig. 19.1 The separation of electrical charges generated at the border between activated and resting myocardium creates moving electric dipoles (*small, solid arrows*). The electrical field generated at the border between activated and resting myocardium ("in front" of the leading edge of activation) is represented by a moving electric dipole, which is the vectorial sum (*large arrow*) of all dipoles

19 Intracardiac Electrograms

Fig. 19.2 A positive potential deflection is recorded when the activation front moves towards the exploring electrode, and a negative deflection is recorded when electrical activation moves away from the electrode

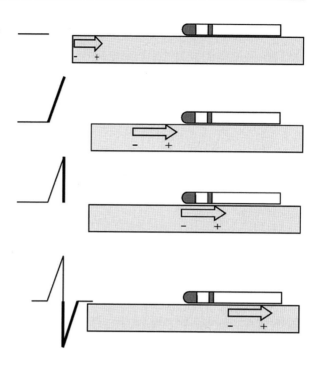

electrode increases. This relationship has been modeled mathematically[†] and in one model it is inversely proportional to the square of the distance.

One corollary of this inverse dependence on distance is the fact that, while a unipolar electrogram represents the sum of local and distant events, the latter contribute less, the farther away they are. Another corollary is that the local electrograms are "sharp," or contain higher-frequency signal, whereas far-field activity generates less sharp, lower-frequency signal.[††]

(Figure 19.3: ventricular signal recorded by a multielectrode catheter located in the atrium is far-field, and therefore, its recorded amplitude and "sharpness" are diminished.)

[†]Mathematical descriptions of electrogram or electrocardiogram recordings have used different physical models. In a model of an electrical dipole in a volume conductor and using principles enounced by Helmholtz in 1853, the amplitude (V) is inversely proportional to the square of the distance ($V = M \times \cos \alpha \times R^{-2}$)[8,9] where M is the moment of the dipole, R is the distance from the recording electrode to the dipole, and α is the angle between the dipole and the distance vector. Using solid angle and dipole moment,[10] the recorded signal amplitude (E) is proportional to the surface area of the excitation front (A) and inversely proportional to the square of the distance (R) [$E = (A/R^2) \times (V/4\pi)$], where V is the voltage across the cell membrane. More complex equations have been used to describe effects of electrical activity in strands or cables (cells, Purkinje fibers).[11]
[††]The "sharpness" of the potential (V) signal can be simplistically described by dV/dt; the distance exponent in the first derivative will be *higher*: if $V \sim$ surface area of excitation front (S) $\times R^{-2}$, then sharpness of electrograms ($\sim dV/dt$) is $\sim S \times (-2) \times (dR/dt) \times R^{-3}$; hence, the slope and sharpness of the recorded signal decrease with increasing distance even more rapidly than the amplitude of the signal.

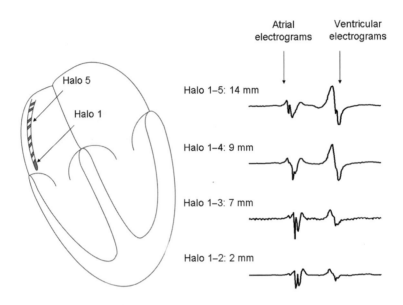

Fig. 19.3 Electrograms illustrating the effect of interelectrode distance and of the distance from the electrode pair to signal (far-field vs. near-field). Atrial and ventricular electrograms are recorded from a multielectrode catheter ("Halo") placed on the lateral wall of the right atrium. Interelectrode distance is given for each pair. Note the low amplitude and low-frequency of the far-field ventricular electrograms in contrast to the near-field atrial electrograms (despite the much stronger raw ventricular signal, related to the mass of tissue that is electrically active). Also note that the duration (width) and amplitude of the ventricular electrograms are proportional to the interelectrode distance

Bipolar electrograms represent the potential difference between two closely spaced electrodes, and they produce a better signal-to-noise ratio. Bipolar signals are calculated as the algebraic difference between the two unipolar electrograms at the two sites, using the same reference. In simple models and as directly derived from the inverse dependence on distance of the unipolar electrogram amplitude, the amplitude of the bipolar electrogram decreases even more rapidly with increasing distance than the unipolar amplitude (the bipolar electrogram approximates the first derivative of the unipolar electrogram; hence, if the unipolar amplitude is inversely proportional to R^2, then the bipolar amplitude is inversely proportional to R^3).[12,13] In addition, the amplitude is proportional to the interelectrode distance: it decreases as electrodes are closer.[†††] The duration of bipolar electrograms is proportional to the distance between the two exploring electrodes; as the electrodes are more closely spaced, the electrogram is narrower (Fig. 19.3). The electrogram duration (width) is also inversely proportional to the conduction velocity: slower conduction between the two electrodes results in widening of the bipolar electrograms.

[†††]This derives from these simple models, because if the distance between electrodes is L, and if $L \ll R$, then $V1-V2 \approx dV$, which is proportional to $d(R^{-n}) = n \times (R^{-n-1}) \times dR = n \times (R^{-n-1}) \times dL \times \cos \alpha$, where α is the angle between the vector of the distance to the signal source dipole and the line between the two electrodes (Fig. 19.4).

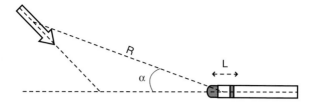

Fig. 19.4 Schematic representation of a moving electric dipole at a distance R from the recording electrode pair. The distance between electrodes is L, and α is the angle between the vector of the distance to the electric dipole and the inter-electrode line

19.1
Characteristics of Unipolar and Bipolar Electrogram Recordings

19.1.1
"Field of View" and Spatial Resolution

The "field of view" is wide for unipolar electrograms, as they record all events occurring between the exploring electrode and the reference electrode. While the contribution of electrical events decreases with their increasing distance from the exploring electrode, far-field activity is frequently recorded. Particularly, when the far-field events involve signals of much higher amplitude than the local signal at the exploring electrode, these may alter it, or "drown" it out, despite being distant. As mentioned, the far-field electrograms are composed of lower frequency signal, which may help discriminating them from the high-frequency local signal. Similarly, unipolar electrograms are exposed to noise from various distant sources. Filtering may improve the electrogram by eliminating noise, but may also alter the useful signal. In addition, the reference electrode is not a true "zero" reference located at infinite distance; therefore, it will also record potentials local to that electrode, i.e., recordings are not truly unipolar.

Bipolar electrograms largely (but not totally) eliminate noise and far-field activity, by virtue of subtraction. Signals and noise that are distant enough (such that $R \gg L$, where R is the distance from signal or noise source to exploring electrodes and L is the distance between electrodes, see Fig. 19.4) will be "seen" quasi-identically by the two electrodes, and eliminated by subtraction. In addition, as discussed above, the amplitude and frequency of signal decrease more steeply with distance from the recording site than with unipolar recordings, further decreasing the effective "field of view." The inter-electrode distance affects the "field of view," which decreases as the inter-electrode distance shortens; conversely, the "field of view" widens as the inter-electrode distance increases, to the extreme case of infinite inter-electrode distance, which results in unipolar recordings.

Spatial resolution refers to the ability to precisely locate the discrete area of excited tissue generating the recorded potentials. The unipolar electrogram reflects, ideally, the potential generated by the tissue in direct contact with the exploring electrode. Far-field activity and noise may interfere, and strategies to address them may be useful (filtering), as described above. In contrast, bipolar electrograms reflect the electrical activity produced by the tissues in contact with and between the electrodes. Spatial resolution increases as the exploring electrodes are smaller and as the distance between the two electrodes of the bipolar recording is decreased. In practice, exploring electrodes of 4 mm are commonly used for mapping, and smaller sizes are used mostly for research; when 8 mm tip catheters (commonly used for ablation) are used, caution should be used in interpreting the spatial information. Commonly used multielectrode catheters have inter-electrode distances of 5–10 mm; more closely spaced electrodes can be used, for better spatial resolution.

19.1.2
Temporal Resolution

While recorded intracardiac electrograms have durations generally in the range of at least 20 ms, and up to more than 150 ms, it is frequently necessary to detect the *local* activation time within a few milliseconds. This is essential when one attempts to identify the earliest activation site, such as the focus of arrhythmia, or the site of an accessory pathway insertion or breakthrough in a line of block. It is also essential in the creation of isochronal activation maps and identification of reentrant arrhythmia circuits.

Local activation is defined by the rapid upstroke of the local transmembrane potential. Multiple experimental studies and mathematical models have searched for the best fiducial points on unipolar and bipolar electrograms that coincide with local activation, using the transmembrane potential as a gold standard (an excellent summary of these studies is available[14]).

For unipolar recordings, the point of maximum downslope (maximum negative dV/dt) corresponds to dV/dt max of the local transmembrane potential with error of less than 1 ms[15–17] (historically, the S wave nadir, R wave peak, and the onset of the fast downstroke have also been considered). Computer algorithms perform automated detection of local activation times by calculating the slope (using, for example, 2, 3, or 5 points on the curve), and using detection thresholds of −0.2 to −2.5 mV/ms, as well as a defined time window in the cardiac cycle. For bipolar recordings, there is less agreement about where to mark local activation. Options that have been proposed and evaluated include the voltage peak (Vmax or absolute Vmax)[12,16,18-21]; maximum absolute slope (dV/dt)[19,20,22]; first elevation >45° from baseline[19,23]; baseline crossing with the steepest slope (BSS)[21,24–26]; and morphological algorithms marking the point of symmetry of the bipolar electrogram.[21,22,27] In models in which the bipolar electrogram is the first derivative of the unipolar electrogram,[12,16] under conditions of uniform wavefront shape and velocity, the maximum absolute peak of the bipolar electrogram should be synchronous with the maximum downslope of the unipolar electrogram. Practically, these have been shown to coincide with reasonable precision in multiple studies[19,20,28] (Fig. 19.5). In addition, the maximum absolute peak is relatively easy to identify visually and by automated software; therefore, it is commonly used.

19.1.3
Directionality

Unipolar electrograms are not dependent on the direction of the wavefront, but are dependent on wavefront origin. If the wavefront originates outside the tissue in contact with the

Fig. 19.5 Local activation time is best estimated by the maximum absolute peak on the bipolar electrogram and by the maximum negative downslope (dV/dt) on the unipolar electrogram

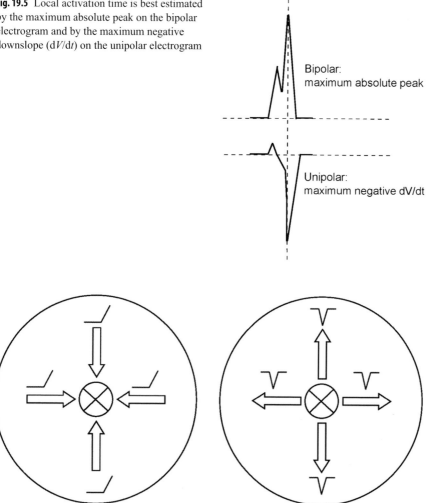

Fig. 19.6 Unipolar electrograms are not dependent on the direction of the wavefront, but are dependent on wavefront origin. If the electric dipole is moving towards the electrode, a positive deflection will be recorded (R wave). If the wavefront originates at the exact location of the electrode, it will move away from it in all directions, generating a QS wave

electrode, it will first approach, then reach, and then move away from the electrode, generating an RS electrogram. On the other hand, if the wavefront originates at the exact location of the electrode, it will move away from it in all directions, generating a QS wave (Figs. 19.6–19.8). This is useful when mapping, for instance, accessory pathway insertion sites and focal tachycardias. However, the accuracy depends on the size of the electrode, and may be affected by movement, contact, etc.; studies have shown that a QS wave can be seen on a 0.5–1 cm radius around the accessory pathway insertion site, and ~1 cm diameter around VT origin.[6]

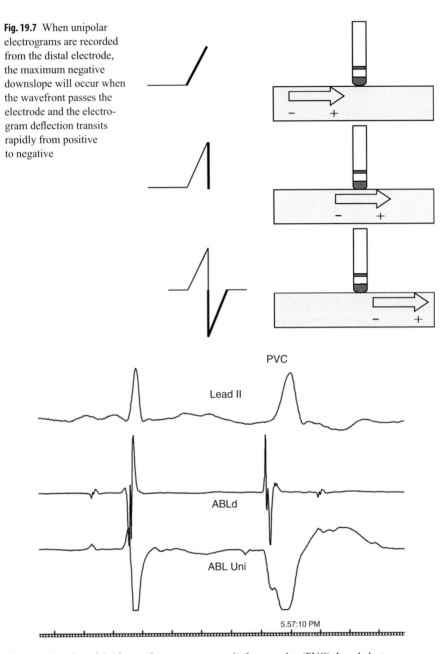

Fig. 19.7 When unipolar electrograms are recorded from the distal electrode, the maximum negative downslope will occur when the wavefront passes the electrode and the electrogram deflection transits rapidly from positive to negative

Fig. 19.8 Mapping of the focus of a premature ventricular complex (PVC). Local electrograms are recorded here from the tip of the ablation catheter at the point of earliest electrical activation during the PVC, which precedes the QRS complex on the surface electrocardiogram (Lead II). Local activation time is at the maximum absolute voltage of the bipolar electrogram (ABLd), and at the maximum negative downslope ($-dV/dt$) in the unipolar electrogram (ABL Uni) – note that these coincide. Also note the QS morphology of the unipolar electrogram at the point of origin of electrical activity during the PVC, in contrast with the rS morphology seen during a sinus beat. Ablation here successfully eliminated the PVC focus

In contrast, bipolar electrogram morphology depends on the direction of propagation of the wavefront, or the angle between the recording pair of electrodes and the wavefront dipole (Fig. 19.4). This can be very useful in practice, particularly when one searches for narrow electrical breakthrough points, such as an accessory atrioventricular pathway, an electrical connection between the atrium and a vein (pulmonary, superior vena cava, coronary sinus), or a discontinuous block or ablation line. From the breakthrough point, the wavefront spreads in both directions. Hence, if a multielectrode catheter is placed parallel to the border between the two narrowly connected areas (atrioventricular valve annulus, pulmonary vein antrum, or ablation line, for example), the recorded bipolar electrograms reverse polarity at the breakthrough point (Fig. 19.9), Some of the practical advantages and disadvantages of unipolar and bipolar electrograms are summarized in Table 19.1.

Other electrogram morphology information:

- *"Fractionated electrograms"* have been qualitatively described as containing multiple low amplitude (typically <1 mV), high-frequency deflections, and they most likely represent distortion of the wavefront by alterations in cell to cell connections. The presence of fractionated electrograms may reflect any of the following: presence of local fibrosis, scar, functional block; complex or disorganized local myocardial architecture

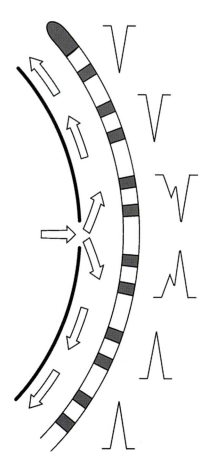

Fig. 19.9 Schematic representation of an activation wavefront breaking through a gap in a line of block. Electrogram polarity reverses at the breakthrough point

Table 19.1 Summary of advantages and disadvantages of unipolar and bipolar electrogram recording

Unipolar	Bipolar
Advantages Good spatial resolution (depending on size of the electrode) Good temporal resolution Independent of the direction of the wave front Repolarization times can be measured for ventricular signals (Activation-recovery times)	*Advantages* Good for visual/manual assessment of activation sequence and cycle length Far field activity and common noise attenuated
Disadvantages Influenced by far field activity Sensitive to electrical noise Reference electrode is not a true "zero" reference and will also record potential local to that electrode (i.e., not really unipolar)	*Disadvantages* Loss of spatial resolution (depending on electrode distance) Loss of temporal resolution Signal dependent on wave front direction (could be an advantage)

SIMPLE ELECTROGRAMS DURING ATRIAL FIBRILLATION

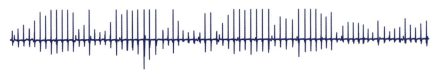

COMPLEX FRACTIONATED ELECTROGRAMS DURING ATRIAL FIBRILLATION

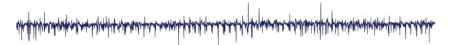

Fig. 19.10 Examples of "simple" and complex fractionated atrial electrograms (CFAEs) during atrial fibrillation

(crista terminalis, venous ostia); or local autonomic discharges, as during atrial fibrillation (CFAE, complex fractionated electrical activity – Fig. 19.10). Electrogram fractionation during atrial fibrillation is frequently transient, thus probably reflecting functional, rather than structural properties. It has been proposed and shown in clinical studies that ablation of areas of CFAE results in cure or an increased chance of cure of atrial fibrillation.[29,30] The underlying mechanisms for the success of CFAE-targeted ablation are still unclear. Attempts have been made to identify "CFAE" in a more quantitative fashion, and this remains an active area of investigation.[31-35]

- Electrogram amplitudes have been used to distinguish scar from normal myocardial tissue. Typically, scar areas are identified if amplitudes are <0.5 mV in the atrium and <1.0 mV in the ventricle; however, these values are somewhat arbitrary. Scar location may be an important guide to catheter ablation and thus scar localization by amplitude criteria has become an important tool. It is important to verify tissue contact during scar mapping, as amplitude may be decreased by poor contact.

- *Artifacts* can be produced at any level of the recording system. At electrode–tissue contact level, tissue injury results in transient repolarization abnormalities and ST segment elevation in unipolar electrograms. Occasionally, myocardial repolarization can introduce mid- or late diastolic potentials. Polarization of electrodes may result in gradual shift of the baseline. Pacing artifacts (Fig. 19.11), motion artifact, poor contact (resulting in decreased ratio of local to far-field signals and also increased power line noise), and 50 or 60 Hz power line noise can also alter the recorded signal (Fig. 19.12).

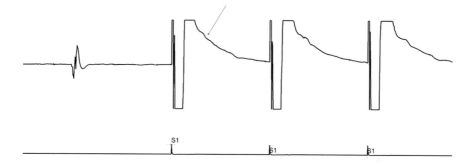

Fig. 19.11 Pacing artifact almost completely masking local electrogram at the pacing electrode. The arrow indicates the local electrogram

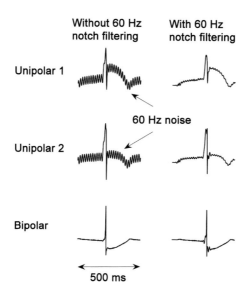

Fig. 19.12 Two unipolar electrograms recorded 5 mm apart and a bipolar electrogram obtained by taking the difference between the two unipolar electrograms. The unipolar electrograms on the *left* have significant 60 Hz interference without 60 Hz notch filtering. The 60 Hz interference is attenuated after notch filtering (result shown on the *right*). The 60 Hz interference is also eliminated in the bipolar recordings by virtue of subtraction

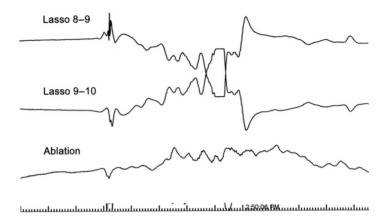

Fig. 19.13 The fluid flow and local heating from externally irrigated ablation catheters produces a low-frequency, low-amplitude noise in the adjacent electrodes during ablation. The noise generated here in the two consecutive lasso electrode pairs is symmetric and helps confirm the location of the ablation catheter near lasso electrode 9

The pacing artifact includes an initial high-frequency component resulting in saturation, generated by the high-frequency, high-voltage (relative to the ~1–10 mV amplitude of electrograms) pacing stimulus, followed by an exponential decay in voltage due to high-pass filtering (Fig. 19.11). Mechanical contact with other catheters can cause high-amplitude, high-frequency signals that are not related to the cardiac cycle. The fluid flow and heating from externally irrigated catheters during ablation can result in a low-frequency, low-amplitude noise in the adjacent electrodes (Fig. 19.13).

19.1.4
Signal Processing

Various catheters with two or more electrodes, as well as electrode arrays, baskets, etc., are available for myocardial unipolar and bipolar recording and stimulation. The electrical signal is transmitted from the electrodes, through wires incorporated in the catheters, to the recording and stimulation system. Multiple processing steps include recording the raw signal, amplification, analog filtering, digital conversion, digital filtering and processing, display, and storage (see diagram in Chap. 1).

Amplification is the initial step in signal processing, as the amplitude of recorded raw signals is generally less than 10 mV. The amplified signal then undergoes *analog filtering*. This is necessary to prevent signal aliasing, caused by sampling the signal at a rate too low for the frequency of the signal (Chap. 2).

The amplified and filtered signal is fed into analog-to-digital (A/D) converters with dynamic input range typically of ±2.5 or ±10 V. The *digitization* process uses sampling rates of at least 600 Hz, generally about 1,000 Hz, which results in an accurate representation of the electrograms with a temporal resolution of 1 ms. The Nyquist rule is that, in order to reproduce a signal without distortion, the maximum frequency component of the signal must be less than half the sampling rate. Thus, pre-digitization analog filtering must eliminate frequencies above 500 Hz, as those above 500 Hz will not be accurately represented (see Fig. 4.9, Chap. 4). In addition, high-pass analog filtering is used prior to digital sampling in order to avoid saturation and clipping of the signal (Fig. 19.14).

Subsequent *digital filtering* is a useful step in the processing of intracardiac electric signals, which attempts to remove unwanted components and improve signal to noise ratio.

Low frequency signals are generated by various sources, including respiratory movements, catheter movement, and variable catheter contact, which create baseline wander (or drift). These have frequencies generally less than 0.05–0.1 Hz. *High-pass filters* attenuate or eliminate signal components with frequencies below the cutoff frequency. In the electrophysiology laboratory, 30–50 Hz high-pass filters are used to eliminate such low-frequency components as myocardial repolarization and baseline drift from bipolar electrograms. In addition, far-field signals are attenuated by high-pass filtering, as the signal frequency decreases with the distance from the recording site (as discussed above).

This type of filtering can distort the morphology of electrograms, which is particularly significant for unipolar recordings (Fig. 19.15). A unipolar recording of a QS wave signifies proximity to the earliest activation site, and this can be altered by high-pass filtering. Thus, unipolar electrograms are generally either not filtered, or are minimally high-pass-filtered at 0.05 Hz.

Most intracardiac signals of interest are below 300 Hz, and *low-pass filtering* at a setting over 400 or 500 Hz is used to eliminate high-frequency noise generated by non-cardiac muscle activity or various electromagnetic sources.[5,36] Given the previous steps in signal processing, low-pass filtering over 500 Hz has little impact. Power line interference commonly contaminates intracardiac signals with 60 Hz noise (50 Hz in Europe). This is addressed with 60 Hz notch filters, which eliminate that specific frequency (Fig. 19.12). Intracardiac electrograms also contain these frequencies, and therefore will inevitably be distorted to some extent in the filtering process.

In all modern systems, filtering is used and can be adjusted in order to optimize the visualization, measurement, and interpretation of the signal of interest. However,

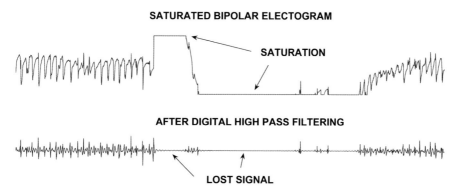

Fig. 19.14 Example of signal saturation and clipping introduced by low-frequency noise (such as baseline wander, movement, etc.). Even if the saturated signal is high-pass filtered to eliminate the low-frequency saturation artifact, the useful signal cannot be recovered, as it has been lost during sampling

Fig. 19.15 Effects of different filter settings on the unipolar electrogram recorded by an electrode in contact with atrial myocardium. Note the changes in amplitude and morphology, as well as in timing of maximum negative downstroke. Minimal filtering (0.05–500 Hz) is commonly used for unipolar electrograms

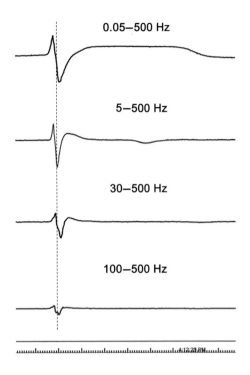

discriminate use and careful interpretation are necessary, as the filtering process can attenuate components of the signal of interest and therefore distort it (Fig. 19.15).

The amount of data that is collected during electrophysiology studies depends on the total duration of the saved clips and the number of channels that are being recorded. Electrophysiologic studies typically use up to 12 surface ECG channels, up to >20 channels of electrograms, one pacing channel, and occasionally a pressure channel, sampled at 1,000 Hz. Thus, generally 50–150 Mb of data accumulate per hour of saved recordings; as some studies can be up to >8–10 h long, the total file sizes and storage requirements are significant. In addition, three dimensional (3D) mapping systems handle additional data related to location and geometry, and thousands of reconstructed virtual channels (in the case of noncontact mapping). Proprietary compression algorithms are used by various recording and mapping systems (Table 19.2).

Several practical consequences and applications of electrogram recording and processing techniques have been introduced in the discussion above. In the following text, we will discuss several additional applications.

19.1.5
Activation Times

Identifying the earliest activation site is commonly used in the practice of clinical cardiac electrophysiology to identify target sites for ablation. For these measurements, fiducial points of reference in the cardiac cycle are chosen on the surface ECG or intracardiac electrograms,

Table 19.2 Using electrogram characteristics to guide electrophysiologic procedures (details in text)

Electrogram analysis	Utility/remarks
Timing	Onset of activation, use of bipolar/unipolar recordings
Morphology	
Sharpness	Far vs. near-field
Amplitude	Scar vs. normal tissue, far vs. near-field
Polarity of bipolar electrograms	At break through sites
QS (unipolar)	Identify sites of origin, or arrhythmia focus
Fractionation	Possibly identify autonomic ganglia, or targets for AF ablation
Sequence, or spatio temporal activation pattern	
Arrhythmia circuit	
Conduction block	Used to assess ablation success in achieving block
Three-dimensional maps	
Activation	Identify arrhythmia circuits, breakthrough or preexcitation sites
Voltage	Identify scar and healthy myocardium
Non-contact	Endocardial (intracavitary), epicardial (noninvasive ECG imaging)
Frequency-domain analysis	Dominant Frequency; identify drivers and degree of fibrillatory arrhythmia organization

with care to notice and avoid variability, which may affect results. Criteria to determine local activation times are described above. This may be difficult to assess accurately in abnormal myocardium, because low-amplitude local signals may be obscured by the larger far-field signals.[6] A unipolar QS morphology typically also identifies the activation origin. Catheter ablation is generally not successful at sites with an RS complex, which are remote from the earliest activation site. However, the area with a QS complex may extend for a 0.5 cm radius around the actual earliest site. Another caveat is that an electrode floating inside the chamber and not in contact with the myocardium may also record a QS complex. This is confirmed by a slow initial down-slope of the electrogram and lack of capture with unipolar pacing. However, most activation mapping is done using bipolar electrograms. Determining activation times from bipolar recordings (peak or baseline crossing) is technically easier than finding the peak negative dV/dt in unipolar recordings. A combined approach using simultaneously recorded unipolar and bipolar recordings is frequently used[6] (Fig. 19.8).

1. Electrogram characteristics at adjacent sites

Breakthrough sites (accessory pathways, ostia, etc.) can be located by identifying the electrodes at which the bipolar electrograms reverse polarity as has been discussed above (Fig. 19.9).

2. Confirming block

After cavotricuspid isthmus block is achieved by ablation, the change in direction of activation results in inversion of bipolar electrograms recorded lateral to the isthmus when pacing from the coronary sinus.

3. Creating maps

Maps are created from multiple recordings obtained either sequentially with one catheter (and relying on stability of the activation sequence) or simultaneously, with multiple electrodes (including basket catheters). Although cardiac electrical activation and arrhythmia are 3D phenomena, particularly in the thick wall of the ventricles, clinical mapping is recorded from only one surface of the chamber (endocardium or epicardium); three-dimensional, volume mapping, using multielectrode needles penetrating the myocardium, is limited to research. For *activation maps*, as an example, detection of local activation times can be performed manually, or computer-assisted for rapid detection of large numbers of electrograms, using various algorithms as described above. For ease of understanding and viewing, color activation maps can then be displayed. Three-dimensional reconstructions of the endocardial surface of the cardiac chamber can be obtained using electroanatomic catheter location systems based on electric or magnetic fields (CARTO, NavX, EnSite, LocaLisa), or ultrasound (RPM). Activation maps can then be merged and displayed on the reconstructed 3D chamber.

Several catheter location systems that are in use are based on measurements of low-amplitude electrical currents at the electrode of interest generated by electrical or magnetic fields emitted from reference locations. The CARTO system uses the fact that currents are generated in a metal coil located in a variable magnetic field. The catheter tip has a magnetic sensor that records three ultra-low energy magnetic fields emitted from separate locations on a unit outside the body. Using amplitude, frequency, and phase information, the 3D location and orientation of the sensor are computed. The EnSite system uses a 5.6 kHz low-amplitude electric signal emitted from three pairs of electrodes located on the skin and recorded from the catheter tips. Using the equations of electrical fields in solid media, catheter location is computed. The Localisa system uses low-amplitude currents (1 mA) applied between reference electrode pairs across the thorax in three orthogonal directions, at three different frequencies (approximately 30 kHz) and voltage is recorded at the catheter tip, thereby permitting the computation of 3D catheter position. Of note, the electric field-based systems are sensitive to changes in impedance that may occur during prolonged mapping procedures, because of changes in the water content of the thoracic tissues, and re-calibration may be necessary. The RPM system uses ultrasonic ranging techniques for catheter localization.

19.1.5.1
Activation Maps: Isochronal and Isopotential Maps

Activation mapping refers to the determination of the timing of the excitation wavefront arrival at multiple locations of the cardiac chamber. This provides essential information about the spread of myocardial excitation during normal and abnormal rhythms, identifies arrhythmia origin or circuits, and provides a basis for therapy (ablation, cardiac resynchronization).

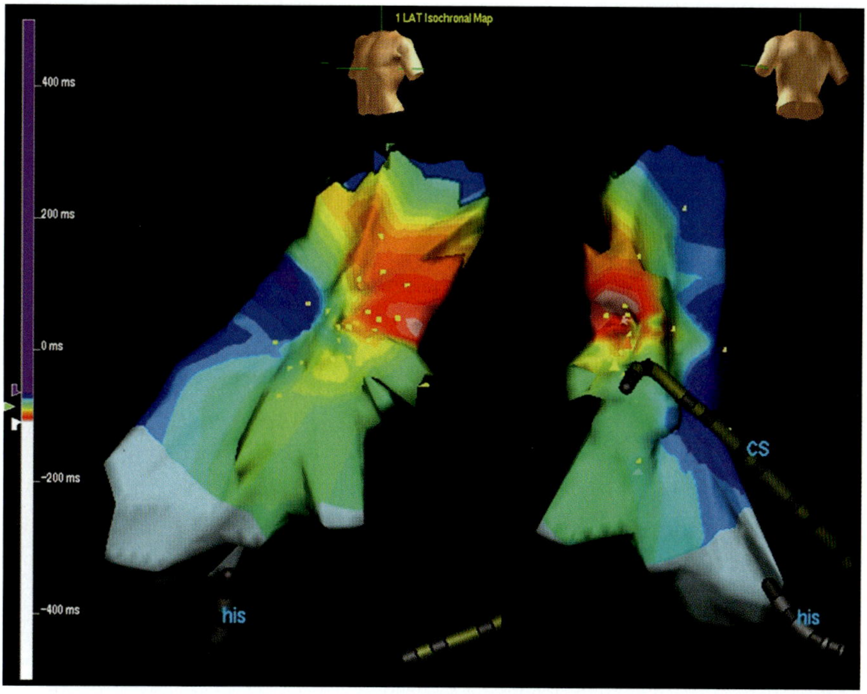

19 Intracardiac Electrograms   335

Fig. 19.16 Isochronal activation map of a premature ventricular depolarization focus in the right ventricular outflow tract – lateral and posterior views. The isochronal color map reflects the spread of electrical activation from a focal source. *White* represents the earliest electrical activation. Ablation in this location successfully eliminated the PVC (Map was obtained with the NavX system and digitally cropped for this illustration.)

This can be displayed graphically in isochronal maps (Fig. 19.16). Activation times are determined for multiple points, either synchronously, using multielectrode catheters or arrays, or sequentially, by moving the recording catheter. Spatial accuracy depends on the availability of a sufficiently large number of recording points. Those activations that occur at the same time point in the cardiac cycle and are spatially contiguous are assumed to form the wavefront at that point in time, which can then be identified by lines (isochrones) and/or color. However, it is essential to realize that this is not necessarily true, and that two adjacent sites can be activated simultaneously by two distinct wavefronts arriving independently: "…the presence of activation times consistent with propagation of an activation front…does not necessarily prove such an activation actually exists…."[37,38]

Isopotential maps are constructed using the instantaneous potential recorded at all points mapped. Different colors are assigned to each voltage. In focal arrhythmias, the area that first displays the most negative unipolar voltage is the area activated first and represents the arrhythmia focus (Fig. 19.17). Surrounding areas that have not been depolarized yet have a positive or less negative potential. Propagation of the wavefront can be visualized by playing the movie of sequential isopotential maps and thus help visualize reentrant arrhythmia circuits.

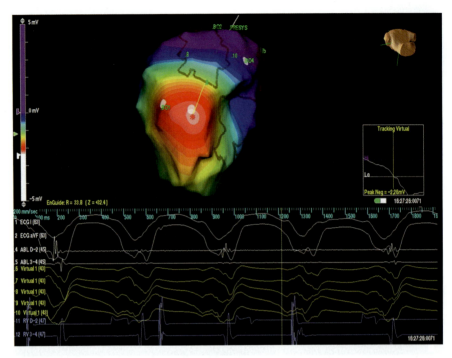

Fig. 19.17 Example of left ventricular isopotential map – obtained with a non-contact mapping technique (EnSite array). The most negative potential at this point in time (the *white area*) reflects the earliest endocardial activation and corresponds to the arrhythmia focus, located in the inferior and lateral aspect of the left ventricle. Virtual (reconstructed) unipolar electrograms (channels 6 through 10 displayed) from the area of the arrhythmia focus have a QS morphology. The voltage in the surrounding areas is positive or less negative, as the tissue is not yet depolarized

19.1.5.2
Voltage Maps

Another type of map is the voltage map, constructed from recordings of electrogram voltage in multiple points. It is used to identify areas of scar or infiltration (fat in ARVD, inflammation in sarcoid, etc.), which are a substrate for reentry or focal arrhythmias. Paths of viable tissue inside the scar, which are potential substrates for circuit reentry, can often be visualized by adjusting the voltage limits set for scar on the color voltage maps, with the caveats that the maps should be sufficiently detailed, and that artifactual paths may be "created" this way. Scar borders, also frequently involved in arrhythmia circuits and targeted for ablation, can be better estimated and visualized in a similar fashion, by adjusting voltage map settings (Fig. 19.18). During epicardial mapping, the epicardial layer of fat can be difficult to distinguish from actual scar, as it also results in low-amplitude electrograms. Electrogram characteristics (low-frequency – as it is relatively "far-field," absence of late signals, inability to capture with pacing) and anatomic location (overlying the main epicardial coronary vessels) may help distinguish it from scar.

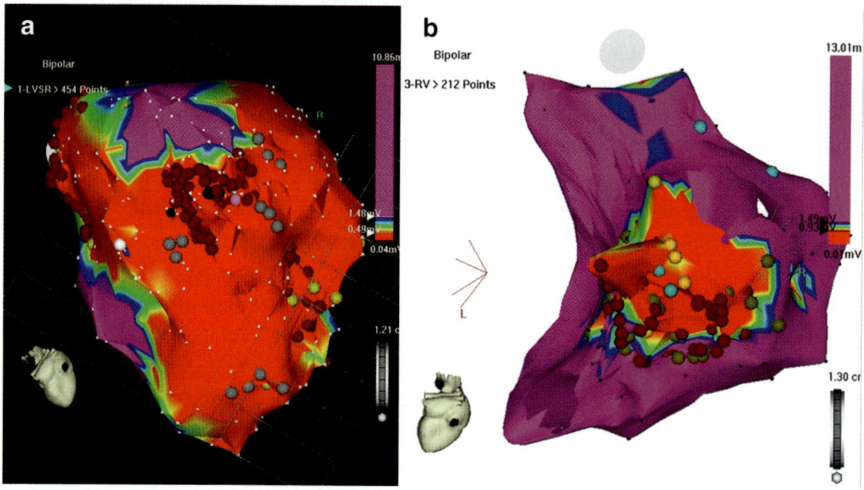

19 Intracardiac Electrograms

Fig. 19.18 Examples of voltage maps. (**a**) The area in red represents points with maximum electrogram voltage less than 0.5 mV in this case, and is consistent with an extensive area of anterior, septal, and lateral left ventricular scar from a previous myocardial infarction. *Purple areas* represent maximum electrogram voltage more than ~1.5 mV, consistent with normal myocardium. (**b**) The area in *red* represents points with maximum electrogram voltage less than 1.0 mV, and is consistent with an area of inferior scar from a previous myocardial infarction. *Purple areas* represent maximum electrogram voltage more than ~1.5 mV, consistent with normal myocardium. In both cases, channels of viable myocardium participating in reentry were identified near scar borders – and ablation (lesions tagged) successfully eliminated the ventricular tachycardia (Maps created with the CARTO system.)

19.1.5.3
Non-Contact Mapping – Principles and Brief Description

Contact mapping techniques are limited by the number of electrodes and catheters that are in direct contact with the mapped surface. Point-by-point mapping of sufficient density, performed with one electrode catheter during multiple arrhythmia cycles, can provide adequate maps. This may not be possible or easily done if the arrhythmia is not sustained, not reliably inducible, or is poorly tolerated hemodynamically. Techniques that can simultaneously acquire electrical activity from the whole endocardial surface with high resolution have been developed using non-contact mapping.

Efforts to model and reconstruct cardiac activation started more than half a century ago with attempts to solve the relationship between cardiac potentials and ECG recordings at the body surface, taking into account the complex cardiothoracic geometry and the electrical properties of the interposed tissues,[9,39] using Laplace's law and principles of current flow in volume conductors initially described by Helmholtz in 1853. Initial approaches involved solving the problem "forward," starting with known epicardial activation and calculating the surface ECG potentials, then validating these calculations by in vitro models with defined geometry and known epicardial and body surface potentials. By then "inverting" the solution, epicardial potentials could be calculated from body surface potentials.

However, this approach was fraught with multiple limitations, including multiplicity of solutions. An alternative approach, first introduced by Taccardi et al in 1987,[40] is to obtain noncontact recordings from endocavitary electrodes. In terms of mathematical modeling and validation, this approach reduced the difficulties introduced by distance and by multiple tissue interfaces – as the intracavitary blood may be considered an electrically inert and uniform medium. The depolarization wavefront is an area formed by a multitude of electric dipoles, and the amplitude of the recorded signal depends on the solid angle that it subtends when viewed from the recording electrode, as well as on the angle of view between the wavefront and the recording dipole, following geometric laws of perspective. In addition, the recorded signal amplitude is inversely proportional to the square of the distance from the recording electrodes and the wavefront. Multiple groups developed the mathematical and technical methods necessary for accurate reconstruction of endocardial electrograms based on noncontact recordings, which have subsequently been clinically validated.[7,40-42] A multi-electrode array deployed on an intracavitary balloon[43] is currently in clinical use. The initial step is to acquire accurate and detailed information about the cardiac *endocardial geometry*. This is performed using a roving catheter emitting an electrical signal at 5.68 kHz which is detected by current-sink electrodes positioned on the shaft, distally and proximally to the array. The locator signal can also be subsequently used to guide the roving catheter to target sites on the virtual geometry. As the geometry is acquired in reference to the array catheter, maintaining its position unchanged is essential for the accuracy of the virtual geometry. Next, the electrical activity of interest is recorded by the 64 electrodes located on the balloon array, located intracavitary. Based on the recorded far-field signals and the known balloon array and endocardial geometry, as well as the electrical properties of intracavitary blood, 3,360 "virtual endocardial electrograms" are reconstructed. Electrogram reconstruction is a mathematical process that essentially computes the inverse solution to Laplace's law, while limiting the solutions by setting boundary conditions based on physiological considerations. Mathematically, problems requiring inverse solutions are "ill-posed problems" and amplify noise and artifacts; hence, the signal is filtered prior to computation, and mathematical methods of "regularization" are used in the calculation. Each electrode on the noncontact array is influenced by all points on the endocardial surface, and the amplitude and frequency of the voltage contribution of each endocardial point depends on its local electrical activity, as well as on its distance from the recording electrode. By processing recordings from multiple neighboring electrodes "viewing" the point of interest but not in contact with it, and weighing each electrode's contribution for its distance from that point, a "virtual electrogram" is "reconstructed." Activation and voltage maps can then be created (Fig. 19.17). Multiple factors can impact the map accuracy, including the settings used for signal filtering, the distance from the electrodes to the myocardium, and the degree of inaccuracy of myocardial geometry. High-pass filtering from 0.05 to 32 Hz is used. The lower cutoffs may be used to include more far-field electrical activity such as that from epicardial locations, whereas higher settings (16–32 Hz) eliminate such far-field signals from epicardium or nearby chambers and better isolate near-field, high-frequency signals particularly when these have low amplitudes (mid-diastolic potentials within scar, Purkinje potentials), and might otherwise be masked by the far-field signal. Low-pass filtering is generally set up to 300 Hz. A more detailed discussion of noncontact mapping can be found elsewhere.[39]

Conversely, reconstructing epicardial electrical activation from a large number of non-invasive electrocardiograms recorded at the body surface ("ECG imaging") is possible, and significant progress has been made in overcoming the difficulties posed by the larger distance to the body surface, as well as by the multiple interposed tissues and tissue interfaces,[44–46] although this technique is not currently in widespread use.

19.2
Frequency Domain Analysis of Atrial Fibrillation

The complex and variable patterns of electrical activity during fibrillatory rhythms (atrial and ventricular) make analysis in the time domain (signal amplitude on y axis and time on x axis) difficult. Spectral techniques have been used for analysis in the frequency domain (signal amplitude on y axis and frequency on x axis) of these complex signals. Any continuous signal can be mathematically decomposed, using the Fourier transform, into a series of sinusoidal functions. The fibrillatory intracardiac electrograms are rendered optimally amenable to Fourier transformation by additional processing (filtering, rectification). Each of the sinusoidal waves that compose the signal has a specific frequency, amplitude, and phase, and their summation results in the actual signal. The sinusoid with the largest amplitude is called the "dominant frequency." The dominant frequency has been used as an estimate of the atrial activation rate during atrial fibrillation. However, there are several factors that interfere with the accurate estimation of atrial activation rates during atrial fibrillation, including low or variable electrogram amplitudes, frequency variability, presence of double potentials, and fractionated activity, noise, and far-field ventricular potentials. These limitations, when present, may require manual analysis for confirmation.

Signals that are perfectly periodic are decomposed into a sinusoid signal with the dominant frequency and additional sinusoids with frequencies that are all multiples, or "harmonics," of the dominant frequency. In contrast, disorganized, irregular signals have additional components, with frequencies that are not multiples (harmonics) of the dominant frequency. Thus, harmonic analysis can be used to quantify the regularity, or organization, of the signal (Fig. 19.19). One proposed "organization index" is the ratio of the power spectral area under the dominant frequency and its multiples, divided by the total signal power.[47–49]

Frequency spectrum analysis for atrial fibrillation may provide insights into its pathophysiology, as well as potential clinical tools for treatment or prognosis.[47] It has been shown that atrial fibrillation can be more easily terminated by shocks or burst pacing when it is associated with more organized signals.[50,51] Interventions such as antiarrhythmic drugs or autonomic manipulation have been shown to result in changes in the frequency spectrum of atrial fibrillation.[52] In human atrial fibrillation, frequency gradients between the left and right atrium have been noted, suggesting that high-frequency sources located in the left atrium drive the AF and may be appropriate targets for ablation. The presence or absence of a frequency gradient may have predictive value for the success of ablation.[53] With further improvements in methodology and recognition of its limitations, dominant frequency analysis may allow the development of additional applications for the understanding and treatment of "fibrillatory arrhythmias."

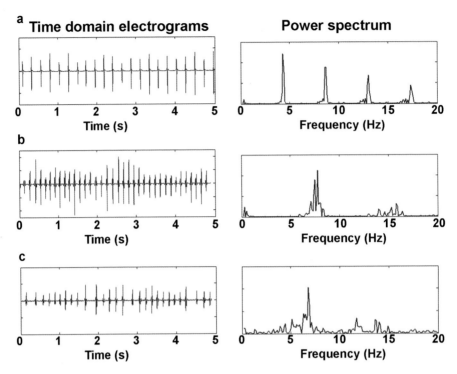

Fig. 19.19 Examples of arrhythmias and their power spectrum. (**a**) Atrial flutter characterized by its regularity. The power spectrum shows the dominant frequency at approximately 4 Hz with multiple peaks at the harmonics of this frequency. (**b**) Atrial fibrillation with some degree of regularity. The power spectrum shows a dominant frequency at 7.5 Hz with a very small harmonic at 15 Hz. (**c**) Atrial fibrillation with more irregularity. No harmonics are seen in the power spectrum

19.2.1
Intracardiac Electrograms Recorded by Implantable Devices (Pacemakers, Defibrillators)

The basic principles of electrogram recording are of course similar in implanted devices to those described for transvenous catheters. However, there are some issues that are unique to implanted devices. Basic functions of implantable cardiac rhythm management devices (pacing, defibrillation, diagnostics) require recording intracardiac electrograms. The electrode tip is in contact with the myocardium (Fig. 19.20). The raw recorded signal is processed as discussed elsewhere in this book, undergoing amplification, band-pass filtering, and rectification. When the processed signal amplitude reaches a set voltage threshold, a sensed event is declared. This is fed into the timing circuits and functioning algorithms.

Unipolar electrograms are recorded using the device can as the reference electrode ("tip-to-can"). Endocardial bipolar electrograms configurations include tip-to-ring (inter-electrode distance usually ~10 mm) or tip-to-coil ("integrated bipolar," used in implantable defibrillators). Epicardial systems can record unipolar (tip-to-can) or bipolar (tip-to-tip) electrograms.

Fig. 19.20 Schematic representation of an intracardiac dual-chamber pacing device system

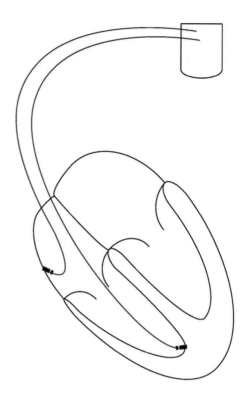

The local activation at the tip coincides with the *intrinsic deflection*, i.e., the "largest and steepest deflection" of the electrogram. Electrogram characteristics, including amplitude, slew rate, and morphology, are determined by all the principles discussed above. The amplitude is determined mainly by the amount of viable myocardium under the electrode, and is typically 5–30 mV for ventricular signals and 1.5–6 mV for atrial signals. The slew rate is the maximum absolute slope (dV/dt_{max}, measured in volts per second) of the intrinsic deflection, with typical values of 2–3 V/s for ventricular and 1–2 V/s for atrial electrograms. In practice, the minimally acceptable slew rates are considered >1.0 V/s for ventricular and >0.3 V/s for atrial electrograms. The slew rate will be lower for far-field or repolarization signals, and increases with shorter inter-electrode distances. Electrogram morphology depends predominantly on the near-field sequence of myocardial activation. The features of the recorded electrogram change after implant, as a result of the local inflammatory response at the electrode-tissue interface, which causes initial edema and subsequently fibrosis. This reaction alters the local electrical properties and increases the distance between the electrode and the tissue which is the source of electrical activity. As a consequence, there is an initial decrease in amplitude and slew rate (the latter being more pronounced), which subsequently increase over days to weeks to chronic levels, as fibrosis develops. Chronic electrogram amplitudes are usually lower by up to ~10% and chronic slew rates are ~30–40% lower compared to the initial, acute parameters.[54,55] Active fixation (screw-in) electrodes display more acute changes than passive fixation (tined) leads. Steroid-eluting electrodes do not significantly affect sensing characteristics, but they do decrease the chronic pacing thresholds. Physiologic (respiratory cycle, exercise, posture, age) and pathologic (metabolic, ischemic or antiarrhythmic drug-related) conditions can alter device electrograms.[56-63] In addition, electrogram parameters change with arrhythmias (premature depolarizations, tachycardia, etc.), with the most extreme examples of variability being atrial and ventricular

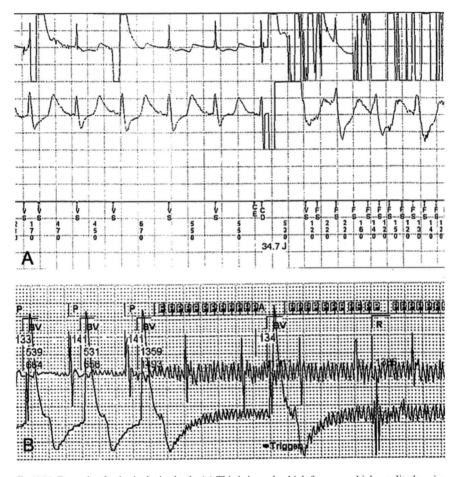

Fig. 19.21 Example of noise in device leads. (**a**) This is irregular, high frequency, high amplitude noise saturating the channel produced by an interruption in the electrical connection (in this case a lead fracture). The marker channel shows ventricular sensed (VS) events and "fibrillation sensed" (FS) events that fall in the rate detection window set for ventricular fibrillation. This noise was (erroneously) interpreted by the implantable defibrillator as ventricular fibrillation and resulted in multiple inappropriate shocks. (One 34.7 J shock was delivered during this tracing, due to prior sensed ventricular fibrillation that was cropped out for this figure.) The *top* channel is the ventricular bipolar electrogram, the middle electrogram is the far-field, coil-to-can electrogram, and marker channels indicating sensed events are at the *bottom*. (**b**) Electromagnetic interference of unknown cause produces high frequency, low amplitude noise in both atrial and ventricular sensing channels. The middle channel is the atrial bipolar electrogram and the *bottom* channel is the ventricular bipolar electrogram

fibrillation. This has important practical implications in normal device functioning and in the sensing and detection of arrhythmias. Electrograms can also be altered by noise produced by various sources: electromagnetic interference, myopotentials, lead fracture (Fig. 19.21), and faulty connections.[64] As discussed above, the "field of view" is wider with increasing inter-electrode distance and widest for unipolar electrograms. Thus, only bipolar electrograms are used for sensing in defibrillators, where noise can result in inappropriate shocks. In addition, systems with large inter-electrode distance (tip-to-coil recording in integrated bipolar systems, tip-to-tip recording in epicardial systems, tip-to-can "unipolar" recordings) are intrinsically more sensitive to noise and far-field signal "oversensing." Further discussion can be found elsewhere.[65]

References

1. Samojloff A. Weitere Beiträge zur Elektrophysiologie des Herzens. *Pflugers Arch*. 1910; 135: 417–468.
2. Faraday M. On electrical decomposition. *Phys Trans R Soc*. 1834.
3. Wilson FN, Johnston FD, Macleod AG, et al. Electrocardiograms that represent the potential variations of a single electrode. *Am Heart J*. 1934;9:447–458.
4. Kadish AH, Morady F, Rosenheck S, et al. The effect of electrode configuration on the unipolar His-bundle electrogram. *Pacing Clin Electrophysiol*. 1989;12(9):1445–1450.
5. Josephson ME. Electrophysiologic investigation: technical aspects. In: Josephson ME, ed. *Clinical Cardiac Electrophysiology*. 4th ed. Philadelphia, PA: Lippincott Williams and Wilkins; 2008.
6. Stevenson WG, Soejima K. Recording techniques for clinical electrophysiology. *J Cardiovasc Electrophysiol*. 2005;16(9):1017–1022.
7. Scher AM, Spach MS. Cardiac depolarization and repolarization and the electrogram. In: Berne RM, ed. *Handbook of Physiology*. Bethesda, MD: American Physiological Society; 1979:372.
8. Wilson FN, MacLeod AG, Barker PS. *The Distribution of the Currents of Action and of Injury Displayed by Heart Muscle and Other Excitable Tissues*. Ann Arbor, MI: University of Michigan Press; 1933.
9. Wilson FN, Bayley RH. The electric field of an eccentric dipole in a homogeneous spherical conducting medium. *Circulation*. 1950;1(1):84–92.
10. Scher AM, Young AC. Ventricular depolarization and the genesis of QRS. *Ann N Y Acad Sci*. 1957;65(6):768–778.
11. Spach MS, Barr RC, Serwer GA, et al. Extracellular potentials related to intracellular action potentials in the dog Purkinje system. *Circ Res*. 1972;30(5):505–519.
12. Durrer D, Van Der Twell LH. Spread of activation in the left ventricular wall of the dog. I. *Am Heart J*. 1953;46(5):683–691.
13. Schaefer H, Trautwein W. Further experiments on the nature of the excitation wave in the myocardium of the dog. *Pflugers Arch*. 1951;253(2):152–164.
14. Biermann M, Shenasa M, Borggrefe M, et al. Interpretation of cardiac electrograms. In: Shenasa M, Borggrefe M, Breithardt G, eds. *Cardiac Mapping*. 2nd ed. Elmsford, NY: Blackwell/Futura; 2003:15–39.
15. Spach MS, Dolber PC. Relating extracellular potentials and their derivatives to anisotropic propagation at a microscopic level in human cardiac muscle. Evidence for electrical uncoupling of side-to-side fiber connections with increasing age. *Circ Res*. 1986;58(3):356–371.

16. Spach MS, Kootsey JM. Relating the sodium current and conductance to the shape of transmembrane and extracellular potentials by simulation: effects of propagation boundaries. *IEEE Trans Biomed Eng*. 1985;32(10):743–755.
17. Steinhaus BM. Estimating cardiac transmembrane activation and recovery times from unipolar and bipolar extracellular electrograms: a simulation study. *Circ Res*. 1989;64(3):449–462.
18. Blanchard SM, Buhrman WC, Tedder M, et al. Concurrent activation detection from unipolar and bipolar electrodes. *Pacing Clin Electrophysiol*. 1988;11:525.
19. Paul T, Moak JP, Morris C, et al. Epicardial mapping: how to measure local activation? *Pacing Clin Electrophysiol*. 1990;13(3):285–292.
20. Pieper CF, Blue R, Pacifico A. Influence of time of sampling onset on parameters used for activation time determination in computerized intraoperative mapping. *Pacing Clin Electrophysiol*. 1991;14(12):2187–2192.
21. Pieper CF, Blue R, Pacifico A. Activation time detection algorithms used in computerized intraoperative cardial mapping. A comparison with manually determined activation times. *J Cardiovasc Electrophysiol*. 1991;2(5):388–397.
22. Kaplan DT, Smith JS, Rosenbaum D, et al. On the precision of automated activation time estimation. *Comput Cardiol*. 1987;14:101–104.
23. Scherlag BJ, Samet P, Helfant RH. His bundle electrogram. A critical appraisal of its uses and limitations. *Circulation*. 1972;46:601–613.
24. Cassidy DM, Vassallo JA, Marchlinski FE, et al. Endocardial mapping in humans in sinus rhythm with normal left ventricles: activation patterns and characteristics of electrograms. *Circulation*. 1984;70(1):37–42.
25. Josephson ME, Horowitz LN, Spielman SR, et al. Role of catheter mapping in the preoperative evaluation of ventricular tachycardia. *Am J Cardiol*. 1982;49(1):207–220.
26. Vassallo JA, Cassidy DM, Marchlinski FE, et al. Abnormalities of endocardial activation pattern in patients with previous healed myocardial infarction and ventricular tachycardia. *Am J Cardiol*. 1986;58(6):479–484.
27. Simpson EV, Ideker RE, Smith WM. An automatic activation detector for bipolar cardiac electrograms. *IEEE Eng Med Biol 10th Ann Int Conf*. 1988;1:113–114.
28. Pieper CF, Blue R, Pacifico A. Simultaneously collected monopolar and discrete bipolar electrograms: comparison of activation time detection algorithms. *Pacing Clin Electrophysiol*. 1993;16(3 pt 1):426–433.
29. Nademanee K, McKenzie J, Kosar E, et al. A new approach for catheter ablation of atrial fibrillation: mapping of the electrophysiologic substrate. *J Am Coll Cardiol*. 2004;43(11):2044–2053.
30. Nademanee K, Schwab MC, Kosar EM, et al. Clinical outcomes of catheter substrate ablation for high-risk patients with atrial fibrillation. *J Am Coll Cardiol*. 2008;51(8):843–849.
31. Calo L, De Ruvo E, Sciarra L, et al. Diagnostic accuracy of a new software for complex fractionated electrograms identification in patients with persistent and permanent atrial fibrillation. *J Cardiovasc Electrophysiol*. 2008;19(10):1024–1030.
32. Kremen V, Lhotska L, Macas M, et al. A new approach to automated assessment of fractionation of endocardial electrograms during atrial fibrillation. *Physiol Meas*. 2008;29(12):1371–1381.
33. Porter M, Spear W, Akar JG, et al. Prospective study of atrial fibrillation termination during ablation guided by automated detection of fractionated electrograms. *J Cardiovasc Electrophysiol*. 2008;19(6):613–620.
34. Scherr D, Dalal D, Cheema A, et al. Automated detection and characterization of complex fractionated atrial electrograms in human left atrium during atrial fibrillation. *Heart Rhythm*. 2007;4(8):1013–1020.
35. Yoshida K, Ulfarsson M, Tada H, et al. Complex electrograms within the coronary sinus: time- and frequency-domain characteristics, effects of antral pulmonary vein isolation, and relationship to clinical outcome in patients with paroxysmal and persistent atrial fibrillation. *J Cardiovasc Electrophysiol*. 2008;19(10):1017–1023.

36. Murgatroyd FD, Krahn AD, Klein GR, et al. Stimulation and electrophysiological monitoring. In: *Handbook of Cardiac Electrophysiology*. London: ReMEDICA; 2002:10–14.
37. Ideker RE, Smith WM, Blanchard SM, et al. The assumptions of isochronal cardiac mapping. *Pacing Clin Electrophysiol*. 1989;12(3):456–478.
38. Durrer D, Van L, Bueller J. Epicardial and intramural excitation in chronic myocardial infarction. *Am Heart J*. 1964;68:765–776.
39. Chow AWC, Schilling RJ, Davies DW, et al. Noncontact cardiac mapping. In: Cabo C, Rosenbaum DS, eds. *Quantitative Cardiac Electrophysiology*. New York: Marcel Dekker, Inc.; 2002:361–383.
40. Taccardi B, Arisi G, Macchi E, et al. A new intracavitary probe for detecting the site of origin of ectopic ventricular beats during one cardiac cycle. *Circulation*. 1987;75(1):272–281.
41. Colli-Franzone P, Guerri L, Viganotti C, et al. Potential fields generated by oblique dipole layers modeling excitation wavefronts in the anisotropic myocardium. Comparison with potential fields elicited by paced dog hearts in a volume conductor. *Circ Res*. 1982;51(3):330–346.
42. Khoury DS, Rudy Y. A model study of volume conductor effects on endocardial and intracavitary potentials. *Circ Res*. 1992;71(3):511–525.
43. Beatty GE, Kagan J, Budd JR. Endocardial Therapeutics, Inc., assignee. Endocardial mapping system. US patent 5297549, 1994.
44. Ghanem RN, Jia P, Ramanathan C, et al. Noninvasive electrocardiographic imaging (ECGI): comparison to intraoperative mapping in patients. *Heart Rhythm*. 2005;2(4):339–354.
45. Ghosh S, Avari JN, Rhee EK, et al. Noninvasive electrocardiographic imaging (ECGI) of epicardial activation before and after catheter ablation of the accessory pathway in a patient with Ebstein anomaly. *Heart Rhythm*. 2008;5(6):857–860.
46. Intini A, Goldstein RN, Jia P, et al. Electrocardiographic imaging (ECGI), a novel diagnostic modality used for mapping of focal left ventricular tachycardia in a young athlete. *Heart Rhythm*. 2005;2(11):1250–1252.
47. Ng J, Goldberger JJ. Understanding and interpreting dominant frequency analysis of AF electrograms. *J Cardiovasc Electrophysiol*. 2007;18(6):680–685.
48. Ng J, Kadish AH, Goldberger JJ. Effect of electrogram characteristics on the relationship of dominant frequency to atrial activation rate in atrial fibrillation. *Heart Rhythm*. 2006;3(11):1295–1305.
49. Ng J, Kadish AH, Goldberger JJ. Technical considerations for dominant frequency analysis. *J Cardiovasc Electrophysiol*. 2007;18(7):757–764.
50. Everett TH, Kok LC, Vaughn RH, et al. Frequency domain algorithm for quantifying atrial fibrillation organization to increase defibrillation efficacy. *IEEE Trans Biomed Eng*. 2001;48(9):969–978.
51. Pachon MJ, Pachon ME, Lobo TJ, et al. A new treatment for atrial fibrillation based on spectral analysis to guide the catheter RF-ablation. *Europace*. 2004;6(6):590–601.
52. Ropella KM, Sahakian AV, Baerman JM, et al. Effects of procainamide on intra-atrial [corrected] electrograms during atrial fibrillation: implications [corrected] for detection algorithms. *Circulation*. 1988;77(5):1047–1054.
53. Lazar S, Dixit S, Callans DJ, et al. Effect of pulmonary vein isolation on the left-to-right atrial dominant frequency gradient in human atrial fibrillation. *Heart Rhythm*. 2006;3(8):889–895.
54. Platia EV, Brinker JA. Time course of transvenous pacemaker stimulation impedance, capture threshold, and electrogram amplitude. *Pacing Clin Electrophysiol*. 1986;9(5):620–625.
55. DeCaprio V, Hurzeler P, Furman S. A comparison of unipolar and bipolar electrograms for cardiac pacemaker sensing. *Circulation*. 1977;56(5):750–755.
56. Goldschlager N, Epstein A, Friedman P, et al. Environmental and drug effects on patients with pacemakers and implantable cardioverter/defibrillators: a practical guide to patient treatment. *Arch Intern Med*. 2001;161(5):649–655.
57. Rajawat YS, Patel VV, Gerstenfeld EP, et al. Advantages and pitfalls of combining device-based and pharmacologic therapies for the treatment of ventricular arrhythmias: observations from a tertiary referral center. *Pacing Clin Electrophysiol*. 2004;27(12):1670–1681.

58. Schuchert A, Kuck KH, Bleifeld W. Stability of pacing threshold, impedance, and R wave amplitude at rest and during exercise. *Pacing Clin Electrophysiol*. 1990;13(12 pt 1):1602–1608.
59. Shandling AH, Florio J, Castellanet MJ, et al. Physical determinants of the endocardial P wave. *Pacing Clin Electrophysiol*. 1990;13(12 pt 1):1585–1589.
60. Rosenheck S, Schmaltz S, Kadish AH, et al. Effect of rate augmentation and isoproterenol on the amplitude of atrial and ventricular electrograms. *Am J Cardiol*. 1990;66(1):101–102.
61. Varriale P, Chryssos BE. Atrial sensing performance of the single-lead VDD pacemaker during exercise. *J Am Coll Cardiol*. 1993;22(7):1854–1857.
62. Chan CC, Lau CP, Leung SK, et al. Comparative evaluation of bipolar atrial electrogram amplitude during everyday activities: atrial active fixation versus two types of single pass VDD/R leads. *Pacing Clin Electrophysiol*. 1994;17(11 pt 2):1873–1877.
63. Furman S, Hurzeler P, De Caprio V. Cardiac pacing and pacemaker. III. Sensing the cardiac electrogram. *Am Heart J*. 1977;93(6):794–801.
64. Pinski SL. Electromagnetic interference and implantable devices. In: Ellenbogen KA, Kay GN, Lau CP, et al., eds. *Clinical Cardiac Pacing, Defibrillation, and Resynchronization Therapy*. 3rd ed. Philadelphia, PA: Saunders; 2007:1149–1176.
65. Ellenbogen KA, Kay GN, Lau CP, et al., eds. *Clinical Cardiac Pacing, Defibrillation, and Resynchronization Therapy*. 3rd ed. Philadelphia, PA: Saunders; 2007.

Advanced Signal Processing Applications of the ECG: T-Wave Alternans, Heart Rate Variability, and the Signal Averaged ECG

20

Ashwani P. Sastry and Sanjiv M. Narayan

20.1
Introduction

A variety of advanced signal processing techniques are already used in contemporary cardiology practice, embedded in widely used commercial tools. This chapter focuses on three such ECG tools that have clinical trial data to support them and that have been incorporated into practice guidelines: T-wave alternans (TWA), heart rate variability (HRV), and the signal averaged ECG (SAECG). TWA is defined as alternate-beat fluctuations in the amplitude or morphology of the ECG T-wave, and reflects dispersion of repolarization.[1] HRV is defined as fluctuations in the interval between consecutive sinus node-initiated beats, and indicates the balance of autonomic influences on the sinus node.[2] The SAECG is derived from multiple beats, aligned by their QRS complexes and averaged to increase the signal-to-noise ratio, to reveal low amplitude signals typically produced by slow conduction.[3] Each tool has been used for several purposes. However, the best validated applications are in predicting the risk for sudden cardiac arrest (SCA) from lethal ventricular arrhythmias, or the risk for major adverse cardiac events following myocardial infarction.

SCA is responsible for over 300,000 deaths per year in the United States, largely from ventricular tachycardia and fibrillation.[4] Patients with left ventricular systolic dysfunction and/or symptomatic heart failure are considered at high risk for SCA, and currently are candidates for prophylactic implantable cardioverter defibrillator (ICD) therapy.[5] However, most ICD recipients receiving devices for such indications do not experience ventricular tachycardia or ventricular fibrillation over the ensuing 2–3 years, suggesting that they may not have required their ICD.[6] Conversely, the majority of individuals at risk for SCA in the general population do not have reduced left ventricular systolic function and are therefore missed by these criteria.[7] As a result, there is a growing concern over the use of systolic function to stratify risk for SCA and a mounting interest in alternative tools.

Studies in animal models[8,9] and patients[10] show that ventricular tachycardia/fibrillation arises predominantly via reentry, which requires three pathophysiologic conditions to be met.

A.P. Sastry (✉)
Division of Cardiology, Duke University Medical Center, Durham, NC
e-mail: ashwani.sastry@duke.edu

First, reentry requires *repolarization dispersion*, which allows a wavefront to block in some myocardial regions while activating others. TWA measures such repolarization dispersion.[1] Second, reentry requires *slow conduction*, which facilitates tissue recovery before an excitation wave attempts to re-excite it. Slow conduction can be detected via the SAECG, particularly if caused by infarct scar.[3] Third, reentry requires unidirectional block for initiation. It is notable that many triggers of ventricular tachycardia/fibrillation may lead to abnormalities in these indices. For example, *stress and anger* may trigger arrhythmias,[11] and attenuate HRV[12] by increasing sympathetic over parasympathetic activity. Volume overload may also exacerbate arrhythmias[13] and, via ventricular stretch, may increase TWA.[14]

While TWA, HRV, and the SAECG, measure distinct tissue properties, they share several signal processing challenges. For example, TWA and the SAECG both measure signals on the order of microvolts despite the fact that ECG signals are typically measured on the order of millivolts. Measuring these signals thus requires accurate signal acquisition (Chap. 1), noise reduction, and analog to digital conversion (Chap. 2). All methods are based on the ECG, and thus require precise detection of QRS onset (Chap. 5) to ensure appropriate alignment for averaging (Chap. 7). Signal resampling is necessary in many implementations of HRV analysis. Finally, all methods can be assessed in the time domain or the frequency domain (Chap. 3).

This chapter will describe the signal processing approaches commonly applied for each index in terms of its proposed pathophysiology, acknowledging the lack of a precise mechanistic understanding for human ventricular arrhythmias, and then describe its clinical utility.

20.2
T-Wave Alternans (TWA)

TWA is an ECG phenomenon where the ST segment, T-wave and/or U-wave oscillate every-other-beat. In the early 1900s, Hering and Sir Thomas Lewis reported TWA that was visible to the naked eye and associated with ventricular arrhythmias.[15,16] Other dramatic examples of TWA include polarity oscillations immediately preceding arrhythmias in long QT syndrome patients,[17] and during active myocardial ischemia. However, contemporary practice measures TWA on the order of microvolts, which has been shown to predict lethal ventricular arrhythmias.[1] This requires the use of advanced signal processing techniques. In routine practice, TWA visible to the unaided eye is rarely encountered.

20.2.1
Physiologic Signal Being Evaluated By TWA

TWA reflects spatial and temporal dispersion of repolarization. As depicted in Fig. 20.1, spatial repolarization dispersion may prevent activation of ventricular regions with longer action potential duration (APD), causing a 2:1 conduction pattern (i.e., alternans). Alternatively, temporal variability of APD from beat to beat may cause TWA.

Although these mechanisms for TWA have been shown in animal models,[18,19] the mechanisms for human TWA remain unclear. Until recently, TWA was felt to result from a tissue

20 Advanced Signal Processing Applications of the ECG: TWA, HRV and SAECG

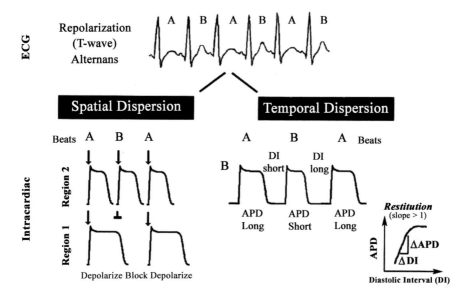

Fig. 20.1 T-wave alternans (TWA) represents dispersion of repolarization. *Left*: *spatial dispersion of repolarization*. Compared to region 2, region 1 has longer action potential duration (APD) and depolarizes every-other-cycle (beats 1 and 3). *Right*: *temporal dispersion of repolarization*. APD alternates between cycles, either from alternans of cytosolic calcium (not shown), or steep APD restitution. APD restitution (inset) is the relationship of APD to diastolic interval (DI), the interval separating the current action potential from the prior one. If restitution is steep (slope >1), DI shortening abruptly shortens APD, that abruptly lengthens the next DI and APD, leading to APD alternans

property (APD restitution slope >1) where small changes in rate caused marked changes in APD. At very rapid rates in animal models, this enables small rate fluctuations to cause large APD oscillations, wavebreak, and ventricular tachycardia/fibrillation.[19–21] However, in clinical practice, TWA predicts outcome only if present at slow heart rates (≤109 beats/min).[22] Accordingly, it has recently been shown to be unlikely that TWA reflects APD restitution slope >1.[23]

As an alternative mechanism in animal models, fluctuations in cytosolic calcium may cause alternans via direct and indirect effects on sarcolemmal ion channels.[19,24–27] Indeed, we have recently provided evidence from combined clinical and modeling studies that TWA at slow rates may reflect oscillations in myocyte calcium handling in patients with systolic dysfunction.[28] This observation requires further study in patients with and without heart failure.

Of additional interest for the optimal detection of TWA is how it relates to the "final common pathway" for potentially lethal ventricular tachycardia/fibrillation. Although TWA reflects pro-arrhythmic substrates (i.e., it has high negative predictive value), it is also a potentially a stable oscillation that may not transit to ventricular tachycardia/fibrillation (i.e., it has modest positive predictive value). The final pathway to arrhythmogenesis is likely the conversion from concordant alternans (that is spatially uniform) to discordant alternans, in which juxtaposed myocardium oscillates with opposite phase (Fig. 20.2) resulting in extreme repolarization dispersion precipitating ventricular tachycardia/fibrillation.[19]

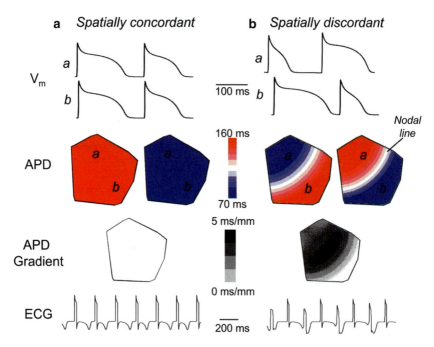

Fig. 20.2 Spatially (**a**) concordant and (**b**) discordant TWA in simulated 2D cardiac tissue. (**a**) *Top traces* show simulated action potentials from sites *a* and *b* that alternate in a long-short pattern. *Second panel* shows that the spatial APD distribution is either long (*blue*) or short (*red*) for each beat. *Third panel* shows minimal spatial APD dispersion (*gray scale*). *Bottom panel* shows simulated ECG with TWA. (**b**) *Top traces*. At a faster rate, site *a* now alternates short-long, whereas at the same time, site *b* alternates long–short. *Second panel* shows the spatial APD distribution, with a nodal line (*white*) with no APD alternation separating the out-of-phase top and bottom regions. *Third panel* shows that the spatial APD dispersion is markedly enhanced, with the steepest gradient (*black*) located at the nodal line. *Bottom panel*: simulated ECG, with T wave and QRS alternans, as observed experimentally (modified, with permission from Weiss et al[19])

At present, it is not clear if the ECG can discriminate discordant alternans. We have reported that TWA shows phase reversal and redistributes later within the T-wave[29] after critically timed premature beats in high risk patients, which improves predictive value above that of traditional TWA.[30] However, this requires further validation. Other potential indices of discordance may include ECG QRS alternans[19] or increased complexity of T-wave oscillations,[31] although these also require further validation.

20.2.2
Basic Description of the Technique

TWA is a dynamic signal derived from multi-lead surface ECG recordings. Noise-free ECG recordings and precise signal processing are needed to provide a high signal-to-noise ratio. Notably, TWA voltage as low as 1 μV may be clinically significant, yet noise is typically on the order of 10 μV. On a standard ECG recording, 1 mm represents 100 μV and QRS amplitude is ~1,000 μV. For a dynamic range (i.e., peak-to-trough amplitude) of 5 mV, 12-bit and 16-bit analog-to-digital converters provide resolutions of 1.2 μV and <0.1 μV, respectively, sufficient for TWA analysis. The typical ECG sampling frequency of 250–1,000 Hz is also sufficient for TWA.[32]

Ideally, the analysis should gracefully handle ectopic and aberrant QRS complexes. As TWA is a dynamic phenomenon, the analysis method should be capable of measuring TWA changes over time, as well as the distribution of TWA within the ST-T segment and changes in TWA phase. From a practical perspective ECG data recordings for TWA should be as simple as possible, and the TWA test should be easily interpretable. Finally, TWA measurement should minimize indeterminacy and provide well-validated accuracy against clinical endpoints.

Many methods are now available to measure TWA.[32] The two most commonly used are the spectral method and the more recently introduced modified moving average (MMA) method (Fig. 20.3). We will discuss the technical details as well as the potential benefits and drawbacks of each.

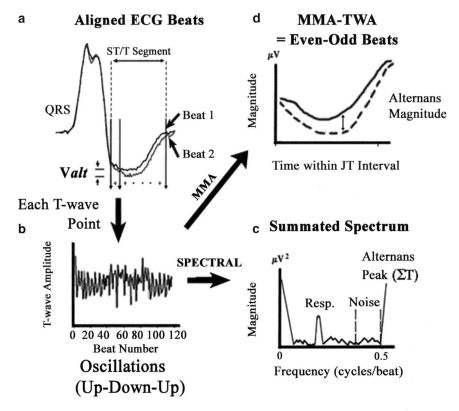

Fig. 20.3 Computation of TWA. (**a**) Beats are aligned by QRS complexes. (**b**) Beat-to-beat oscillations reflect alternans at each timepoint in the aligned T-waves (*arrows* in (**a**)). (**c**) Spectral analysis applies fast Fourier transformation to yield a power spectrum in which alternans is the peak at the frequency of half the heart-rate (0.5 cycles/beat).[33] Alternatively (**d**) modified moving average (MMA) analysis uses a non-linear filter to quantify the maximum difference between the means of "even" vs. "odd" beats in an alternating sequence[49]

20.2.3
Key Signal Processing Techniques 1 – The Spectral Method

Martinez and Olmos recently developed a comprehensive "unified framework" for computing TWA from the surface ECG, in which they classified TWA detection into preprocessing, data reduction, and analysis stages.[32] We will adopt this framework to describe the spectral and MMA methods for TWA detection.

20.2.3.1
Basic Description

The spectral method uses discrete Fourier transformation (DFT) to compute TWA magnitude and is the basis for the widely applied commercial CH2000 and HeartWave systems (Cambridge Heart Inc., Bedford, MA). It has also been used successfully in non-proprietary methods to examine TWA mechanisms in relation to clinical events.[1]

Essentially, this approach uses spectral analysis to quantify alternation in ST-T segment voltage from beat-to-beat. The magnitude of beat-to-beat alternans for each ST-T segment time point is determined from the DFT between beats at that point. This process is repeated for each time point, and results are added to measure the average voltage of alternation within the ST-T segment. The voltage of alternation is compared with noise estimates to determine the noise-subtracted alternans voltage and the degree of confidence in the alternans measurement (Fig. 20.3).

20.2.3.2
Preprocessing

The ECG is recorded from the Frank orthogonal leads in X, Y, Z axes and the precordial V1–V6 leads. The ECG signal is amplified and then filtered. Low-pass filtering is performed to eliminate high frequency components that typically represent noise, as well as to avoid aliasing from subsequent analog to digital conversion (see Chap. 2). High-pass filtering with a cutoff of 0.04–0.1 Hz is used to eliminate low frequency wander. The signal is then digitized, with sampling frequencies of 500 Hz or greater.

From the incoming beat series, QRS complexes are detected and fiducial points are determined and used for alignment (Chap. 5). Aligned beats are corrected to baseline voltage, using the T-P segment as an isoelectric baseline. The segments of interest for TWA are the ST segment and T wave, identified within a certain time window from QRS onset. In this way, the ECG data stream is "parsed" into a beat series, aligned by their QRS complexes and each with a defined ST-T segment.

Beats or signal regions not suitable for analysis because of aberrant QRS complexes or poor signal quality must now be rejected. This is done in two stages: (1) premature (early) or postmature (late) beats are eliminated, defined as beats with an RR interval differing from the median by more than 10 ms, and (2) ectopic beats are eliminated. Ectopic beats may be identified as those with a cross-correlation coefficient <0.95 relative to the average of all beats. Depending on the actual implementation, ectopic beats may be simply deleted or replaced with a template beat (typically the average of all beats). It is important to note that removal or substitution of beats may significantly affect TWA because of changes in TWA phase[33] (see below).

20.2.3.3
Data Reduction

To reduce processing time, data reduction (or undersampling) is commonly performed by decimation. For example, with a 500 Hz rate of analog to digital conversion and a hypothetical ST segment of 500 ms, each ST-T segment of interest includes 250 points. At this stage choosing an evenly spaced sampling of points improves computational speed and may minimally impact the final result. In most implementations of the spectral method, 7–75 evenly spaced points within the ST-T segment are typically retained.

20.2.3.4
Actual Calculation of TWA

After data reduction, we are left with a sub-series of retained beats, whose ST-T segments are represented by a small number of points. Alternans is calculated at each point from the waveform characteristics across-beats (Fig. 20.4).

As an example, at a particular point in the ST-T segment, voltage may vary from beat to beat (in µV) as shown in Fig. 20.4a 2,4,2,4,2,4,2,4.

At this time point in the ST-T segment, there is perfect alternant behavior. More realistically, in the presence of superimposed random noise, this alternating series may appear (in µV) as in Fig. 20.4c, e 1,4,3,5,1,4,3,6.

The DFT enables the alternating component of each series to be extracted, as shown in Fig. 20.4b, d, f. Skipping the mathematical details, the voltage series over time at a particular point in the ST-T segment is $V_1, V_2, V_3, V_4 \ldots V_n$.

The magnitude of the 0.5 cycle/beat component in the DFT spectrum of this series is computed by

$$DFT[0.5 \ cycles \ / \ beat] = V_1 - V_2 + V_3 - V_4 \ldots V_n. \qquad (20.1)$$

This can also be written as

$$DFT[0.5 \ cycles \ / \ beat] = (V_1 + V_3 + V_5 \ldots) - (V_2 + V_4 + V_6 \ldots)$$
$$= \frac{n}{2} \text{Average(odd beats)} - \frac{n}{2} \text{Average(even beats)}, \qquad (20.2)$$

where n is the number of beats being considered.

Thus, calculating the DFT at 0.5 cycles/beat is mathematically equivalent to taking the average of the odd beats and subtracting the average of the even beats. This relationship is the basis for the time domain analysis of TWA, to which we will return shortly.

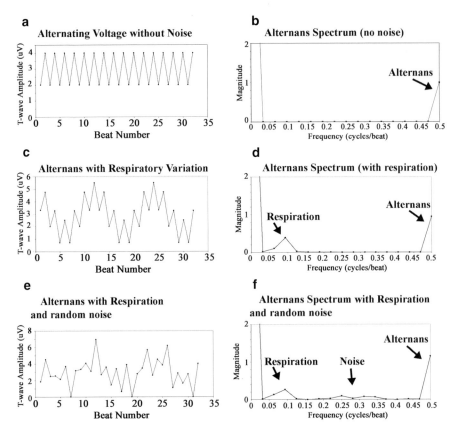

Fig. 20.4 Effect of noise on the spectral computation of TWA. This figure shows that the addition of noise results in spectral components that are distinct from the alternate beat (0.5 cycles/beat) peak of TWA. (**a**) *T-wave amplitude voltage, showing perfect alternans* from beat to beat. Voltage of alternation is 2 μV. (**b**) *Fourier transformation* of perfectly alternant beat series from (**a**). The large peak at the extreme *left* (frequency zero) represents the average voltage across the whole series. The other signal is at 0.5 cycles/beat, representing alternans (*arrow*), with magnitude 1 μV (microvolt) corresponding to $V_{alt} = 2$ μV. (**c**) *Respiratory variation superimposed* on perfectly alternating beat series from (**a**). (**d**) *Fourier transformation* of the beat series in (**b**). In addition to the alternans signal (0.5 cycles/beat), there is a signal at 0.09 cycles/beat representing respiratory variation. (**e**) *Representative physiologic alternans signal* that adds random noise to the beat series in (**b**). (**f**) *Fourier transformation* of the beat series in (**e**). This shows small signals between 0.15 and 0.4 cycles/beat representing noise, distinct from the large alternans signal and the signal at 0.09 cycles/beat (respiration)

As an example, if the time series alternates perfectly with amplitude 2 μV between successive beats as in our first example above, then DFT magnitude at 0.5 cycles/beat is $(n/2)*2 = n$ (μV).

The calculated DFT is typically normalized so that length of the beat series does not affect the final result. The calculation of $DFT[0.5 cycles / beat]$ (i.e., magnitude of alternation) is repeated for each point in the ST-T segment, and the results are summed to determine the total voltage of alternation for the entire ST-T segment, $DFT_{cumulative}[0.5\ cycles / beat]$, that is used to report TWA magnitude.

In practice, there are highly efficient algorithms to compute the DFT over all frequencies from 0 to 0.5 cycles/beat, so that the calculation of $DFT[0.5\ cycles/beat]$ (i.e., magnitude at the alternans frequency) is not performed using Eq. (20.1) above. The advantage of computing the DFT over all frequencies is that this provides a means of determining noise levels at neighboring frequencies, and thus estimating confidence in the TWA measurement. For this process, the DFT values at all other frequencies between 0 and 0.5 cycles/beat are also summed over all ST-T segment points to determine a cumulative DFT spectrum. This cumulative DFT spectrum is used to estimate the mean and standard deviation of noise, providing one of the main strengths of the spectral method.

Leaving aside the mathematical details, the following formulae are used to determine whether or not TWA is present. The $V_{alt.cum}$ is TWA magnitude corrected for noise. V_{alt} is the final average noise subtracted peak-to-peak magnitude of alternation in the ST-T segment, determined from $V_{alt.cum}$ by correcting for the number of points, P (typically 7–75), in the ST-T segment, which are examined. The alternans ratio, also known as the κ-score, is a measure of the signal-to-noise ratio of the measurement.

$$V_{alt.cum} = 2\sqrt{DFT_{cumulative}[0.5\ cycles/beat] - \mu_{noise}}, \qquad (20.3)$$

$$\text{Alternans ratio} = \kappa = \frac{DFT_{cumulative}[0.5\ cycles/beat] - \mu_{noise}}{\sigma_{noise}}, \qquad (20.4)$$

$$V_{alt} = 2\sqrt{\frac{DFT_{cumulative}[0.5\ cycles/beat] - \mu_{noise}}{P}} \qquad (20.5)$$

where μ_{noise} is the noise average and σ_{noise} is the noise standard deviation.

20.2.3.5
Data Storage

File sizes for TWA data are large, reflecting the need to store ECG data with sufficient precision to define subtle T-wave oscillations, continuously for multiple minutes and in several leads. Thus, files are typically megabytes in size, but the exact size depends upon the TWA method implemented and compression methods. Files may be larger for the spectral method than for the MMA method, which is based on ambulatory ECG data.

20.2.3.6
Noise in Spectral TWA Analysis

There is no standard method for calculating spectral noise (μ_{noise} in Eqs. (20.3)–(20.5)). Noise may be biological, representing signals that are not of interest from skeletal muscles or breathing, or non-biological, from other electronic equipment or suboptimal electrode contact with the skin. Interestingly, some noise may create alternans – for instance, patients tend to pedal on bicycle ergometers at a rate of one-half-of-heart-rate![22] Thus, if bicycle exercise is used to elicit TWA, the patient must be prevented from cycling at this rate. In general, noise is defined to exclude physiologically meaningful signals, such as respiratory variations that typically occur at 0.1–0.3 cycles/beat, or the alternans signal itself (0.5 cycles/beat). Typically, the noise average, μ_{noise} and standard deviation, σ_{noise}, are computed from ~8 points in a band adjacent to the alternans magnitude, such as 0.34–0.44 cycles/beat, or 0.39–0.49 cycles/beat. Alternative frequency ranges and numbers of points may be used for noise estimation (Fig. 20.4).

Traditionally, long beat windows (64–128 beats) assure a good signal-to-noise ratio and are the preferred approach. Of course, this effectively averages TWA over these periods, reducing the ability to resolve TWA for shorter periods that may be clinically relevant.[31] Conversely, while using shorter windows (i.e., averaging fewer samples) improves temporal resolution, this also reduces signal-to-noise ratio. Because the spectral method equally weights the contribution of each beat to TWA, i.e., it is linear whether a beat is normal or ectopic, the spectral method may result in significantly higher noise relative to *non-linear* methods of analysis (see below) for shorter beat windows.

Premature or ectopic beats may reverse the phase of TWA (i.e., change ABABAB… oscillations to BABABA…) in simulations[33] and clinical ECGs.[29] For example, Fig. 20.5 shows a long ECG sequence with a single premature beat at its midpoint (Fig. 20.5a). TWA occurs on either side of this ectopic (Fig. 20.5b) with a clear spectral peak at the alternans frequency (0.5 cycles/beat).

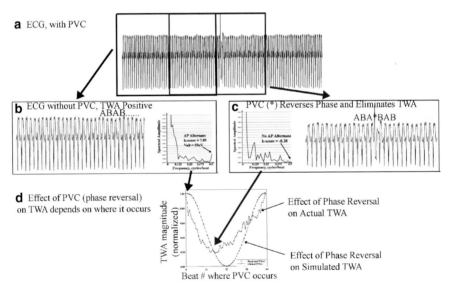

Fig. 20.5 Impact of ectopic and premature beats on the spectral computation of TWA. (**a**) *ECG sequence with a single premature ventricular complex (PVC) half-way through.* (**b**) *TWA is observed spectrally prior to the PVC*, with V_{alt} =59 µV in the magnitude spectrum. This point is the baseline for normalization (in (**d**)). (**c**) *TWA is not observed for the sequence centered on the PVC.* As shown, the PVC reverses phase, so that ABABA… becomes ABA*B…. Spectrally, this results in two equal length segments of opposite phase that cancel algebraically and result in minimal alternans. (**d**) *Impact of PVC position on TWA*, where PVCs at the end of the sequence have minimal impact, while those at the center extinguish TWA. This panel shows the impact on simulated TWA that is extinguished as stated. Actual TWA was not extinguished, suggesting that TWA was not uniform throughout the sequence and likely dominated in the left-hand segment[33]

Notably, the impact of a premature ventricular complex (PVC) or irregular beat depends upon its location. A PVC at the end of the sequence being analyzed may have little impact. In contrast, a PVC at the mid-point of the sequence being analyzed may have a profound effect on measured alternans. Figure 20.5d shows a segment of ECG data where a PVC occurs at the midpoint of the segment, reversing alternans phase such that ABABAB... becomes BABABA ..., producing equal-length segments on either side of the PVC with opposite phase of alternans. This cancels algebraically (Eq. (20.1)), thus extinguishing TWA for the entire segment. This effect is shown in Fig. 20.5d for the actual sequence (red arrow) and in simulations.[33]

A short beat window tends to minimize this problem, as TWA recovers quickly within a few beats of a phase reversal, but at the cost of reduced signal to noise ratio. For these reasons, alternative methods such as MMA (see below), have been proposed to use shorter beat windows to improve time resolution and resilience to phase reversal.

20.2.3.7
Measuring Variations in Spectral TWA

The actual beats selected for TWA analysis influence the result, which may vary over time. Thus, a sliding beat window of fixed length may indicate the variation in alternans voltage over time in the raw ECG (see, for example, Fig. 2 in Ref.[34]). These dynamics may provide clinical information above and beyond single time points, and commercial equipment (e.g., from Cambridge Heart) plots TWA magnitude over time.

20.2.4
Interpretation of Spectral TWA Tests

Criteria for interpreting TWA from the most widely used commercial system (Cambridge Heart, Bedford, MA) are well-described,[22] and have been simplified by recent recommendations to use the diagnosis from the automated reader. *Positive TWA* (Fig. 20.6) is defined as TWA sustained for ≥ 1 min with $V_{alt} \geq 1.9$ µV and κ-score >3.0 in any vector (X, Y, Z) or two precordial ECG leads, if onset heart rate <110 beats/min. Positive TWA must also have <10% bad beats and <2 µV spectral noise *without* artifactual alternans. *Negative TWA* is the absence of positive TWA as long as a heart rate >105 beats/min is achieved, while *indeterminate TWA* classifies all other results.

20.2.5
Interpreting Noisy and Indeterminate TWA Tests

The handling of TWA noise, as well as how to interpret indeterminate tracings, is controversial. Current recommendations minimize this issue by immediately retesting patients with indeterminate TWA tests.[35] However, if TWA remains indeterminate, as seen in 9–47% of reported studies, recent studies provide guidance. Commercial systems using the spectral method for TWA analysis (Cambridge Heart, Bedford, MA) categorize noise from various

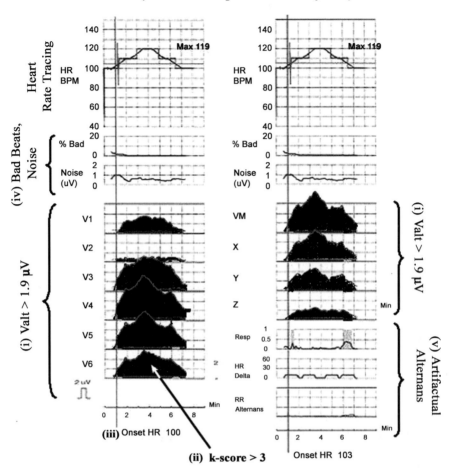

Fig. 20.6 Interpretation of spectral TWA. This tracing from a commercial system (Cambridge Heart, Bedford, MA) shows positive TWA. (i) $V_{alt} \geq 1.9$ µV in two precordial or one vector lead (here $V_{alt} \approx 4$–6 µV in V3–V6) with (ii) k-score ≥ 3 (*gray shading*) for >1 min (here ≈ 5 min), at (iii) onset rate <110 beats/min (here 100 beats/min), with (iv) <10% bad beats and <2 µV noise, without (v) artifactual alternans (see text). *Black horizontal bars* indicate periods when conditions for positive TWA are met

sources. This enables each source to be independently assessed. Excessive ventricular ectopy or failure to achieve target heart rate likely reflects adverse pathophysiology,[35] and such causes of indeterminate TWA[35,36] may be grouped with positive TWA as "abnormal TWA." On the other hand, indeterminate TWA due to respiratory noise, artifact, or poor ECG electrode contact is likely of little prognostic value and should not be grouped into "abnormal TWA."[35]

20.2.6
Clinical Use of Spectral TWA

Recent American Heart Association/ American College of Cardiology (AHA/ACC) guidelines provided a class IIa indication for the use of spectral TWA to predict the risk for life-threatening ventricular arrhythmias.[37] These guidelines were on the basis of numerous studies showing that TWA has a high negative predictive value for cardiac arrest and ventricular tachycardia/fibrillation in patients with ischemic[30,38,39] and non-ischemic[40-42] cardiomyopathy. Moreover, recent studies suggest that spectral TWA may also have value in risk-stratifying patients with preserved left ventricular ejection fraction (LVEF) (>40%) post-myocardial infarction.[43,44] Many of these results were recently summarized in a meta-analysis.[45]

Conversely, two notable recent studies question the utility of TWA for predicting SCA.[46,47] It remains to be determined whether this reflects the inadequacy of ICD therapy as a surrogate for life-threatening SCA (as the ratio of ICD therapy to true SCA may be as high as 5:1), the fact that arrhythmias in the TWA substudy of the SCA in heart failure trial occurred late, thus reducing the apparent effectiveness of TWA when assessed over the entire follow-up period,[47] or other technical limitations.

20.2.7
Key Signal Processing Technique 2 – The Modified Moving Average (MMA)

The MMA method for TWA analysis attempts to address some weaknesses of the spectral method. As illustrated in Eq. (20.2), the DFT magnitude at 0.5 cycle/beat is equivalent to subtracting the average of the even from the odd beats. Thus, in principle, taking the difference between the moving average of even and odd beats enables the exact calculation of alternans magnitude at 0.5 cycles/beat. This reduces computational complexity, but at the expense of no longer determining the full DFT spectrum from which to estimate noise. The MMA method introduces non-linearity into the averaging process to limit the impact of noise and aberrant beats. In this way, it is theoretically possible to reliably estimate TWA from short beat windows with improved time resolution and reduced susceptibility to phase reversals.

The MMA method is described as follows.[48] The raw data stream is amplified, filtered, and digitized; QRS complexes are detected and voltage corrected, and ST-T segments are defined as in the spectral method. Filtering of aberrant and ectopic beats need not be as stringent as in the spectral method, although segments of excessive ECG noise are removed. The remaining beats form an n beat series.

The beat series is divided into two, one consisting of the even beats (E_n), and the other consisting of the odd beats (O_n). The MMA is then created iteratively for each series, by adapting the moving average (or "rolling mean") to incorporate each successive beat. To avoid skewing the moving average by noisy or outlying beats, this is not done linearly. Rather, a non-linear updating factor is used to weight the moving average, on the basis of differences between the new beat and the current average. The actual difference is used if it lies between −1 and −32 μV or +1 and +32 μV. If the difference is >32 μV, then 32 μV is used; if the difference is <-32 μV, then -32 μV is used.[49] Differences between -1 and 0 μV are amplified to -1 μV, and differences between 0 and $+1$ μV are amplified to 1 μV.

Scaling leads to amplification of the difference between the prior MMA and the next original ECG beat when the difference is small and to attenuation when the difference is large. Theoretically, this non-linearity minimizes the effects of noise and ectopy, and amplifies small yet potentially meaningful variations in the ST-T segment.

The final TWA measurement is taken as the maximum absolute value of the point by point difference between even and odd MMAs across the JT interval. For this reason MMA does not correlate with the spectral method, which averages alternans at each JT point – although one could easily modify the MMA method to report the average over the JT segment of the differences between the even/odd moving averages, to more closely parallel results from the spectral method.

20.2.8
Measurement of Variations in MMA-TWA Over Time

The beat window over which to calculate MMA varies in the literature from 16 to 64 beats. As in the spectral method, a longer window decreases noise but at the expense of reduced time resolution and increased sensitivity to phase changes. A second parameter in the MMA method is the factor by which to scale changes in the MMA with each beat – this updating factor is typically 8. A larger factor will decrease the given contribution of any one beat to the calculated MMA, and vice versa.

Notably, the MMA method does not estimate the average or standard deviation of noise, and therefore does not provide an estimate of confidence in the TWA measurement.

20.2.9
Clinical Utility of MMA-TWA

The primary stated strength of the MMA method is reduced susceptibility to noise and phase reversals when short beat windows are used, as well as improved time resolution. Because of these factors and lower computational complexity, the MMA method has been applied retrospectively to ambulatory ECGs.

In a retrospective case controlled study of low risk post-myocardial infarction patients, MMA TWA analysis on ambulatory ECG recordings identified a 4–7 fold higher risk of life threatening arrhythmias in patients in the 75th compared with the 25th percentile.[48] This was supported by a study of low-risk patients undergoing stress ECG testing, in whom MMA-TWA >65 μV predicted arrhythmic, cardiovascular, and all-cause mortality compared to those with lower levels of MMA-TWA.[50] MMA has also been validated in a higher risk population of individuals with left ventricular ejection fractions $<50\%$ following acute myocardial infarction, in which MMA-TWA (and spectral-TWA) alone, and in combination with other risk factors, predicted cardiovascular and arrhythmic mortality.[44]

However, the utility of MMA-TWA has yet to be conclusively demonstrated in the traditional target population for risk stratification – patients with left ventricular ejection fractions <35–40% who are currently indicated for ICD implantation although they may not experience ventricular tachycardia/fibrillation in the medium term. Another problem with MMA-TWA is that no well-accepted cutpoint yet exists for an "abnormal" test. Furthermore, some of the suggested advantages of the MMA method are not necessarily intrinsic to MMA, and could be incorporated in the spectral method by appropriate methodologic alterations.

20.2.10
Comparing MMA and Spectral Methods of Computing TWA

Few studies directly compare the MMA and spectrally derived TWA. One formal comparison used ROC curves to determine an optimal MMA cutoff value to predict spontaneous ventricular tachycardia/fibrillation in patients with left ventricular dysfunction.[51] This had not been previously defined. The optimum cutoff value for MMA-TWA was 10.75 µV, an order of magnitude higher than the 1.9 µV used for spectral TWA. MMA-TWA trended to identify patients with cardiac death or ventricular tachycardia/fibrillation on long term follow-up from those without ($p=0.06$), while the spectral method successfully separated these groups ($p=0.02$). A recent large study in post-MI patients with LVEF <50% showed that both spectral and MMA-TWA (threshold 5 µV) predicted arrhythmic events.[44] In contrast, a recent preliminary study compared MMA-TWA to spectral-TWA on identical ECGs using the respective commercial systems, and found that MMA-TWA did not correlate with spectral-TWA and did not predict events.[52]

Further clinical studies are needed to better define the utility of MMA-computed TWA, particularly in patients who currently are indicated for ICD implant, and to compare MMA-TWA with spectral-TWA.

20.2.11
Future Directions in TWA Analysis

Definition of the mechanisms for human TWA may help to improve methods to risk-stratify for SCA in patients who are currently outside the ICD indicated population – i.e., with relatively well preserved left ventricular ejection fraction (>40%). Similarly, it would be helpful to develop indices of imminent ventricular tachycardia/fibrillation propensity, rather than the current method of actuarial risk. Studies on the impact of premature beats on TWA or methods to reveal subtle QRS alternans (as a surrogate for discordant alternans) may be fruitful in this regard. Recent studies that complex T-wave oscillations precede spontaneous ventricular tachycardia/fibrillation[31] suggest that non-alternating periodicity (other than 0.5 cycles/beat) should be explored in more detail. Finally, the impact of autonomic tone on TWA should be explored to better link a measure of arrhythmic substrate (TWA) with an adverse neurohormonal milieu.

20.3 Heart Rate Variability (HRV)

20.3.1 Basic Description

HRV measures variation in R–R intervals during sinus arrhythmia (denoted as "N–N" intervals). HRV thus reflects the influence of autonomic nervous inputs upon the sinus node that, beyond intrinsic sinus node rate, reflects parasympathetic and sympathetic activity (Fig. 20.7). Health is associated with large HRV oscillations while many disease states may depress HRV. In particular, depressed HRV has been associated with adverse outcome in patients with myocardial infarction and with heart failure.[53]

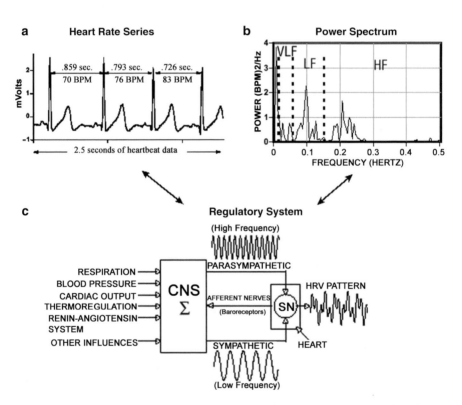

Fig. 20.7 Heart rate variability (HRV). (**a**) Sinus beats showing beat-to-beat variations in RR interval. (**b**) Fourier analysis of the RR intervals (typically analyzed over 24 h) reveals discrete peaks attributable to distinct mechanisms. The high frequency band may selectively examine parasympathetic activity, and the low frequency band may reflect sympathetic innervation while the very low frequency band may reflect activity of the renin-angiotensin-aldosterone system. (**c**) Schematic of regulatory system in CNS

20.3.2
Physiologic Signal Being Evaluated by HRV

HRV reflects the influence of the autonomic nervous system upon the sinus node. Although the sinus node has an intrinsic rate, revealed after blockade of the autonomic nervous system,[54] physiologic sinus arrhythmia reflects parasympathetic and sympathetic activity. Parasympathetic nervous system activity increases HRV, for example in response to respiratory cycles, while sympathetic nervous system activity decreases HRV.

HRV can be measured in the time and frequency domains. In the time domain, HRV is well represented using simple methods determining the standard deviation of different groups of sinus intervals. The most frequently used time domain estimates of HRV are the standard deviation of NN (SDNN) intervals, the standard deviation of the averages of the NN (SDANN) intervals, the root mean squared successive differences (RMSSD), and the HRV triangular index (TINN) (see below).

In the frequency domain, HRV can be classified into distinct bandwidths of high (HF 0.15–0.40 Hz), low (LF 0.04–0.15 Hz), very low (VLF 0.0033–0.04 Hz), and ultralow (ULF <0.0033 Hz) frequencies. Vagal activity modulates HRV in all frequency bands,[53] although certain frequencies may be more selective for specific physiological components. The high frequency (HF) component of HRV at 0.15–0.40 Hz predominantly reflects respiratory sinus variation from vagal activity that predominates in health and is abolished by atropine. Low frequency (LF) activity at 0.04–0.15 Hz largely reflects sympathetic activity (particularly if normalized to total spectral power) that increases in disease states such as heart failure. Notably, non-normalized LF activity may better reflect both autonomic limbs. VLF at 0.0033–0.04 Hz reflects parasympathetic activity but may also indicate activation of the renin-angiotensin-aldosterone system. ULF (below 0.0033 Hz) is of uncertain physiologic significance.

Despite more active interest in frequency domain analysis of HRV, there is a close analog between the time domain indices and frequency bandwidths. An ~80% correlation exists for SDNN with total spectral power, SDANN with ULF power, and average of SDNN intervals every 5 min (ASDNN) with VLF power. Thus, time and frequency domain methods likely measure the same physiologic phenomena.

Non-linear analyses of HRV have also been proposed,[2] such as the inverse power-law slope and fractal scaling. These indices are often independent of time and frequency domain analyses. However, their physiologic significance is unclear. Deterministic chaos is not thought to account for pathologic patterns of HRV, although loss of complexity is a feature of several disease states.

Many pathological states attenuate HRV. For instance, HRV may be depressed following a myocardial infarction due to autonomic denervation, reduced upstroke velocity of systolic arterial pressure, or distortion of sensory nerve endings from altered myocardial geometry. HRV is also depressed in heart failure patients, in whom the magnitude of HRV depression predicts ventricular tachycardia/fibrillation as well as long-term outcome. HRV also falls in states with cardiac denervation, such as after cardiac transplantation and with diabetic neuropathy. Several ambulatory ECG systems that record the ECG for prolonged periods provide indices of HRV that have been used in several clinical applications. Figure 20.7 indicates schematically how an ECG time series and spectral measures of HRV may relate to regulatory systems in the central nervous system.

20.3.3
Key Signal Processing Techniques

A European Society of Cardiology and North American Society of Pacing and Electrophysiology Position Statement (1996) discussed time domain, frequency domain, and non-linear analyses of HRV.

20.3.3.1
Data Acquisition and Signal Pre-Processing

Signal requirements for HRV are simplified by the fact that the precise morphology of QRS complexes and ST-T segments are not directly analyzed, unlike analyses for TWA and the SAECG. Thus, raw ECG data and the analog to digital conversion steps for HRV analysis must be sufficient only for the accurate timing of QRS complexes. Digitization of raw ECG data at 250 Hz is typically sufficient. Second, although beats must be classified as "normal" ("N," as opposed to ectopic) to be assessed in HRV, their shape does not have to be accurately resolved (unlike the need for microvolt level resolution in TWA and the SAECG). Thus, 10 bit digitization of ECG voltage at each time point is sufficient.

The first step in computing HRV is to annotate beats from long term ECG recordings. The ambulatory ECG series is parsed into "normal sinus beats" (typically designated "N"), supraventricular beats (often designated "SVE," or "S"), and ventricular beats (typically designated "V"), usually using cross-correlation techniques. As HRV processes inter-beat (RR) intervals, ectopic beats which introduce sudden and dramatic changes in the inter-beat interval relative to sinus beats can have a significant effect on HRV calculations. Ectopic beats may be handled in a number of ways, depending on whether time or frequency domain methods are used (see below).

20.3.3.2
Time Domain Indices of HRV

In the time domain, the most frequently used estimates of HRV are the SDNN intervals (SDNN), the SDANN intervals, the RMSSD, and the HRV triangular index (TINN). If the NN intervals in a 24-h ambulatory recording are given by the series

$$R[t]|_{t=1...T}$$

then

$$\text{SDNN} = \sigma_{NN} = \sqrt{\frac{1}{T-1}\sum_{t=1}^{T}(R[t]-\mu_{NN})}, \quad (20.6)$$

where μ_{NN} is the average of all NN intervals. Similarly,

$$\text{RMSSD} = \sigma_{RMS} = \sqrt{\sum_{t=1}^{T}(R[t+1]-R[t])^2}, \quad (20.7)$$

$$h(\lambda,\phi,t) = \int_{-H}^{0} \frac{\rho(\lambda,\phi,z,t) - \rho_{ref}(\lambda,\phi,z)}{\rho_{ref}(\lambda,\phi,z)} dz, \tag{20.8}$$

where B is the number of 5 min intervals in the entire series $R[t]$, $R_{5\min}[b]$ is the series of averages of $R[t]$ over each of the B 5 min intervals, and μ_{ANN} is the mean of $R_{5\min}[b]$.

When using time domain methods, ectopic beats can be handled by simple deletion, as frequency and phase considerations do not come directly into play in HRV determinations. For example, in the beat series,

$$N1, N2, S1, N3, N4, \tag{20.9}$$

(where "N" beats are normal sinus beats and the "S" beat is supraventricular) the RR intervals "N2–S1" and "S1–N3" would be deleted, leaving only the RR intervals N1–N2 and N3–N4 in the series of RR intervals subject to HRV analysis. This largely eliminates the influence of ectopic beats.

Low frequency, long-term components are best estimated by the standard deviation of 5-min averages of NN intervals (SDANN), while the square roots of the mean squared differences of successive NN intervals (RMSSD) best reflect short-term, high frequency components.

20.3.3.3
Heart Rate Turbulence (HRT)

HRT is a modified approach to HRV that focuses on sinus nodal rate after the ectopic beats[55] that are excluded from traditional HRV analysis. HRT is typically measured in the time domain. High HRT (after the post-ectopic pause) reflects a normal acceleration in sinus node rate followed by oscillations before steady-state is re-achieved. Conversely, depressed HRT may predict adverse cardiovascular outcome and the risk for ventricular tachyarrhythmias.[56] Although not considered in detail in this chapter, a recent consensus document from the International Society for Holter and Noninvasive Electrophysiology outlines standards for measuring HRT, and reviews the literature supporting its conclusions.[57]

20.3.3.4
Spectral Indices of HRV

By subjecting consecutive N–N intervals to Fourier analysis (see Chap. 3), HRV may be described in distinct bandwidths of high (HF 0.15–0.40 Hz), low (LF 0.04–0.15 Hz), very low (VLF 0.0033–0.04 Hz), and ultralow (ULF <0.0033 Hz) frequencies. Physiologic studies in humans and a variety of animal models have correlated these frequencies with different limbs of the autonomic nervous system,[53] as described above (The Physiologic Signal Being Measured).

20.3.3.5
Resampling

In order to calculate HRV in the frequency domain, ambulatory ECG data must be *resampled* at a constant frequency.[58] The ambulatory ECG contains QRS complexes at variable rather than fixed time intervals. Each measurement of the RR interval occurs at the time of a QRS complex, resulting in a series of data points (RR intervals) that are sampled non-uniformly in time.

In order to correctly apply standard frequency domain techniques (such as the FFT) to this data, additional time points must be added to the original beat series to make the sampling times uniform. We must then interpolate appropriate RR intervals for these points. Figure 20.8 illustrates one method to achieve this. Any frequency faster than the highest heart rate detected in the recorded ECG data can be used as the resampling frequency, though often a convenient frequency significantly greater than the heart rate (such as 4 Hz, corresponding to 240 samples/min) is used for resampling.

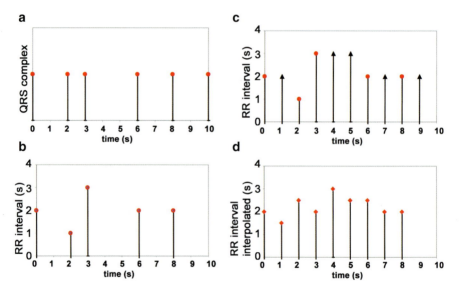

Fig. 20.8 Resampling required for the spectral analysis of HRV. (**a**) *Raw ECG data* show six QRS complexes at irregular intervals. (**b**) *Amplitude at each QRS.* Reformatting the raw ECG data from (**a**) with the amplitude at each QRS complex equal to the RR interval between the given beat and the next beat, i.e., the first and second QRS complexes are 2 s apart so the amplitude of the first QRS complex is given value 2. (**c**) *Adding data points.* Resampling at 1 Hz first requires adding data points (*triangles*) so that points are consistently 1 s apart. As an intermediate step, the amplitude of the added points is taken from the amplitude of the preceding "real" QRS complex. (**d**) *Interpolation.* The appropriate amplitude of each point in the resampled series is determined by linear interpolation. The amplitude of each data point in (**d**) is calculated as the average of the amplitudes of the adjacent points from (**c**)

20.3.3.6
Ectopic Beats

An additional difficulty with using frequency domain techniques is that ectopic beats cannot be handled by simple deletion. Simple deletion will disturb the results from FFT analysis in unpredictable ways.[58] One solution is to replace intervals generated by ectopic beats with RR interval(s) generated by averaging the preceding and succeeding RR intervals. In Eq. (20.9), "N2–S1" and "S1–N3" would be deleted and replaced by a number of intervals of duration 1/2 ("N1–N2"+"N3–N4"). Another alternative is to use higher order interpolation – for example choosing two sinus intervals preceding and two sinus intervals following the ectopic interval and fitting these intervals using a cubic equation in order to better estimate the intervals to be interposed.[59]

20.3.4
Clinical Utility

Current guidelines for the management of patients at risk for SCA state "heart rate variability ... may be useful for improving the diagnosis and risk stratification of patients with ventricular arrhythmias or who are at risk of developing life threatening ventricular arrhythmias" as a class IIb indication.[37]

These guidelines are based on several studies that link depressed HRV with adverse cardiovascular outcome. Many groups have demonstrated that in patients following myocardial infarction, depressed HRV provides a sensitivity of 30–40% and specificity of 80–90% for ventricular tachycardia or ventricular fibrillation.[60] In fact, depressed HRV is a robust marker of adverse prognosis in multiple settings such as after a myocardial infarction, in patients with heart failure, and in responders to cardiac resynchronization therapy.[61] However, in DINAMIT (Defibrillator in Acute Myocardial Infarction Trial),[62] patients with depressed autonomic tone (either reduced HRV or elevated resting heart rate) and left ventricular ejection fraction <35% measured 6–40 days after a myocardial infarction showed no survival improvement when treated with an ICD. It remains unclear to what extent this reflects an inability to identify patients at high risk for ventricular tachycardia/fibrillation very soon after myocardial infarction, when pro-arrhythmic substrates may still be maturing, or the failure of the risk stratification methods used.

Intriguing recent data suggest that autonomic activity may alter immediately preceding spontaneous ventricular tachycardia/fibrillation. In patients with pre-existing ICDs, HRV fell dramatically in the minutes preceding spontaneous ventricular tachycardia or ventricular fibrillation onset.[63] In the frequency domain, this was accompanied by increased LF and reduced HF, reflecting a shift from vagal to sympathetic predominance. Further studies are required.

In general, HRV is best utilized through its negative predictive value. The positive predictive value of HRV is increased if several indices are combined (such as ULF and VLF), or if HRV is used in combination with left ventricular systolic dysfunction and other risk factors. Successful cardiac resynchronization therapy elevates HRV, as do exercise training and beta-blockade. However, it remains to be shown if increased HRV from other interventions improves clinical outcome.

20.3.5
Technical Considerations and Data Storage

The duration of recordings affects the clinical utility of HRV. Twenty-four hour records have been analyzed for time domain parameters, although recent work shows that 5-min analyses can be used to study HRV "transients." In the frequency domain, short recordings minimize the effects of temporal variations (non-stationarity), although recording duration should exceed 10 times the longest wavelength (1/lowest frequency component) of interest.

File sizes for HRV data are relatively small. Even though HRV data are acquired for prolonged periods, the data consist only of the times of normal sinus beats in one lead. A representation of the actual voltage-time series of the ECG is not required.

20.3.6
Future Directions for HRV

Reduced HRV may predict the risk for ventricular tachyarrhythmias following myocardial infarction, particularly when combined with other non-invasive tests. Studies are needed to show whether patients who are treated appropriately for myocardial infarction or heart failure are at higher risk for ventricular tachycardia/fibrillation and other events if HRV does not rise, compared to those in whom HRV does rise. Assessment of short-term fluctuations in HRV, including heart rate turbulence (HRT) that is measured after ectopic beats may help to assess dynamic risk for ventricular tachycardia/fibrillation. In addition, dynamic modulations of P–P and P–R intervals and periodicities in blood pressure and respiration may reveal pro-arrhythmic interactions between autonomic and hemodynamic mechanisms.

20.4
Signal Averaged ECG (SAECG)

20.4.1
Basic Description

The SAECG detects subtle abnormalities in the QRS complex (i.e., ventricular depolarization) or P-wave (i.e., atrial depolarization) in a carefully acquired surface ECG. By averaging successive ECG complexes, this method increases the signal-to-noise ratio and enables the detection of microvolt-level signals that may otherwise fall below the noise floor (Chap. 7). This chapter will focus on use of the SAECG to detect small-amplitude signals at the QRS terminus ("late potentials") that may predict SCA, although there is also growing interest in using the SAECG to uncover P-wave prolongation as a marker for atrial fibrillation.[64]

20.4.2
Physiologic Signal Being Evaluated by the SAECG

Figure 20.9 shows an abnormal SAECG with *late potentials* at the end of the QRS. Late potentials are low-amplitude, high frequency signals that reflect slow and fragmented conduction through infarct scar or pathology such as arrhythmogenic right ventricular cardiomyopathy.[65] Slowly conducting regions are substrates for reentry and while late potentials do not always reflect the critical isthmus of ventricular tachycardia circuits,[66] late potentials are present in 70–92% of patients with coronary disease and ventricular tachycardia.[67] Late potentials empirically predict arrhythmic outcome, particularly when combined with measures of left ventricular ejection fraction, autonomic activity, ventricular ectopy on ambulatory ECG, and ischemia on exercise testing.[68]

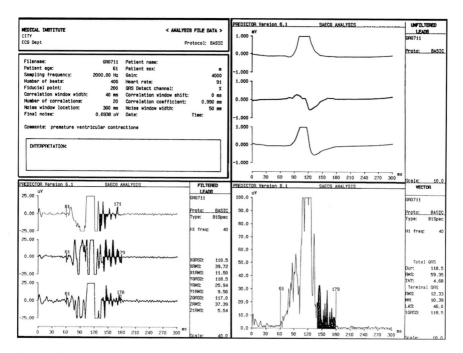

Fig. 20.9 Time-domain analysis of signal-averaged electrocardiogram (SAECG). Data are recorded from a patient with a healed myocardial infarction and a history of sustained ventricular tachycardia. Averaged X, Y, Z ECGs (*upper right panel*) are amplified and filtered (*lower left panel*), and combined into a vector magnitude (*lower right panel*). Endpoints of analysis include the filtered QRS duration (total QRS duration: 118.5 ms), root-mean-square voltage of the terminal 40 ms of the filtered QRS (terminal QRS RMS: 12.33 μV), and the duration that the filtered QRS complex that remains below 40 μV (terminal QRS LAS: 46.0 ms). The terminal 40 ms of the processed X, Y, Z, and vector magnitude QRS complexes has been shaded. *The SAECG is abnormal* and meets criteria for ventricular late potentials. Other measurements (*upper left panel*) include the noise level after averaging (0.6938 μV) and the number of beats averaged (406)

20.4.3
Measurement Techniques

The electrical fingerprint of delayed conduction through ventricular scar is very small in relation to the QRS complex. Although amplification of the ECG may reveal them, this approach also amplifies the very noise that obscures these signals and may not improve detection. On the other hand, averaging multiple QRS complexes "reinforces" consistent ventricular signals as opposed to variable noise, thus improving signal-to-noise ratio by a factor related to the square-root of the number of beats averaged (Chap. 7).

20.4.3.1
Data Acquisition and Signal Pre-Processing

The SAECG is typically recorded using three orthogonal Frank X, Y, and Z leads. The acquired signal is digitized, often with a sampling frequency of 500–1,000 Hz to 10–12 bit resolution (1,024–4,096 digital levels). In the case of the QRS-SAECG (described in this section), QRS complexes are identified and fiducial points are determined for accurate beat alignment, which is crucial for avoiding misalignment that may obscure late potentials (Fig. 20.10). Alignment can be achieved by many methods that typically aim to maximize the numerical cross-correlation (minimize the error) between aligned beats. Averaged QRS complexes should also exclude ectopic, aberrantly conducted, or grossly "noisy" beats. To achieve this, beats are cross-correlated against a representative beat within the series, to ensure that only beats of a similar morphology are included. These beats are then averaged.

20.4.3.2 Temporal Signal Averaging

The typical SAECG is generated by averaging QRS complexes over time (temporal averaging). While methods differ in how they determine the number of beats to average, one method is to aim for a pre-specified "noise floor" of 0.5–0.7 µV. ECG beats are then averaged until the voltage of an isoelectric region (the TP segment) falls to this noise floor. Typically, this requires the averaging of 200–400 QRS complexes (i.e., 3–7 min). An alternative approach is to average to a pre-specified number of beats (e.g., 150 beats), then report the noise level. If the noise level exceeds the desired noise floor, a different consecutive set of beats from the original ECG recording can be used until the noise floor is reached.

Multiple sources of noise may exist. Noise may be biological, referring to signals other than those of interest predominantly from skeletal muscles or breathing. Noise may also be non-biological, including electronic noise from the power line and other electronic equipment (including noise from sophisticated mapping systems used in electrophysiologic studies), noise from suboptimal electrode contact with the skin, or even noise introduced from the recording system.

The resultant average QRS complex is then filtered – typically with a bi-directional filter, which is usually a variation of a Butterworth filter. High-pass filtering, typically at 25–40 Hz, removes low frequency activity (e.g., baseline ECG drift and low frequency ST/T components). Low pass filtering, typically at 250 Hz, removes high frequency noise.

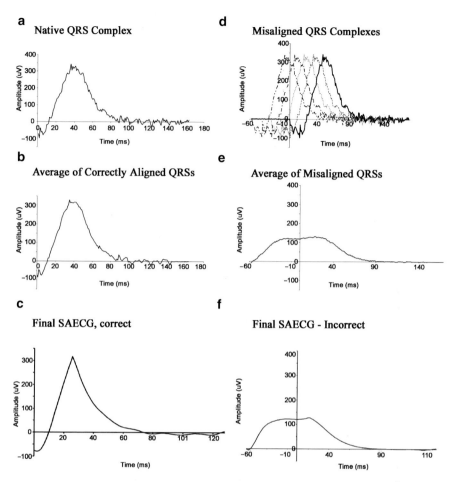

Fig. 20.10 QRS averaging and effects of misalignment on SAECG. (**a**) Representative QRS complex from recorded ECG data. (**b**) Serial QRS complexes from a given patient are averaged until a "noise floor" is reached. Signal to noise ratio is greatly enhanced. (**c**) Application of bi-directional filtering yields the final SAECG, which is abnormal in this case. (**d**) QRS and fiducial point detection errors can result in significant QRS misalignment. (**e**) Averaging of misaligned QRSs (**d**) causes smoothing, misrepresenting the true QRS complex (compare with (**b**)). This figure is constructed by averaging 60 misaligned QRSs, only five of which are shown in (**d**). (**f**) Application of bi-directional filtering to (**e**) results in an SAECG without a late potential. The late potential is lost due to the effects of misalignment

20.4.3.3
Spatial Signal Averaging

Spatial ECG averaging is a less common approach that summates and then averages potentials that are recorded simultaneously from multiple pairs of closely spaced electrodes.[69] Because this is not performed over time, this method provides real-time, *beat-by-beat* analysis of successive QRS complexes and can therefore assess irregular rhythms, unlike temporal averaging. Spatial averaging is the basis for body surface potential mapping that has been used to detect the risk for SCA[70] and other arrhythmias.[71]

20.4.3.4
Spectral Analysis

As described in Chap. 3, spectral analysis treats the QRS complex (and/or P-wave) as if it were composed of multiple sinusoidal waveforms. Spectral analysis decomposes the ECG into components of varying magnitude, frequency, and phase[72] using Fourier analysis, wavelet transformation, or other methods.[3] The SAECG can also be analyzed using a combination of time and frequency domains (spectrotemporal analysis).[73] This procedure shifts the Fourier transformation of multiple ECG segments in time to indicate the timecourse of component frequencies and, while not widely used, may reveal fractionation within the QRS complex (e.g., in patients with bundle branch block). However, at the current time, definitions for spectral (frequency domain) or spectro-temporal analyses of late potentials have not been standardized.

20.4.3.5
Criteria for Abnormal Temporally Averaged SAECG

Late potentials are defined by three criteria – a prolonged total filtered QRS duration, low voltage in the terminal portion of the QRS (usually the last 40 ms), and a prolonged duration of the terminal QRS that lies *below* a particular amplitude (usually 40 µV). Each of these measurements varies with the exact filtering parameters applied to the averaged ECG data (Fig. 20.11). Using the 40-Hz bi-directional filter, a Task Force Committee of the European Society of Cardiology, the AHA, and the ACC suggested the following definition of late potentials[72]:

- Filtered QRS duration >114 ms
- Terminal (last 40 ms) QRS root mean square voltage <40 µV
- Low amplitude (<40 µV) late potential duration >38 ms

The SAECG shown in Fig. 20.9 meets all three of these criteria for late potentials, and is therefore abnormal.

This approach has some limitations. First, late potentials can be detected only when fragmented signals outlast the QRS complex. In patients with bundle branch block, late potentials may be obscured by the delayed activation of otherwise normal myocardium. The SAECG therefore is not defined in the presence of bundle branch block. Second, the SAECG only enhances signals with a fixed relationship to averaged complexes (and the alignment fiducial). Late potentials that vary between beats will be attenuated by averaging. Similarly, misalignment of QRS complexes will have a dramatic effect on observed late potentials (Fig. 20.10). Lastly, as mentioned above, the filter used to remove noise and

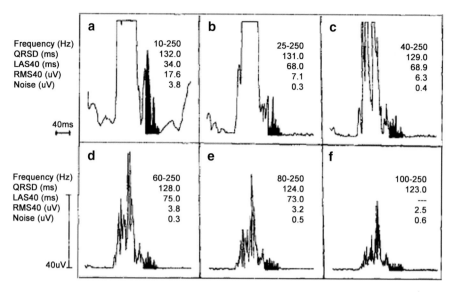

Fig. 20.11 Effects of filter parameters on SAECG. SAECG from a patient with inducible monomorphic VT. From (**a**) through (**f**), the high-pass filter frequency is progressively increased from 10 Hz (**a**) to 100 Hz (**f**). The QRS duration shows a slight gradual decrease at higher filter cutoffs, from 132 ms at 10 Hz, to 123 ms at 100 Hz. The RMS40 shows a significant nonlinear decrease with higher filter cutoffs. The duration of low amplitude signals <40 μV (LAS40) increases from (**a**) through (**d**) and then shows a slight decrease in (**e**). This patient has a positive SAECG per criteria defined for a 40 Hz bi-directional filter (**c**) (QRSD >114 ms, RMS40 <40 μV, LAS40 >38 ms). Similar criteria are not defined for the other filter settings

low frequency wander significantly impacts the SAECG. This limitation is only partially avoided by using filter specific criteria for each parameter, and filter selection still has a significant effect on the results of SAECG analysis in a given individual.

20.4.4
Clinical Utility

Current AHA/ACC guidelines for the management of patients at risk for SCA state that "the SAECG… may be useful for improving the diagnosis and risk stratification of patients with ventricular arrhythmias or who are at risk of developing life threatening ventricular arrhythmias," and list the SAECG as a class IIb indication.[37]

The strongest evidence that late potentials identify risk for ventricular tachycardia/fibrillation is provided by a major substudy of the multicenter unsustained tachycardia trial (MUSTT). In 1925 patients with coronary disease and left ventricular ejection fraction <40%, filtered QRS duration >114 ms (i.e., late potentials) independently predicted the endpoint of arrhythmic death or cardiac arrest.[74] The 5-year rates of the primary end point (28% vs. 17%, $p=0.0001$), cardiac death (37% vs. 25%, $p=0.0001$), and total mortality

(43% vs. 35%, $p=0.0001$) were significantly higher in those patients when compared to those without an abnormal SAECG. Moreover, the combination of ejection fraction <30% with an abnormal SAECG identified a very high-risk cohort for both arrhythmic death (36% at 5 years) and cardiac death (44% at 5 years).

Although not part of the AHA/ACC guidelines, both the spectral[72] and spectrotemporal analyses[73] have been shown in small clinical studies to improve the predictive value for arrhythmias above that of traditional late potentials.

20.4.5
Data Storage

Files for SAECG data have to store ECG shapes, i.e., the voltage-time series, for a few minutes in each lead. Files are typically megabytes in size, depending upon the exact implementation and the type of data compression.

20.5
Conclusions

Advanced signal processing techniques have proven value in risk stratifying patients for adverse cardiovascular outcomes, as reflected by their inclusion in AHA/ACC guidelines for patient management. These tools exemplify many of the principles outlined in this volume, and their wide commercial availability, their utility between centers in various clinical trials, and routine clinical use illustrate their robustness. Future refinements will come from a more precise understanding of the mechanisms linking specific disease processes, such as myocardial infarction or heart failure, with specific adverse outcomes, such as ventricular tachycardia or fibrillation. In the case of risk stratification for SCA, methods should in the future be targeted at screening the wider population without systolic dysfunction.

Acknowledgement Supported, in part, by grants to SMN from the Doris Duke Charitable Foundation and the National Heart, Lung, and Blood institute (HL 70529, HL83359).

References

1. Narayan SM. T-wave alternans and the susceptibility to ventricular arrhythmias: state of the art paper. *J Am Coll Cardiol*. 2006;47:269–281.
2. Stein PK, Domitrovich PP, Huikuri HV, et al. Traditional and nonlinear heart rate variability are each independently associated with mortality after myocardial infarction. *J Cardiovasc Electrophysiol*. 2005;16:13–20.
3. Cain ME, Anderson JL, Arnsdorf MF, et al. Signal-averaged electrocardiography: ACC consensus document. *J Am Coll Cardiol*. 1996;27:238–249.
4. Zheng Z-J, Croft JB, Giles WH, et al. Sudden cardiac death in the United States, 1989 to 1998. *Circulation*. 2001;104:2158–2163.

5. Epstein AE, Dimarco JP, Ellenbogen KA, et al. ACC/AHA/HRS 2008 guidelines for device-based therapy of cardiac rhythm abnormalities. A report of the American College of Cardiology/American Heart Association Task Force on Practice Guidelines (writing committee to revise the ACC/AHA/NASPE 2002 guideline update for implantation of cardiac pacemakers and anti-arrhythmia devices) developed in collaboration with the American Association for Thoracic Surgery and Society of Thoracic Surgeons. *J Am Coll Cardiol.* 2008;51:e1-e62.
6. Goldenberg I, Vyas AK, Hall WJ, et al. Risk stratification for primary implantation of a cardioverter-defibrillator in patients with ischemic left ventricular dysfunction. *J Am Coll Cardiol.* 2008;51:288–296.
7. Sawhney NS, Narayan SM. Sudden cardiac arrest in patients with preserved systolic function: the clinical dilemma. *Heart Rhythm.* 2009;6:S15–21.
8. El-Sherif N, Scherlag BJ, Lazzara R, et al. Reentrant ventricular arrhythmias in the late myocardial infarction period. I. Conduction characteristics in the infarction zone. *Circulation.* 1977;55:686–702.
9. El-Sherif N, Scherlag BJ, Lazzara R, et al. Reentrant ventricular arrhythmias in the late myocardial infarction period. II. Patterns of initiation and termination of re-entry. *Circulation.* 1977;55:702–719.
10. Kuo C-S, Munakata K, Reddy CP, et al. Characteristics and possible mechanism of ventricular arrhythmia dependent on the dispersion of action potential durations. *Circulation.* 1983;67:1356–1367.
11. Steinberg JS, Arshad A, Kowalski M, et al. Increased incidence of life-threatening ventricular arrhythmias in implantable defibrillator patients after the World Trade Center attack. *J Am Coll Cardiol.* 2004;44:1261–1264.
12. Kleiger RE, Miller JP, Thanvaro S, et al. Relationship between clinical features of acute myocardial infarction and ventricular runs 2 weeks to 1 year after infarction. *Circulation.* 1981;63:64–70.
13. Verma A, Kilicaslan F, Martin D, et al. Preimplantation B-type natriuretic peptide concentration is an independent predictor of future appropriate implantable defibrillator therapies. *Heart.* 2006;92:190–195.
14. Narayan SM, Drinan DD, Lackey RP, et al. Acute volume overload elevates T-wave alternans magnitude. *J Appl Physiol.* 2007;102:1462–1468.
15. Hering H. Experimentelle Studien an Saugentieren uber das Electrocardiogram. *Z Exp Med.* 1909;7:363.
16. Lewis T. Electrical alternation. *Heart.* 1909;10:262.
17. Schwartz P, Malliani A. Electrical alternation of the T-wave: clinical and experimental evidence of its relationship with the sympathetic nervous system and with the long Q-T syndrome. *Am Heart J.* 1975;89:45–50.
18. Walker ML, Rosenbaum DS. Cellular alternans as mechanism of cardiac arrhythmogenesis. *Heart Rhythm.* 2005;2:1383–1386.
19. Weiss JN, Karma A, Shiferaw Y, et al. From pulsus to pulseless: the Saga of cardiac alternans [review]. *Circ Res.* 2006;98:1244–1253.
20. Banville I, Gray RA. Effect of action potential duration and conduction velocity restitution and their spatial dispersion on alternans and the stability of arrhythmias. *J Cardiovasc Electrophysiol.* 2002;13:1141–1149.
21. Koller ML, Maier SKG, Gelzer AR, et al. Altered dynamics of action potential restitution and alternans in humans with structural heart disease. *Circulation.* 2005;112:1542–1548.
22. Bloomfield DM, Hohnloser SH, Cohen RJ. Interpretation and classification of microvolt T-wave alternans tests. *J Cardiovasc Electrophysiol.* 2002;13:502–512.
23. Narayan SM, Franz MR, Kim J, et al. T-wave alternans, restitution of ventricular action potential duration and outcome. *J Am Coll Cardiol.* 2007;50:2385–2392.
24. Pruvot EJ, Katra RP, Rosenbaum DS, et al. Role of calcium cycling versus restitution in the mechanism of repolarization alternans. *Circ Res.* 2004;94:1083–1090.

25. Eisner D, Li Y, O'Neill S. Alternans of intracellular calcium: mechanism and significance. *Heart Rhythm*. 2006;3:743–745.
26. Livshitz LM, Rudy Y. Regulation of Ca^{2+} and electrical alternans in cardiac myocytes: role of CAMKII and repolarizing currents. *Am J Physiol Heart Circ Physiol*. 2007;292:H2854–H2866.
27. Laurita KR, Rosenbaum DS. Mechanisms and potential therapeutic targets for ventricular arrhythmias associated with impaired cardiac calcium cycling. *J Mol Cell Cardiol*. 2008;44:31–43.
28. Narayan SM, Bayer J, Lalani G, et al. Action potential dynamics explain arrhythmic vulnerability in human heart failure: a clinical and modeling study implicating abnormal calcium handling. *J Am Coll Cardiol*. 2008;52:1782–1792.
29. Narayan SM, Lindsay BD, Smith JM. Demonstrating the pro-arrhythmic preconditioning of single premature extrastimuli using the magnitude, phase and temporal distribution of repolarization alternans. *Circulation*. 1999;100:1887–1893.
30. Narayan SM, Smith JM, Schechtman KB, et al. T-wave alternans phase following ventricular extrasystoles predicts arrhythmia-free survival. *Heart Rhythm*. 2005;2:234–241.
31. Shusterman V, Goldberg A, London B. Upsurge in T-wave alternans and nonalternating repolarization instability precedes spontaneous initiation of ventricular tachyarrhythmias in humans. *Circulation*. 2006;113:2880–2887.
32. Martinez JP, Olmos S. Methodologic principles of T-wave alternans analysis: a unified framework. *IEEE Trans Biomed Eng*. 2005;52:599–613.
33. Narayan SM, Smith JM. Spectral analysis of periodic fluctuations in ECG repolarization. *IEEE Trans Biomed Eng*. 1999;46:203–212.
34. Narayan SM, Smith JM. Exploiting rate hysteresis in repolarization alternans to optimize the sensitivity and specificity for ventricular tachycardia. *J Am Coll Cardiol*. 2000;35:1485–1492.
35. Kaufman E, Bloomfield D, Steinman R, et al. "Indeterminate" microvolt T-wave alternans tests predict high risk of death or sustained ventricular arrhythmias in patients with left ventricular dysfunction. *J Am Coll Cardiol*. 2006;48:1399–1404.
36. Grimm W, Christ M, Bach J, et al. Noninvasive arrhythmia risk stratification in idiopathic dilated cardiomyopathy: results of the marburg cardiomyopathy study. *Circulation*. 2003; 108: 2883–2891.
37. ACC/AHA/ESC. ACC/AHA/ESC 2006 guidelines for management of patients with ventricular arrhythmias and the prevention of sudden cardiac death – executive summary. A report of the American College of Cardiology/American Heart Association Task Force and the European Society of Cardiology Committee for Practice Guidelines (writing committee to develop guidelines for management of patients with ventricular arrhythmias and the prevention of sudden cardiac death). *J Am Coll Cardiol*. 2006;48:1064–1108.
38. Rosenbaum DS, Jackson LE, Smith JM, et al. Electrical alternans and vulnerability to ventricular arrhythmias. *N Engl J Med*. 1994;330:235–241.
39. Bloomfield DM, Steinman RC, Namerow PB, et al. Microvolt T-wave alternans distinguishes between patients likely and patients not likely to benefit from implanted cardiac defibrillator therapy: a solution to the multicenter automatic defibrillator implantation trial (MADIT) II conundrum. *Circulation*. 2004;110:1885–1889.
40. Klingenheben T, Zabel M, D'Agostino RB, et al. Predictive value of T-wave alternans for arrhythmic events in patients with congestive heart failure [letter]. *Lancet*. 2000;356:651–652.
41. Bloomfield DM, Bigger JT, Steinman RC, et al. Microvolt T-wave alternans and the risk of death or sustained ventricular arrhythmias in patients with left ventricular dysfunction. *J Am Coll Cardiol*. 2006;47:456–463.
42. Salerno-Uriarte JA, De Ferrari GM, Klersy C, et al. Prognostic value of T-wave alternans in patients with heart failure due to nonischemic cardiomyopathy: results of the ALPHA study. *J Am Coll Cardiol*. 2007;50:1896–1904.
43. Ikeda T, Yoshino H, Sugi K, et al. Predictive value of microvolt T-wave alternans for sudden cardiac death in patients with preserved cardiac function after acute myocardial infarction; results of a collaborative cohort study. *J Am Coll Cardiol*. 2006;48:2268–2274.

44. Exner DV, Kavanagh KM, Slawnych MP, et al. Noninvasive risk assessment early after a myocardial infarction the REFINE study. *J Am Coll Cardiol.* 2007;50:2275–2284.
45. Gehi AK, Stein RH, Metz LD, et al. Microvolt T-wave alternans for risk stratification of ventricular tachyarrhythmic events: a meta-analysis. *J Am Coll Cardiol.* 2005;46:75–82.
46. Chow T, Kereiakes DJ, Onufer J, et al. Does microvolt T-wave alternans testing predict ventricular tachyarrhythmias in patients with ischemic cardiomyopathy and prophylactic defibrillators? The MASTER (Microvolt T wave alternans testing for risk stratification of post-myocardial infarction patients) trial. *J Am Coll Cardiol.* 2008;52:1607–1615.
47. Gold MR, Ip JH, Costantini O, et al. Role of microvolt T-wave alternans in assessment of arrhythmia vulnerability among patients with heart failure and systolic dysfunction: primary results from the T-wave alternans sudden cardiac death in heart failure trial substudy. *Circulation.* 2008;118:2022–2028.
48. Verrier RL, Nearing BD, La Rovere MT, et al. Ambulatory electrocardiogram based tracking of t wave alternans in postmyocardial infarction patients to assess risk of cardiac arrest or arrhythmic events. *J Cardiovasc Electrophysiol.* 2003;14:705–711.
49. Nearing BD, Verrier RL. Modified moving average analysis of T-wave alternans to predict ventricular fibrillation with high accuracy. *J Appl Physiol.* 2002;92:541–549.
50. Nieminen T, Lehtimäki T, Viik J, et al. T-wave alternans predicts mortality in a population undergoing a clinically indicated exercise test. *Eur Heart J.* 2007;28:2332–2337.
51. Cox VL, Patel M, Kim J, et al. Predicting arrhythmia-free survival using spectral and modified-moving average analyses of T-wave alternans. *Pacing Clin Electrophysiol.* 2007;30:352–358.
52. Oshodi GO, Costantini O, Amit G, et al. Detecting T wave alternans: do the modified moving average and spectral exercise methods measure the same thing? *Heart Rhythm.* Abstract.
53. Lahiri MK, Kannankeril PJ, Goldberger JJ. Assessment of autonomic function in cardiovascular disease: physiological basis and prognostic implications. *J Am Coll Cardiol.* 2008;51:1725–1733.
54. Jose A, Collison D. The normal range and determinants of the intrinsic heart rate in man. *Cardiovasc Res.* 1970;4:160-167.
55. Schmidt G, Malik M, Barthel P, et al. Heart-rate turbulence after ventricular premature beats as a predictor of mortality after acute myocardial infarction. *Lancet.* 1999;353:1390–1396.
56. Iwasa A, Hwa M, Hassankhani A, et al. Abnormal heart rate turbulence predicts the initiation of ventricular arrhythmias. *Pacing Clin Electrophysiol.* 2005;28:1189–1197.
57. Bauer A, Malik M, Schmidt G, et al. Heart rate turbulence: standards of measurement, physiological interpretation, and clinical use: International Society for Holter and Noninvasive Electrophysiology Consensus. *J Am Coll Cardiol.* 2008;52:1353–1365.
58. Clifford GD, Tarassenko L. Quantifying errors in spectral estimates of HRV due to beat replacement and resampling. *IEEE Trans Biomed Eng.* 2005;52:630–638.
59. Lippman N, Stein KM, Lerman BB. Comparison of methods for removal of ectopy in measurement of heart rate variability. *Am J Physiol.* 1994;267:H411–H418.
60. Copie X, Hnatkova K, Staunton A, et al. Predictive power of increased heart rate versus depressed left ventricular ejection fraction and heart rate variability for risk stratification after myocardial infarction. *J Am Coll Cardiol.* 1996;27:270–276.
61. Adamson PB, Smith AL, Abraham WT, et al. Continuous autonomic assessment in patients with symptomatic heart failure: prognostic value of heart rate variability measured by an implanted cardiac resynchronization device. *Circulation.* 2004;110:2389–2394.
62. Hohnloser SH, Kuck KH, Dorian P, et al. Prophylactic use of an implantable cardioverter-defibrillator after acute myocardial infarction. *N Engl J Med.* 2004;351:2481–2488.
63. Pruvot E, Thonet G, Vesin J-M, et al. Heart rate dynamics at the onset of ventricular tachyarrhythmias as retrieved from implantable cardioverter-defibrillators in patients with coronary artery disease. *Circulation.* 2000;101:2398–2404.

64. Darbar D, Hardy A, Haines JL, et al. Prolonged signal-averaged P-wave duration as an intermediate phenotype for familial atrial fibrillation. *J Am Coll Cardiol.* 2008;51:1083–1089.
65. Kenigsberg D, Kalahasty G, Grizzard J, et al. Images in cardiovascular medicine. Intracardiac correlate of the epsilon wave in a patient with arrhythmogenic right ventricular dysplasia. *Circulation.* 2007;115:e538–e539.
66. Hood MA, Pogwizd SM, Peirick J, et al. Contribution of myocardium responsible for ventricular tachycardia to abnormalities detected by analysis of signal-averaged ECGs. *Circulation.* 1992;86:1888–1901.
67. Denes P, Santarelli P, Hauser RG, et al. Quantitative analysis of the high frequency components of the terminal portion of the body surface QRS in normal subjects and in patients with ventricular tachycardia. *Circulation.* 1983;67:1129.
68. Farrell TG, Bashir Y, Cripps T, et al. Risk stratification for arrhythmic events in postinfarction patients based on heart rate variability, ambulatory electrocardiographic variables and the signal-averaged electrocardiogram. *J Am Coll Cardiol.* 1991;18:687–697.
69. El-Sherif N, Mehra R, Gomes JAC, et al. Appraisal of a low noise electrocardiogram. *J Am Coll Cardiol.* 1983;1(2 Pt 1): 456–67.
70. Kavesh NG, Cain ME, Ambos HD, et al. Enhanced detection of distinguishing features in signal-averaged electrocardiograms from patients with ventricular tachycardia by combined spatial and spectral analyses of entire cardiac cycle. *Circulation.* 1994;90:254–263.
71. SippensGroenewegen A, Lesh MD, Roithinger FX, et al. Body surface mapping of counterclockwise and clockwise typical atrial flutter: a comparative analysis with endocardial activation sequence mapping. *J Am Coll Cardiol.* 2000;35:1276–1287.
72. Cain ME, Ambos HD, Witkowski FX, et al. Fast Fourier analysis of the signal-averaged electrocardiograms for identification of patients prone to sustained ventricular tachycardia. *Circulation.* 1984;69:711–720.
73. Vazquez R, Caref EB, Torres F, et al. Improved diagnostic value of combined time and frequency domain analysis of the signal-averaged electrocardiogram after myocardial infarction. *J Am Coll Cardiol.* 1999;33:385–394.
74. Gomes JA, Cain ME, Buxton AE, et al. Prediction of long-term outcomes by signal-averaged electrocardiography in patients with unsustained ventricular tachycardia, coronary artery disease, and left ventricular dysfunction. *Circulation.* 2001;104:436-441.

Digital Stethoscopes

21

Indranil Sen-Gupta and Jason Ng

21.1 Introduction

Stethoscopes are universally employed in clinical practice for the auscultation of body sounds including Korotkoff sounds for blood pressure measurement as well as sounds produced by the heart, lung, bowel, and other vasculature. The majority of stethoscopes clinically used today are still conventional (acoustic) stethoscopes – that is, they operate by direct mechanical transmission of acoustic energy. In recent years, however, technological advancements in electronic stethoscopes have resulted in their increased popularity among cardiologists and clinicians alike. This chapter will briefly address the development of stethoscopes and their general principles of operation, and then focus chiefly on electronic stethoscopes with regard to technical considerations, advantages over conventional stethoscopes, challenges involved in construction and adoption into mainstream clinical practice, and present as well as future cardiovascular applications.

21.2 Development and Principles of Operation

The stethoscope was invented in 1816 by a young French physician named Rene Laennec. Too embarrassed to place his ear directly against a female patient's chest, as was the common auscultatory practice of that time, he rolled up sheets of paper into a cone, placing one end to his ear and the other end to the woman's chest. He found that not only were sounds transmitted through the paper, but that they were also amplified in the process. Laennec then constructed a similar device out of wood, which would become the first monaural stethoscope. This device underwent numerous modifications and ultimately evolved into the conventional, flexible binaural stethoscope of modern-day use.

I. Sen-Gupta (✉)
Division of Neurology, Feinberg School of Medicine,
Northwestern University, Chicago, IL, USA
e-mail: neilsg@md.northwestern.edu

A figure detailing the parts of a modern acoustic binaural stethoscope is shown in Fig. 21.1. The chestpiece of the acoustic stethoscope usually consists of two sides – a diaphragm (plastic disc) and bell (hollow cup) – either of which can be placed against the patient's body for auscultation. Transmission of sounds from the chestpiece to the listener occurs via the hollow rubber tubing connecting into binaurals and earpieces. The diaphragm, which accentuates higher-frequency sounds and attenuates the lows, must be placed in firm contact with the patient for optimal functioning. Vibration of the diaphragm by body sounds creates acoustic waves that are then transmitted to the listener. Conversely, the bell, which accentuates lower-frequency sounds and attenuates the highs, needs to be placed lightly against the patients skin; otherwise, the patient's skin will act as a diaphragm and the lower-frequency sounds will be suppressed. With the bell, acoustic waves produced by vibration of the patient's skin are directly transmitted to the listener.

An example of an electronic stethoscope is shown in Fig. 21.2. The external parts are essentially identical to those of an acoustic stethoscope, with the exception that the device is battery-powered and the chestpiece generally consists of only a diaphragm-type adapter. When using the electronic stethoscope, the user can switch between "diaphragm" and "bell" modes at the push of a button; the stethoscope will accordingly select the proper set of internal electronic filters permitting operation in either mode.

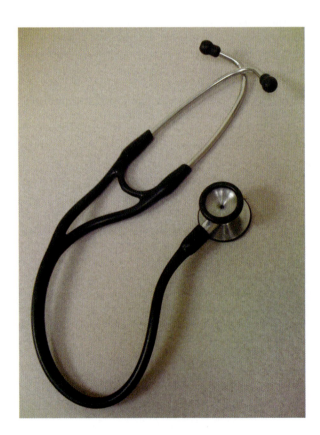

Fig. 21.1 Example of a conventional stethoscope

Fig. 21.2 Example of a digital stethoscope (3M™ Littmann® Electronic Stethoscope Model 3100[1])

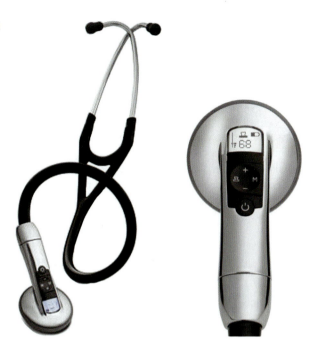

Electroacoustic transduction is first required to convert mechanical sound waves detected by the diaphragm into an electrical signal that can then be appropriately filtered and amplified. At least several different methods have been used to accomplish this, including (1) microphone placement directly inside the chest piece, which is the least effective method and severely impacted by ambient noise, (2) diaphragm coupling to a piezoelectric crystal mechanism, and (3) creating the diaphragm with a conductive inner surface such that it behaves like a capacitor, which has the advantage of enabling sound waves to interact with the diaphragm analogously to an acoustic stethoscope, while simultaneously permitting direct conversion of the sound waves to electrical signals in the process.

A major advantage of electronic stethoscopes is their ability to amplify sounds far better than their acoustic counterparts. However, this feature also makes them more susceptible to noise artifacts. Thus, electronic filtering and other techniques must be used to appropriately reduce noise. Only then can subsequent filtering based on "bell" or "diaphragm" mode settings and amplification based on user-adjustable volume level be performed. Following these steps, the electrical signal is once again converted back to mechanical sound waves that arrive at the auscultator's ears. It should be noted that many electronic stethoscopes also have inner ear protection mechanisms that regulate the maximum sound amplitude output by the device.

Electronic stethoscopes often have digital recording capability, which enables recordings to be transferred to devices like other electronic stethoscopes and computers without loss of fidelity. This in turn allows for possibilities such as playback on other electronic stethoscopes, offline graphical and/or custom analysis along with possible computer-aided diagnosis, telemedicine applications, and construction of teaching archives.

21.3 Electronic Stethoscopes

21.3.1 Technical Considerations and Challenges

Most common auscultatory sounds lie in the 20–2,000 Hz frequency range, with most important cardiovascular murmurs lying in the 30–1,000 Hz range.[8] Some common auscultatory sounds and their frequency ranges can be seen in Fig. 21.3.

The fact that these sounds lie in the lower portion of the normal human hearing spectrum (20–20,000 Hz) poses an inherent problem. As seen in Fig. 21.4, the human ear is progressively less sensitive to lower frequencies, meaning that lower frequencies will require

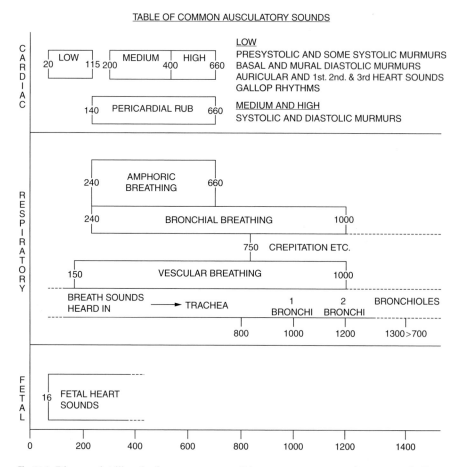

Fig. 21.3 Diagram detailing the frequency ranges of the most common auscultatory sounds (from Durand et al[4]). The *x*-axis is frequency in Hz

21 Digital Stethoscopes

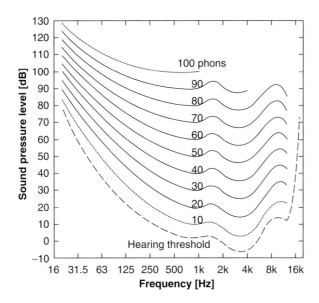

Fig. 21.4 Diagram showing equal loudness contours for the human ear. (Copied with permission from Suzuki et al.[14]). An equal-loudness contour is a measure of sound pressure level (SPL) over the frequency spectrum for which a listener perceives a constant loudness (measured in units called phons) when presented with pure steady tones. Note higher SPLs (in decibels, dB) are generally required at lower frequencies for perception of the same loudness in phons, indicating lower sensitivity of human ear to lower frequencies. Electronic stethoscope filters must therefore account for this and amplify different frequency ranges accordingly to ensure that a variety of physiologic sounds are audible to the examiner

greater amplification in order to be perceived by the auscultator. Thus, filtering for "diaphragm mode" and "bell mode" can both be implemented as low-pass filters (Fig. 21.5).

Another major problem that electronic stethoscopes must combat is the issue of noise. The problem of noise reduction becomes paramount given that electronic stethoscopes are capable of amplifying sounds far beyond the capabilities of their conventional counterparts. In fact, the development of effective noise reduction techniques has been felt to be one of the reasons why electronic stethoscopes are currently becoming more and more popular despite initially facing slow adoption into clinical practice.

Sources of noise in electronic stethoscopy can be thought of in the following categories:
1. *External Noise:* Environmental noise characteristically resides in the 300–3,000 Hz frequency range. Given its components of frequencies higher than that of body sounds, and the increased sensitivity of human hearing to these higher frequencies, this type of noise can still be perceived to be dominant despite some attenuation by the stethoscope chestpiece.
Possible Solutions: At the most basic level, use of low-pass filters as described for "diaphragm" and "bell" modes helps to minimize this problem. However, solely using electronic filtering for this purpose may also filter out important body sounds. Purely mechanical means to deal with this issue include having two different inlets for external

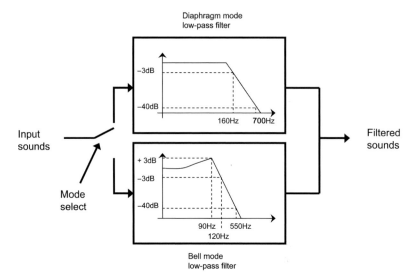

Fig. 21.5 Filters for diaphragm and bell mode (adapted from Durand et al.[4]). Both are low-pass filters. In diaphragm mode, the low pass filter still results in relative amplification of the higher frequencies, as the equal loudness contours indicate lower human ear sensitivity to lower frequencies. In bell mode, these higher frequencies are filtered by the low-pass filter, allowing the human ear to focus only on the lower frequencies

noise, such as implemented by 3M's Ambient Noise Reduction (ANR) technology. ANR technology utilizes the fact that some of the ambient noise inevitably travels through the patient's body and is then transmitted via the chestpiece. Therefore, by creating an additional opening further inside the chestpiece for ambient noise to enter the unit directly from the environment, some degree of noise cancellation is achieved through destructive interference caused by interaction of the ambient noise waves entering from two spatially disparate locations. Note that this noise reduction process is purely mechanical in nature, and occurs prior to electroacoustic transduction.

Noise reduction could also be accomplished through electronic means, as described for example in the patent by Scalise el al.[13] While this patent primarily describes an electronic adapter that could be coupled to the chestpiece of a conventional stethoscope (rather than utilizing an electronic stethoscope per se), the signal processing concepts are nonetheless similar. The authors describe the potential use of two electronic transducers – one for body sounds (along with inherent noise components), and another specifically for external noise – that could achieve noise reduction via simple signal subtraction and/or implementation of adaptive noise filtering. However, the authors note that the two transducers must be fairly close to each other for this approach to be most effective, as there is minimal noise coherence at >1 kHz between transducers separated by more than several centimeters within a diffuse noise field, as shown by Darlington et al.[2] The authors of this patent also suggest methods for noise reduction using a single transducer. In this approach, the transduced signal is seen as the sum of both physiological sounds and noise components. Subsequently, this signal can undergo noise estimation and subtraction, or noise estimation with adaptive filtering, before being passed to the listener.

2. *Auscultation-related noise:* This can be related to manipulation of the stethoscope prior to auscultation, as well as movements (both perceptible and imperceptible) of the listener and/or patient during auscultation itself.

3. *Stethoscope manipulation prior to auscultation:* Inadvertent striking of the chestpiece during this period can theoretically result in sounds loud enough to damage the inner ear.

Possible Solution: Many electronic stethoscopes have protection mechanisms that limit the maximum sound output to the earpieces when the electrical signal obtained through electroacoustic transduction exceeds a certain amplitude.

4. *Movements of listener and/or patient during auscultation:* Anti-tremor filters may be implemented to minimize effects.

5. *Noise due to the stethoscope's internal electronics:* While this can pose a problem if certain components are placed too close to one another, proper circuit design and layout can significantly minimize its effects.

6. *Other biological noises from the patient's body:* Numerous possibilities exist, including, for example, hearing pulmonary sounds while attempting to auscultate the heart.

Possible Solutions: Generally the listener must tolerate these sources of noise, although filters may be implemented for very specific cases (e.g., filters to minimize noise from mechanical heart valves).

21.3.2
Advantages over Conventional Stethoscopes, and Barriers to Clinical Adoption

Electronic stethoscopes have several advantages over their conventional counterparts. Their primary advantage is the superior amplification of body sounds due to electronic volume control abilities, which is a feature that may help clinicians in detecting diseases earlier in their course. Further, the ability to digitally record body sounds makes possible other applications such as offline analysis and telemedicine. In terms of offline analysis, software to visually display digitally recorded body sounds may actually enable clinicians to suspect pathology based on visual correlates even if these sounds were not physically audible with the electronic stethoscope.

Conventional stethoscopes in general suffer from poor sound amplification compared to electronic ones. Further, they demonstrate attenuation of sound transmission in proportion to frequency, have specific extrema in their frequency responses because of tubular resonance properties, and display different sound transmission profiles among different models as shown in the study by Grenier et al.[9] A sample frequency response of an older acoustic stethoscope is shown (Fig. 21.6).

Filtering in electronic stethoscopes can be designed to overcome these limitations, and also to account for the decreased and variable sensitivity of the human ear as a function of frequency to most sounds in the auscultatory range. However, as mentioned earlier, the increased amplification capabilities of electronic stethoscopes (along with their electric components) also make them more susceptible to noise – particularly from physical manipulation artifacts, internal electronics, and the environment.

While several techniques to minimize these sources of noise have already been discussed, it should be noted that some of these developments are still fairly recent. In fact,

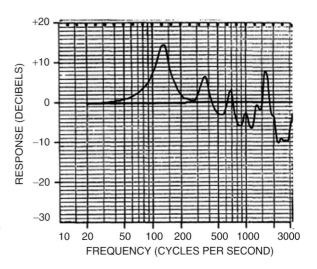

Fig. 21.6 Sample frequency response of an older acoustic stethoscope demonstrates significant variability and numerous extrema within the clinical auscultatory frequency range. (Copied with permission from Ertel et al[7])

the time that has been required to construct sufficiently noise-resistant electronic stethoscopes has been postulated by Grenier et al[9] to be one of the primary reasons for their slow adoption into clinical practice. Further, in addition to electronic stethoscopes generally costing more than their acoustic counterparts, many practicing clinicians may be somewhat reluctant to switch from the acoustic stethoscopes they have grown accustomed to and with which they were initially trained. Despite this, however, recent studies suggest that clinicians do in fact favor many auscultatory features of electronic stethoscopes over those of acoustic ones.

21.3.3
The Phonocardiogram

The phonocardiogram is the electronic recording of the auscultatory sounds from the heart. The use of the phonocardiogram has not been widely used as phonocardiographic signals are not easy to interpret visually while other modalities such as ultrasound imaging (Chapter 14) are able to noninvasively provide more intuitive and detailed images to evaluate function of the heart valves. Nevertheless, the phonocardiogram is a useful means of understanding and visualizing the origins of heart sounds.

Figure 21.7 shows an example of simultaneous recordings of the electrocardiogram, phonocardiogram, and pressure from the left atrium, left ventricle, and aorta. The first heart sound, labeled S1 in the figure, occurs during the closure of the tricuspid and mitral valves. The second heart sound (S2) occurs with the closure of the aortic and pulmonary valves. The third heart sound (S3) occurs during diastole but rarely. The S3 usually is faint and has a low pitch and may represent an abnormality in heart function. The fourth heart sound (S4) occurs immediately before S1 and may also indicate a pathologic state.

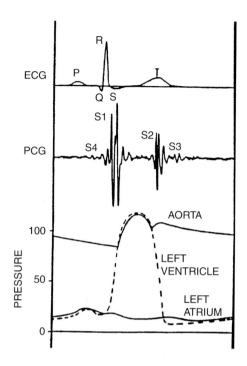

Fig. 21.7 Simultaneous recording of an electrocardiogram (*top*), a phonocardiogram (*middle*), and aortic, left ventricular, and left atrial blood pressures (*bottom*). (Copied with permission from Durand and Guardo[5])

21.3.4
Present Cardiovascular Applications and Future Directions

Cardiovascular applications of electronic stethoscopy are still fairly recent. As mentioned earlier, the ability to digitally record anatomical sounds permits applications such as creation of teaching libraries, digital playback and transfer to other electronic stethoscopes as well as computerized devices for offline analysis, and possibly even telemedicine where recorded sounds can be digitally transferred to colleagues in remote locations.

There is also much interest in coupling electronic stethoscopy with computer-aided analysis and diagnosis, especially for the possibility of detecting a potentially pathological process earlier in its disease course. However, the optimal signal processing techniques (e.g., Fourier transforms, Wavelet transforms, etc.) for accomplishing this are still the subject of much active research.

An example of research involving cardiovascular recordings obtained electronically and computer-aided characterization and/or diagnosis include a study by Degroff et al,[3] which utilized artificial neural networks to characterize electronically recorded innocent versus pathological childhood murmurs with 100% sensitivity and specificity after optimization of network settings. Another study by Noponen et al[12] found that innocent murmurs generally had lower frequencies and more harmonic spectral characteristics than pathological ones, and the authors were able to devise diagnostic criteria achieving 90% specificity and 91% sensitivity.

A study by Herold et al[10] used wavelet filtering to calculate the envelope of recorded heart sounds and investigated whether aortic valve stenosis could be distinguished from other valvular murmurs and nonpathological recordings. The authors found that the correlation of the mean envelope within the aortic valve stenosis group was significantly higher than the correlation between those with aortic valve stenosis vs. those with other valvular murmurs, or those with aortic valve stenosis vs. those without valvular disease. The authors postulated that these findings could enable automated diagnosis of aortic valve stenosis without requiring more expensive testing to establish the diagnosis (e.g., echocardiogram). Similarly, a separate study by Kim et al[11] found that the length of recording segments having spectral components greater than 300 Hz correlated significantly with the peak pressure gradient in patients with aortic stenosis. These findings could provide rapid, noninvasive, inexpensive insight into the severity of aortic stenosis by electronic stethoscopy recording and the use of a computer alone.

With regards to clinical practice, several software toolkits are available for the recording and display of heart sounds. These products allow real-time recording, display, and storage of heart sounds onto a personal computer. Some toolkits can also synchronize the phonocardiogram with the electrocardiogram, which can assist the user in determining the phase of the cardiac cycle during which the given heart sounds occur. Such software toolkits therefore have several potential advantages over either conventional or electronic stethoscopy alone. First, the ability to zoom in on phonocardiograms could enable visual detection of pathological heart sounds that may have otherwise gone unnoticed during auscultation. This in turn could lead to earlier detection of disease processes. Another advantage is diagnostic assistance: the ability to visualize waveform characteristics, as well as comparison with older patient files may lend insight into diagnostic possibilities that would otherwise not have been considered. The creation of permanent teaching libraries or electronic patient "folders" for longitudinal tracking is another useful benefit, as well as telemedicine applications (including, for example, the ability to email digitally recorded information, phonocardiograms, etc. to colleagues).

With further developments in technology and continued research, the adoption of electronic stethoscopes in clinical practice is likely to continue increasing, and will probably be accompanied by more widespread use of computer-aided analysis and/or diagnosis as algorithms continue to improve.

References

1. 3M. 3M™ Littmann® Electronic stethoscope model 3100. <http://solutions.3m.com/wps/portal/3M/en_US/Littmann/stethoscope/electronic-auscultation/model-3000/>; 2003 Accessed 27.10.09.
2. Darlington P, Wheeler PD, Powell A. Adaptive noise reduction in aircraft communication systems. In: *Proceedings of IEEE Conference on Acoustics, Speech and Signal Processing*. Tampa, Florida; 1985;2:716–719.

3. DeGroff CG, Bhatikar S, Hertzberg J, Shandas R, Valdes-Cruz L, Mahajan RL. Artificial neural network-based method of screening heart murmurs in children. *Circulation.* 2001;103: 2711–2716.
4. Durand J, Durand L-G, Grenien M-C. U.S. Patent No. 5,602,924. US Patent and Trademark Office, Washington, DC; 1997.
5. Durand L-G, Guardo R. A model of the heart thorax acoustic system. In: *Applications of Computers in Medicine.* Piscataway, NJ: IEEE Engineering in Medicine and Biology Society; 1982:29.
6. Durand L-G, Pibarot P. Digital signal processing of the phonocardiogram: review of the most recent advancements. *Crit Rev Biomed Eng.* 1995;23:163–219.
7. Ertel PY, Lawrence M, Brown RK, Stern AM. Stethoscope acoustics: II. Transmission and filtration patterns. *Circulation.* 1966;34:899–909.
8. Fuster V, O'Rourke RA, Walsh RA, Poole-Wilson P. *Hurst's the Heart manual of Cardiology.* 12th ed. (Paperback) McGraw, 2009.
9. Grenier M-C, Gagnon K, Genest J Jr, Durand J, Durand L-G. Clinical comparison of acoustic and electronic stethoscopes and design of a new electronic stethoscope. *Am J Cardiol.* 1998; 81:653–656.
10. Herold J, Schroeder R, Nasticzky F, et al. Diagnosing aortic valve stenosis by correlation analysis of wavelet filtered heart sound. *Med Biol Eng Comput.* 2005;43:451–456.
11. Kim D, Tavel ME. Assessment of severity of aortic stenosis through time-frequency analysis of murmur. *Chest.* 2003;124:1638–1644.
12. Noponen A-L, Lukkarinen S, Angerla A, Sepponen R. Phono-spectrographic analysis of heart murmur in children. *BMC Pediatr.* 2007;11:7–23.
13. Scalise SJ, Rainone AS, Davis DW (1998). U.S. Patent No. 5,812,678. Washington, D.C.: U.S. Patent and Trademark Office.
14. Yôiti Suzuki et al. Precise and full-range determination of two-dimensional equal loudness contours. Technical report, Tohoku University, Japan, 2003.

Index

A

Amplifiers, 5
Analog filters, 33–35, 330
Analog signals
   analog-to-digital conversion, 11–15
   definition, 9
   tape players, 10
   thermometer, 9
Analog-to-digital convertors
   analog signals
      quantization, 13–15
      sampling, 11–13
   data compression, 80
   definition, 6
Angiography
   computed tomography
      appropriateness criteria, 295
      body mass index (BMI), 296
      detectors, 281
      limitation, 295
      patient selection and preparation, 287
      prospectively gated axial (PGA), 283
   3-D modeling technique
      arterial segment length evaluation, 170–171
      assist on-line PCI procedure, 173–175
      cone-beam back-projection technique, 163–164
      coronary analysis, quantitative, 169–170
      coronary arterial tree skeleton calculation, 166, 169, 170
      curvature and torsion calculation, 182
      curve function, 181
      deformation algorithm, 179–181
      discrete flexion point evaluation, 172–174
      flexion point identification, 177, 179
      gantry orientation, 165
      image acquisition and selection, 165–166
      left coronary arterial (LCA) tree, PCI, 177, 178
      luminal volume calculation, 181–182
      segmentation of, 166, 167
      single-plane imaging system, 163
      stent and hinge points, 175–177
      structure determination, 164
      tortuosity of artery evaluation, 171–172
      transformation calculation, 166, 168
Antialiasing filter, 5, 6, 32–33, 40
Arterial tonometry, 150
Audio-visual superimposition ECG presentation (AVESP), 311
Auscultation, blood pressure measurement, 145–146
Autocorrelation, cardiac rate estimation
   simple square wave, 58–59
   sine wave, 57–60

B

Baseline wander, signal-to-noise ratio improvement, 30–31
Bicubic interpolation, 94, 110
Bilinear interpolation, 93, 110
Bipolar electrogram
   activation time, 333
   activation times, 333
   advantages and disadvantages, 328
   artifacts, 329
   directionality, 327
   field of view, 323
   implantable device, 340, 342, 343
   inter-electrode distance, 332
   signal processing, 311, 330, 331
   spatial resolution, 323–324
   temporal resolution, 324, 325

Blood pressure measurement, noninvasive
  ambulatory blood pressure monitoring, 150–151
  arterial tonometry, 150
  Doppler ultrasonic flowmeter, 149–150
  finapres and portopres, 149
  oscillometry, 146–149
  palpation and auscultation, 145–146
  pulse oximetry
    limitation, 152–153
    motion artifact reduction, 155
    principles, 151–152
    signal processing, 154–155
    uses, 151, 154
Body mass index (BMI), 296
Brightness, image processing, 94–95, 110

C

Cardiac magnetic resonance (CMR) images
  automated contouring, 268–270
  automated infarct quantification, 271
  delayed enhancement, 270
  image analysis, 264–266
  volumes and mass quantification, 266–268
Color flow Doppler, 202
Comet tail, echocardiography, 204, 206
Complex fractionated atrial electrograms (CFAEs), 328
Computed tomography (CT)
  artifacts, pitfalls and solutions, 288–289
  coronary vessels
    appropriateness criteria, 295
    calcification, 295–296
    coronary artery disease, 294–295
    coronary calcium scoring, 290–294
    heart rate, 296
    indications, 295
    obesity, 296
  CTA (*see* Computed tomography angiography)
  curved planar reformations (CPR), 289–291
  image acquisition and protocols
    ECG dose modulation, 283–284
    image acquisition and reconstruction, 284
    prospective gating, 282–283
    retrospective gating, 282
  maximum-intensity projection (MIP), 290
  multidetector computed tomography (*see* Multidetector computed tomography)
  multiplanar reconstruction (MPR), 289
  non-coronary cardiac
    myocardial masses, 298
    myocardial scar and viability, 297–298
    pulmonary veins, 299
    valvular structures, 296–297
  patient selection and preparation, 287–288
  radiation and dose
    reduction strategies, 286–287
    stochastic and deterministic, 285
  volume rendering techniques (VRT), 290, 292
  X-ray (*see* X-ray)
Computed tomography angiography (CTA)
  appropriateness criteria, 295
  body mass index (BMI), 296
  detectors, 281
  limitation, 295
  patient selection and preparation, 287
  prospectively gated axial (PGA), 283
Constrictive pericarditis, intravascular pressure measurement, 140
Continuous wave Doppler, 201–202
Contrast echocardiography, 210–211
Contrast, image processing, 94–95, 110
Coronary angiography
  coronary catheterization, 157
  3-D modeling technique
    application, 173–179
    arterial segment length evaluation, 170–171
    cone-beam back-projection technique, 163–164
    coronary analysis, quantitative, 169–170
    coronary arterial tree skeleton calculation, 166, 169, 170
    discrete flexion point evaluation, 172–174
    gantry orientation, 165
    image acquisition and selection, 165–166
    segmentation of, 166, 167
    single-plane imaging system, 163
    structure determination, 164
    tortuosity of artery evaluation, 171–172
    transformation calculation, 166, 168
  limitations, 2-D quantitative analysis
    foreshortening, 159
    percutaneous coronary intervention (PCI), 160–163
    stenotic segment identification, 158–159

Index

D

Data compression
  curve fitting, 84–85
  data transformation, 85–86
  differencing
    binary digits required, 84
    definition, 83
  downsampling, 80–81
  loss-less compression, 79
  lossy compression, 79–80
  quantization, 81
  template subtraction, 84
  variable length codes, 82–83
Differencing, data compression
  binary digits required, 84
  definition, 83
Digital filters
  definition, 35
  filter coefficients, 35
  linear filters, 36
  median filter, 36–38
  three-point moving average filter, 35, 36
  two-point differentiator, 36
Digital imaging and communications in medicine (DICOM) standard
  magnetic resonance imaging (MRI), 271
  PET studies, 247
  SPECT studies, 246–247
Digital signals
  advantages, 10
  analog-to-digital conversion
    quantization, 13–15
    sampling, 11–13
  frequency domain
    discontinuity, 23–25
    fast Fourier transform (FFT), 22
    resolution, 23
    time domain signal length, 23
    windowing, 25
    zero-padding, 23
  transmission through noisy channel, 10–11
Digital stethoscopes
  developments and principles, 379–381
  electronic stethoscopes
    advantages, 381
    auscultatory sounds and frequency ranges, 382
    cardiovascular applications, 387–388
    electroacoustic transduction, 381
    noise reduction techniques, 383–385
    phonocardiogram, 386–387
    vs. conventional stethoscopes, 385–386
Dominant frequency, 68. *See also* Rate estimation techniques
Doppler echocardiography
  color flow Doppler, 202
  continuous wave Doppler, 201–202
  principles, 199
  pulsed wave Doppler, 199–201
  shift, 199
  tissue Doppler imaging, 215–216
Doppler ultrasonic flowmeter, 149–150

E

ECG. *See* Electrocardiography
Echocardiography
  applications
    contrast echocardiography, 210–211
    intracardiac echocardiography, 214
    intravascular ultrasound, 213–215
    three-dimensional structures, 211–213
    tissue Doppler imaging, 215–216
  beam adjustment, 192–193
  data storage
    conversion, 209
    selection and compression, 209–210
  display
    modes, 195–196
    phased array transducer, 197–198
    pulser, 194–195
    time gain compensation, 197–198
    two-dimensional image, 195–197
  Doppler echocardiography
    color flow Doppler, 202
    continuous wave Doppler, 201–202
    principles, 199
    pulsed wave Doppler, 199–201
    shift, 199
  principle, 187
  resolution
    axial, 193
    contrast, 194
    definition, 192
    lateral, 193
    temporal, 194
  signal quality
    artifact, 204–208
    noise, 202–204
  transducer, 190–191
  ultrasound
    attenuation, 189–190

definition, 187
frequency, 188
longitudinal wave, 188
reflection, scattering and absorption, 189
velocity, 187–189
Echo-planar images (EPI), 260
Edge detection, image processing, 107–108
Electrocardiography (ECG), 304
  accuracy and precision requirment, 119–120
  analog signal filtering, 120–121
  analog to digital conversion, 123–124
  artifacts
    asymptomatic artifacts, 314–315
    data recording and processing artifacts, 314
    erroneous pacemaker stimuli, 314–315
    noise, 314
    patient-related artifacts, 314
  augmented limb leads, 118–119
  axis, 117
  common mode rejection, 122–123
  computerized analysis, 126
  continuous recorder (*see also* Holter recorders)
    cassette tape recorder, 303
    digital recording system, 303, 305
    solid-state memory systems, 303
  data storage and compression, 129–130
  digital signal filtering, 121–122
  electrical activity of heart
    action potential, 113–114
    automaticity, 114
    recording by electrodes in heart surface, 114–115
    recording by electrodes in skin surface, 116
  event recorders, 305
  heart rate variability (HRV)
    definition, 347
    parasympathetic and sympathetic activity, 362
    signal processing techniques, 364–368
    time and frequency domains, 363
  implantable recorders, 306
  low pass (high frequency) filtering, 122
  LTECG (*see* Long term electrocardiographic recording)
  mobile cardiac outpatient telemetry (MCOT) systems, 305
  potential artifacts, 128–129
  real time monitoring, 306
  reliability of interpretive algorithms, 127–128
  signal averaged ECG (SAECG), 368
    clinical studies, 373–374
    data acquisition and signal pre-processing, 370
    data storage, 374
    definition, 347
    late potentials, 372–373
    spatial signal averaging, 371–372
    spectral analysis, 372
    temporal signal averaging, 370–371
    time-domain analysis, 369
  telemetry (*see* Telemetry)
  template formation
    fiducial points identification, 125–126
    signal averaging, 124–125
  T-wave alternans (TWA)
    computation, 351
    definition, 347
    mechanisms, 348–349
    modified moving average (MMA), 359–361
    signal-to-noise ratio, 350
    spatial and temporal dispersion, 349
    spatially concordant and discordant, 349–350
    spectral method (*see* T-wave alternans)
    ventricular arrhythmias, 348
  ventricular activation, 116–117
  Wilson central terminal (WCT), 117–118
Electron beam computed tomography (EBCT)
  coronary calcium deposits, 291, 293
  scanner design, 280
Electronic stethoscope
  advantages, 381
  auscultatory sounds and frequency ranges, 382
  cardiovascular applications, 387–388
  electroacoustic transduction, 381
  noise reduction techniques, 383–385
  vs. conventional stethoscopes, 385–386
Event and feature detection techniques
  amplitude
    fiducial points, 45–46
    jitter, 45
    waveform, 44–45
  purpose and challenges, 43–44
  slope
    baseline wander, 48
    differential signal advantages, 48
    double-peaked waveform, 46–47

template matching
  advantages and limitations, 51
  baseline wander, 49
  matched filters, 50–51
  maximum slope criteria, 48
  white noise, 49
waveform offset estimation, 52–55
waveform onset detection, 51–52

F
Fast Fourier transform (FFT), 22
Fiducial points, 45–46, 55
Filters
  aliasing prevention, 32–33
  analog filters, 33–35
  digital filters
    definition, 35
    filter coefficients, 35
    linear filters, 36
    median filter, 36–38
    three-point moving average filter, 35, 36
    two-point differentiator, 36
  noise, 27
  phase distortion
    five-point median digital filter, 38–39
    sinusoidal components, 40
  principle, 5
  signal-to-noise ratio improvement
    baseline wander, 30–31
    electrical noise, 60 Hz interference, 28
    low and high pass filters, 28–30
    low-pass cut-off frequency, 32
    notch filtering, 30
    white noise, 30–32
Finapres, blood pressure measurement, 149
Finite residual filter (FRF), 309, 310
Flexion point, angiography, 177, 179
Fractionated electrograms, 327–328
Frequency domain
  digital signals
    discontinuity, 23–25
    fast Fourier transform (FFT), 22
    resolution, 23
    time domain signal length, 23
    windowing, 25
    zero-padding, 23
  Fourier transform, 18–20
  loudness, tone, 17
  time domain signal transformation, 21–22

uses, frequency domain plots
  number of days estimation, 21
  visual and quantitative sense analysis, 19–21
Windows media player signal, 18, 19

H
Heart rate variability (HRV)
  definition, 347
  parasympathetic and sympathetic activity, 362
  signal processing techniques
    clinical applications, 367
    considerations and data storage, 368
    data acquisition and signal pre-processing, 364
    ectopic beats, 367
    future aspects, 368
    heart rate turbulence (HRT), 365
    resampling, 366
    spectral indices, 365
    time domain indices, 364–365
    time and frequency domains, 363
Holter recorders
  audio-visual superimposition ECG presentation (AVESP), 311
  cassette tape recorder, 303
  digital recording system, 303, 305
  R-R histogram generation, 311
  solid-state memory systems, 303
  template matching, 311

I
Image processing technique
  color images, 109
  contrast and brightness, 94–95
  edge detection, 107–108
  filtering, 100–103
  frequency domain images, 96–97
  image resizing, 92–94
  quantization, 92
  sampling, 90–92
  signal averaging, 104–105
  signal-to-noise ratio, 97–99
  template matching, 105–107
Intracardiac dual-chamber pacing device, 341
Intracardiac echocardiography, 214
Intracardiac electrograms
  activation times
    block confirmation, 334
    catheter ablation, 333

electrogram characteristics, 333
    map creation, 334
bipolar electrogram (*see* Bipolar
        electrogram)
contact mapping techniques, 337–339
directionality
    artifacts, 329–330
    bipolar electrogram, 327
    fractionated electrograms, 327–328
    unipolar electrogram, 324–326
electric dipoles, 320–321
frequency domain analysis, atrial
        fibrillation
    arrhythmias, power spectrum, 340
    dominant frequency analysis, 339
    implantable devices, 340–343
isochronal maps, 335
isopotential maps, 335–336
recording electrodes, 319
signal processing
    amplification, 330
    analog filtering, 330
    digital filtering, 331
    digitization, 330–331
    electrophysiology studies, 332, 333
    high-pass filters, 331
    low-pass filtering, 331
unipolar electrogram (*see* Unipolar
        electrogram)
voltage maps, 336–337
Intracardiac pressure measurement.
        See Intravascular pressure
        measurement
Intravascular pressure measurement
    aliasing effect, 136
    aortic root pressure, 141–142
    constrictive pericarditis, 140
    errors, 143–144
    kymograph, 133
    low pass filtering, 141
    micromanometer, 134–135
    power spectra, 138–139
    pressure, definition, 133–134
    sampling rate, 134–137
    signal processing, 142–143
    transducer, 138
    transfer function determination, 139–140
Intravascular ultrasound (IVUS),
        213–215
Isochronal maps, 335
Isopotential maps, 335–336

J
Jitter, 45, 55

K
Kymograph, 133

L
Linear filters, digital system, 36
Long term electrocardiographic (LTECG)
        recording
    AVSEP analysis, arrhythmia, 311–312
    data storage, 313
    ischemia analysis, 312–313
    recorder (*see* Electrocardiography)
Loss-less compression, 79
Lossy compression, 79–80

M
Magnetic resonance imaging (MRI)
    artifacts
        phase mismapping, 264–265
        phase wrap, 263–264
    cardiac gated scans, 261–262
    CMR
        automated contouring, 268–270
        automated infarct quantification, 271
        delayed enhancement, 270
        image analysis, 264–266
        volumes and mass quantification,
            266–268
    data storage, 271–272
    filtering
        echo-planar images (EPI), 260
        field of view, 260
        k-space and image space, 260
        real time imaging, 260
        steady state free precession (SSFP)
            images, 261
        time to acquire an image (TA), 260
    Fourier transform
        k-space, 255–259
        multiple FIDs, 255
        precessional frequency, 256
        spatial gradient, 256
    image formation, 272–273
    magnetic resonance image acquisition, 251
    physiologic parameters
        Larmor equation, 251
        precessional frequency, 253
    signal-to-noise ratio (SNR), 262–263
    technique

free induction decay (FID), 254
image creation, 254–255
magnetic fields, 253
signal decays, 254
signal strength, 253
transverse relaxation rate, 254
water atoms, magnetization, 253
Median filter, digital system, 36–38
Median waveforms, signal averaging, 73–77
Micromanometer, 134–135. *See also*
Intravascular pressure measurement
Microprocessor, 6
Mobile cardiac outpatient telemetry (MCOT) systems, 305
Modified moving average (MMA). *See* T-wave alternans
Morse code, data compression, 82–83
Multidetector computed tomography (MDCT)
artifacts, 288
calcium scoring, 293
coronary artery calcification, 295
detectors, 280
image quality, 279
non-coronary cardiac
myocardial masses, 298
myocardial scar and viability, 297–298
pulmonary veins, 299
valvular structures, 296–297
radiation and dose, 284, 286
retrospective gating, 282
scanner design, 280

N

Nearest neighbor interpolation, 93
Noise
reduction, signal averaging
dart board, 69–70
limitations, 72–74
median waveforms, 73–77
procedure, 70–72
Notch filtering, signal-to-noise ratio, 30
Nyquist sampling rule, analog-to-digital conversion, 12

O

Oscillometry, blood pressure measurent
accuracy and environmental motion effect, 147
block diagram, 148
cuff pressure, 147–148
improved algorithm, 146–147
principle and limitations, 146
signal processing method, 149

P

Palpation, blood pressure measurement, 145–146
Percutaneous coronary intervention (PCI), angiography
2-D analysis
challenging anatomical subsets, 160
comorbidities, 161–162
complications, 161
high quality care, 161
outcomes Improvement, 162–163
3-D analysis, 173–175
Phase distortion
five-point median digital filter, 38–39
sinusoidal components, 40
Phonocardiogram, 386–387
Physiologic recorders
amplifiers, 5
analog-to-digital convertors, 6
antialiasing filter, 6
block diagram, 4
calibration, 6
filters, 5
microprocessor, 6
reference, 6
transducers, 3–5
Piezoelectric crystal, echocardiography, 190
Portopres, blood pressure measurement, 149
Positron emission tomography (PET)
absolute activity, 236
attenuation, 224
attenuation correction, 236
cardiac and respiratory motion, 238
clinical protocols, 229
data storage, 247
detection, 226, 228
filtered backprojection (FBP), 231–232
flow variation, 239–240
forward projection, 229–231
hot *vs.* cold spot optimization, 243–244
image artifacts
transmission/emission misalignment, 243, 244
volume artifact, 241–242
iterative reconstruction, 231–234
limitation, 226
metabolic variation, 241
noise artifacts

detector system, 238
  radiotracer decay, 237–238
photon detection, 223
physiologic signals
  flows spans, 221
  metabolism, 221–223
  radioactive tracer decay, 220
  spatial resolution, 221
physiologic variation
  flow, 238–239
  metabolism, 240
simple backprojection, 229–231
SPECT (*see* Single photon emission
    computed tomography)
temporal images, dynamic imaging, 221
tracer
  concentration, 220
  decay, 220, 227, 228
  properties, 228
Pressure, 133–134. *See also* Intravascular
    pressure measurement
Pulsed wave Doppler, 199–201
Pulse oximetry
  limitation, 152–153
  motion artifact reduction, 155
  principles, 151–152
  signal processing, 154–155
  uses, 151, 154
Pulse repetition frequency (PRF),
    echocardiography, 191, 199–200
Pulse repetition period (PRP),
    echocardiography, 191

Q

Quantization
  analog-to-digital conversion
    peak-to-peak amplitude signal, 13–14
    saturation, 15
  data compression, 81
  image processing, 92

R

Rate estimation techniques
  autocorrelation
    simple square wave, 58–59
    sine wave, 57–60
  frequency domain estimation, 60
  frequency variability, 61–63
  noise, 60–61
  phase change, 64–65
  waveform morphology, 65–67

Red–green–blue (RGB) color, image
    processing, 109
Resizing, image, 92–94
Resolution, echocardiography
  axial, 193
  contrast, 194
  definition, 192
  lateral, 193
  temporal, 194
Reverberation, echocardiography,
    204, 206

S

Sampling process
  analog-to-digital conversion
    aliasing, 12–13
    Nyquist sampling rule, 12
    principle, 11
  image processing, 90–92
Signal averaging
  electrocardiography (SAECG)
    clinical studies, 373–374
    data acquisition and signal pre-processing,
      370
    data storage, 374
    late potentials, 372–373
    principle, 368
    spatial signal averaging, 371–372
    spectral analysis, 372
    temporal signal averaging, 370–371
    time-domain analysis, 369
  image processing, 104–105
  noise reduction
    dart board, 69–70
    limitations, 72–74
    median waveforms, 73–77
    signal improvement, 71–72
    waveform alignment, 70, 72
    window choosing, 70–71
Signal extraction technology (SET),
    Masimo, 153
Signal-to-noise ratio (SNR)
  definition, 40
  improvement, filters
    baseline wander, 30–31
    electrical noise, 60 Hz interference, 28
    high and high pass filters, 28–30
    low-pass cut-off frequency, 32
    notch filtering, 30
    white noise, 30–32
  magnetic resonance imaging, 262–263

Index 399

Single photon emission computed tomography (SPECT). *See also* Positron emission tomography
  attenuation correction, 226
    Chang multiplicative method, 234–235
    impacts, 235
    scatter correction, 235–236
  clinical protocols, 226, 227
  collimator septa, 225
  data storage, 246–247
  dual-head camera, 225
  flow variation, 239
  forward projection, 229
  image artifacts
    attenuation artifact, 243
    volume artifact, 241–242
  metabolic variation, 240–241
  photon detection, 223
  scanner system, 223
  spatial resolution, 221
  tracer properties, 225
Spectral TWA. *See* T-wave alternans
Steady state free precession (SSFP) images, 261
Stent and hinge points, angiography, 175–177
Stethoscopes
  acoustic stethoscope, 380
  electronic stethoscope
    advantages, 381
    auscultatory sounds and frequency ranges, 382
    cardiovascular applications, 387–388
    conventional stethoscopes, 385–386
    electroacoustic transduction, 381
    noise reduction techniques, 383–385
  invention, 379
  phonocardiogram, 386–387

T

Telemetry
  artifactual ST segment deviation, 308
  components, 307
  definition, 306
  Holter monitoring, 308–309
  IR system, 306–307
  motion correction/noise reduction, 309, 310
  physiologic signal, 308
  recorder (*see* Electrocardiography)
  signal processing techniques, 309
  ultrasonic system, 307

Template matching
  event and feature detection techniques
    advantages and limitations, 51
    baseline wander, 49
    matched filters, 50–51
    maximum slope criteria, 48
    white noise, 49
  image processing, 105–107
Three-dimensional angiography. *See* Angiography
Three-dimensional echocardiography, 211–213. *See also* Echocardiography
Three-point moving average filter, digital filters, 35, 36
Tissue Doppler imaging (TDI), 215–216
Tissue harmonic imaging method, 202–204
Transducers
  definition, 3
  echocardiography, 190–191
  phased array transducers, 214
  reference, 3–5
T-wave alternans (TWA)
  computation, 351
  definition, 347
  mechanisms, 348–349
  modified moving average (MMA)
    beat series, 359
    clinical applications, 360–361
    future aspects, 361
    parameter variations, 360
    vs. spectral method, 361
  signal-to-noise ratio, 350
  spatial and temporal dispersion, 349
  spatially concordant and discordant, 349–350
  spectral method
    calculation, 353–355
    clinical studies, 359
    data reduction, 353
    data storage, 355
    discrete Fourier transformation (DFT), 352
    indeterminate and noisy, 357–358
    interpretation, 357
    noise, 355–357
    parameter variation, 357
    preprocessing, 352–353
  ventricular arrhythmias, 348
Two-point differentiator, digital filters, 36

U

Unipolar electrogram
  activation time, 333
  advantages and disadvantages, 328
  amplitude, 320–321
  artifacts, 329
  directionality
    distal electrode, 326
    premature ventricular complex (PVC), 326
    wavefront origin, 324–325
  field of view, 323
  filter setting effects, 332
  implantable devices, 340, 343
  signal processing, 331, 332
  spatial resolution, 323
  temporal resolution, 324, 325

W

Waveform offset estimation
  amplitude, 52
  cumulative area, 53–55
  slope, 53
  tangent line projection, 52–53

Waveform onset detection, 51–52
White noise, signal-to-noise ratio, 30–32
Wilson central terminal (WCT), ECG, 117–118
Windowing, frequency domain, 25

X

X-ray
  hardware
    generator, 275–276
    X-ray tube, 276
  production
    detectors, 280–281
    dual energy, 281
    image acquisition and reconstruction, 278
    image display and storage, 278–279
    image quality, 279–280
    linear attenuation, 278
    scanner design, 280
    X-ray interactions and detectors, 277

Z

Zero-padding, frequency domain, 23